NEW DIRECTIONS IN CHILD ABUSE AND NEGLECT RESEARCH

Committee on Child Maltreatment Research, Policy, and Practice for the Next Decade: Phase II

Anne C. Petersen, Joshua Joseph, and Monica Feit, *Editors*

Board on Children, Youth, and Families

Committee on Law and Justice

INSTITUTE OF MEDICINE *AND*
NATIONAL RESEARCH COUNCIL
OF THE NATIONAL ACADEMIES

THE NATIONAL ACADEMIES PRESS
Washington, D.C.
www.nap.edu

THE NATIONAL ACADEMIES PRESS   500 Fifth Street, NW   Washington, DC 20001

NOTICE: The project that is the subject of this report was approved by the Governing Board of the National Research Council, whose members are drawn from the councils of the National Academy of Sciences, the National Academy of Engineering, and the Institute of Medicine. The members of the committee responsible for the report were chosen for their special competences and with regard for appropriate balance.

This study was supported by Contract/Grant No. HHSP23320110010YC between the National Academy of Sciences and the Administration for Children and Families, U.S. Department of Health and Human Services. Any opinions, findings, conclusions, or recommendations expressed in this publication are those of the author(s) and do not necessarily reflect the views of the organizations or agencies that provided support for the project.

International Standard Book Number-13:   978-0-309-28512-4
International Standard Book Number-10:   0-309-28512-7

Additional copies of this report are available for sale from the National Academies Press, 500 Fifth Street, NW, Keck 360, Washington, DC 20001; (800) 624-6242 or (202) 334-3313; http://www.nap.edu.

Suggested citation: IOM (Institute of Medicine) and NRC (National Research Council). 2014. *New directions in child abuse and neglect research*. Washington, DC: The National Academies Press.

THE NATIONAL ACADEMIES
Advisers to the Nation on Science, Engineering, and Medicine

The **National Academy of Sciences** is a private, nonprofit, self-perpetuating society of distinguished scholars engaged in scientific and engineering research, dedicated to the furtherance of science and technology and to their use for the general welfare. Upon the authority of the charter granted to it by the Congress in 1863, the Academy has a mandate that requires it to advise the federal government on scientific and technical matters. Dr. Ralph J. Cicerone is president of the National Academy of Sciences.

The **National Academy of Engineering** was established in 1964, under the charter of the National Academy of Sciences, as a parallel organization of outstanding engineers. It is autonomous in its administration and in the selection of its members, sharing with the National Academy of Sciences the responsibility for advising the federal government. The National Academy of Engineering also sponsors engineering programs aimed at meeting national needs, encourages education and research, and recognizes the superior achievements of engineers. Dr. C. D. Mote, Jr., is president of the National Academy of Engineering.

The **Institute of Medicine** was established in 1970 by the National Academy of Sciences to secure the services of eminent members of appropriate professions in the examination of policy matters pertaining to the health of the public. The Institute acts under the responsibility given to the National Academy of Sciences by its congressional charter to be an adviser to the federal government and, upon its own initiative, to identify issues of medical care, research, and education. Dr. Harvey V. Fineberg is president of the Institute of Medicine.

The **National Research Council** was organized by the National Academy of Sciences in 1916 to associate the broad community of science and technology with the Academy's purposes of furthering knowledge and advising the federal government. Functioning in accordance with general policies determined by the Academy, the Council has become the principal operating agency of both the National Academy of Sciences and the National Academy of Engineering in providing services to the government, the public, and the scientific and engineering communities. The Council is administered jointly by both Academies and the Institute of Medicine. Dr. Ralph J. Cicerone and Dr. C. D. Mote, Jr., are chair and vice chair, respectively, of the National Research Council.

www.national-academies.org

Consultants

GREGORY A. AARONS, University of California, San Diego
RICHARD P. BARTH, University of Maryland
REBECCA BERTELL, University of Maryland
CINDY CHRISTIAN, The Children's Hospital of Philadelphia
HOWARD DUBOWITZ, University of Maryland
DEBORAH HARBURGER, University of Maryland
STANLEY J. HUEY, JR., University of Southern California
KENT P. HYMEL, The Children's Hospital of Dartmouth
NANCY KELLOGG, University of Texas Health Science Center
JOHN LANDSVERK, Rady Children's Hospital of San Diego
LAWRENCE PALINKAS, University of Southern California
MATHEW URETSKY, University of Maryland
ALLISON WEST, University of Maryland
KRISTEN WOODRUFF, University of Maryland
FRED WULCZYN, Chapin Hall at the University of Chicago

Study Staff

MONICA FEIT, Study Director[1]
JOSHUA JOSEPH, Study Director[2]
MICHAEL McGEARY, Senior Program Officer[3]
TARA MAINERO, Research Associate[4]
ALEJANDRA MARTÍN, Research Associate[5]
KAREN CAMPION, Research Assistant[6]
AMANDA PASCAVIS, Research Assistant[7]
WENDY KEENAN, Program Associate
SAMANTHA ROBOTHAM, Senior Program Assistant
PAMELLA ATAYI, Administrative Assistant
KATHLEEN McGRAW-SHEPHERD, Intern[8]
KIMBER BOGARD, Director, Board on Children, Youth, and Families
ARLENE LEE, Director, Committee on Law and Justice

---

[1]Through January 2013.
[2]Starting January 2013.
[3]Starting January 2013 through March 2013.
[4]Starting September 2013.
[5]Through September 2013.
[6]Starting December 2012 through August 2013.
[7]Starting November 2013.
[8]Starting May 2012 through August 2012.

Acknowledgments

This report reflects contributions from numerous individuals and groups. The committee takes this opportunity to recognize those who so generously gave their time and expertise to inform its deliberations.

To begin, the committee would like to thank the sponsor of this study. Support for the committee's work was provided by the U.S. Department of Health and Human Services, Administration for Children and Families, Administration on Children, Youth and Families, Children's Bureau, Office on Child Abuse and Neglect. We wish to thank Joe Bock, Melissa Brodowski, Catherine Nolan, Bryan Samuels, and Dori Sneddon for their guidance and support.

The committee greatly benefited from the opportunity for discussion with individuals who made presentations at and attended the committee's workshops and meetings (see Appendix B). The committee is thankful for the useful contributions of these many individuals.

The committee could not have done its work without the support and guidance provided by the Institute of Medicine (IOM)/National Research Council (NRC) project staff: Karen Campion, Monica Feit, Joshua Joseph, Wendy Keenan, Tara Mainero, Alejandra Martín, Kathleen McGraw-Shepherd, Amanda Pascavis, and Samantha Robotham. The committee gratefully acknowledges Kimber Bogard of the Board on Children, Youth, and Families and Arlene Lee and Jane Ross of the Committee on Law and Justice for their guidance on this study.

Many other staff within the IOM/NRC provided support to this project in various ways. The committee would like to thank Pamella Atayi, Patrick Burke, Laura DeStefano, Chelsea Frakes, Faye Hillman, Nicole Joy, Michael McGeary, Abbey Meltzer, and Patti Simon. Finally, Rona Briere and Alisa Decatur are to be credited for the superb editorial assistance they provided in preparing the final report.

Reviewers

This report has been reviewed in draft form by individuals chosen for their diverse perspectives and technical expertise, in accordance with procedures approved by the National Research Council's Report Review Committee. The purpose of this independent review is to provide candid and critical comments that will assist the institution in making its published report as sound as possible and to ensure that the report meets institutional standards for objectivity, evidence, and responsiveness to the study charge. The review comments and draft manuscript remain confidential to protect the integrity of the deliberative process. We wish to thank the following individuals for their review of this report:

Dolores Subia BigFoot, University of Oklahoma Health Sciences Center
Jeanne Brooks-Gunn, Columbia University
Mark J. Chaffin, University of Oklahoma Health Sciences Center
Diana English, University of Washington
Sally Flanzer, U.S. Department of Health and Human Services (Retired)
Joan Kaufman, Yale University
Jill E. Korbin, Case Western Reserve University
Richard D. Krugman, University of Colorado at Denver
Kristen Shook Slack, University of Wisconsin–Madison
Charles H. Zeanah, Tulane University

Although the reviewers listed above have provided many constructive comments and suggestions, they were not asked to endorse the report's conclusions or recommendations, nor did they see the final draft of the report before its release. The review of this report was overseen by **Robert S. Lawrence,** Johns Hopkins University, and **Nancy E. Adler,** University of California, San Francisco. Appointed by the National Research Council and the Institute of Medicine, they were responsible for making certain that an independent examination of this report was carried out in accordance with institutional procedures and that all review comments were carefully considered. Responsibility for the final content of this report rests entirely with the authoring committee and the institution.

Contents

SUMMARY   **1**

1 INTRODUCTION   **15**
The 1993 Report, 16
Trends Since 1993, 16
The Current Study, 18
Study Approach, 19
Research Advances in Child Abuse and Neglect, 23
A Systems Framework for Child Abuse and Neglect, 25
The Unique Role of Social and Economic Stratification, 27
Conclusion, 28
Organization of the Report, 29
References, 29

2 DESCRIBING THE PROBLEM   **31**
Definitions, 32
Incidence Rates and the Problem of Underreporting, 38
Incidence Trends, 48
Determination of Child Abuse and Neglect, 53
Conclusions, 61
References, 62

3 CAUSALITY   **69**
Establishing a Causal Connection, 70
Candidate Explanatory Factors for Child Abuse and Neglect, 72

Protective Factors, 95
Methodological Challenges, 96
Conclusions, 97
References, 101

4   CONSEQUENCES OF CHILD ABUSE AND NEGLECT   111
Cascading Consequences, 112
Background, 113
Neurobiological Outcomes, 117
Cognitive, Psychosocial, and Behavioral Outcomes, 128
Health Outcomes, 141
Adolescent and Adult Outcomes, 144
Individual Differences in Outcomes, 148
Economic Burden, 152
Conclusions, 154
References, 155

5   THE CHILD WELFARE SYSTEM   175
Overview of the Child Welfare System, 176
Major Policy Shifts in Child Welfare Since 1993, 191
System-Level Reforms Intended to Improve Practice and
    Outcomes, 196
Research on Key Policy and Practice Reforms, 201
Focus on Well-Being Outcomes, 210
Issues That Remain to Be Addressed, 213
Conclusions, 234
References, 235

6   INTERVENTIONS AND SERVICE DELIVERY SYSTEMS   245
Treatment Programs, 247
Prevention Strategies, 253
Common Issues in Improving Program Impacts, 265
Building an Integrated System of Care, 276
Conclusions, 281
References, 283

7   RESEARCH CHALLENGES AND INFRASTRUCTURE   297
Components of the Child Abuse and Neglect Research
    Infrastructure, 297
Challenges in Child Abuse and Neglect Research, 326
Existing Opportunities to Create an Integrated Child Abuse and
    Neglect Research Infrastructure, 332

Conclusions, 340
References, 341

8 CHILD ABUSE AND NEGLECT POLICY 349
The Policy Landscape, 352
Federal Laws and Policies, 354
State Laws and Policies, 364
Conclusions, 380
References, 380

9 RECOMMENDATIONS 385
Guiding Principles, 386
Recommendations, 389
Final Thoughts, 405
References, 406

APPENDIXES
A WORKSHOP OPEN SESSION AGENDAS 407
B RESEARCH RECOMMENDATIONS AND PRIORITIES FROM
THE 1993 NATIONAL RESEARCH COUNCIL REPORT
UNDERSTANDING CHILD ABUSE AND NEGLECT 411
C BIOSKETCHES OF COMMITTEE MEMBERS 421

Summary

In the two decades since the National Research Council (NRC) issued its 1993 report *Understanding Child Abuse and Neglect*, a new science of child abuse and neglect has been launched, yielding findings that delineate a serious public health problem. Fully 6 million children are involved in reports to child protective services, and many more cases go undetected. Nationally, about three-quarters of cases are classified as neglect, and the majority of reports involve children under the age of 5. Important findings on the consequences of child abuse and neglect reveal the problem is not confined to children and childhood; rather, the effects of child abuse and neglect cascade throughout the life course, with costly consequences for individuals, families, and society. These effects are seen in all aspects of human functioning, including physical and mental health, and in important arenas such as education, work, and social relationships. Addressing this public health problem will require an immediate, coordinated research response that is grounded in the complex environments and systems within which child abuse and neglect occurs and that has high-level federal support.

This study was conducted in response to a request from the Administration on Children, Youth and Families (ACYF) within the U.S. Department of Health and Human Services to update the research highlighted in the 1993 NRC report (see Appendix B for research recommendations from that report). ACYF asked that the updated report "provide recommendations for allocating existing research funds and also suggest funding mechanisms and topic areas to which new resources could be allocated or enhanced resources could be redirected." Specifically, ACYF asked the expert committee appointed to undertake this study to

- build on a review of the literature and findings from the evaluation of research on child abuse and neglect;
- identify research that provides knowledge relevant to the programmatic, research, and policy fields;
- recommend research priorities for the next decade, including new areas of research that should be funded by public and private agencies; and
- identify areas that are no longer a priority for funding.

The Institute of Medicine (IOM) and the NRC within the National Academies appointed a committee with expertise across a broad array of disciplines associated with child abuse and neglect to carry out this study. The committee commissioned a number of background papers that summarized research findings and detailed research infrastructure needs in key areas of child abuse and neglect research. It held four face-to-face meetings, including two public sessions, and numerous conference calls to review the literature; discuss the current understanding of the extent, causes, and consequences of child abuse and neglect and the effectiveness of intervention programs; and deliberate on its findings, conclusions, and recommendations. The committee also held a workshop on "Research Issues in Child Abuse and Neglect" (IOM and NRC, 2012).

Publications on child abuse and neglect have increased more than threefold over the past two decades, documenting significant advances in the field. Among the findings reported are the following: (1) research on the consequences of child abuse and neglect has demonstrated that they are serious, long-lasting, and cumulative through adulthood; (2) the consequences include effects on the brain and other biological systems, as well as on behavior and psychosocial outcomes; and (3) rigorous research has been conducted on interventions to address the problem. Yet despite these gains in grasping the scope and scale of the problem, as well as identifying some general preventive approaches with proven effectiveness, much of the research evidence also underscores how much remains unknown. The causes of child abuse and neglect need to be understood with greater specificity if the problem is to be prevented and treated more effectively. Also needed is a better understanding of what appear to be significant declines in physical and sexual child abuse but not neglect; why children have differential sensitivity to abuse of similar severity; why some child victims respond to treatment and others do not; how different types of abuse impact a child's developmental trajectory; and how culture, social stratification, and associated contextual factors affect the causes, consequences, prevention, and treatment of child abuse and neglect.

DESCRIBING THE PROBLEM

A critical step in devising effective responses to child abuse and neglect is reasonable agreement on the definition of the problem and its scope. A key definition of child abuse and neglect is contained in Section 3 of the Child Abuse Prevention and Treatment Act (CAPTA) (42 U.S.C. § 5101 note).

> At a minimum, any recent act or set of acts or failure to act on the part of a parent or caretaker, which results in death, serious physical or emotional harm, sexual abuse or exploitation, or an act or failure to act, which presents an imminent risk of serious harm.

This definition, enshrined in federal legislation, establishes the basis on which all states, as well as American Samoa, the Commonwealth of the Northern Mariana Islands, the Commonwealth of Puerto Rico, the District of Columbia, Guam, and the Virgin Islands, develop laws requiring certain professionals to report instances of child abuse or neglect to child protective service agencies.

While the CAPTA definition is a useful benchmark for describing what one looks for in determining instances of child abuse and neglect, child abuse and neglect are defined differently across the various purposes for which information on the problem is collected. Achieving clarity in the area of child abuse and neglect has therefore been a challenge. Legal definitions vary across states; researchers apply diverse standards in determining incidence and prevalence rates in clinical and population-based studies; and substantial obstacles challenge efforts to learn about children's, especially young children's, experiences with caregiver-inflicted abuse or neglect. As a result, the characteristics of the problem and determinations regarding its scope will differ depending on the data source used for analysis. This challenge is articulated in the 1993 NRC report and continues to impede a full understanding of the nature of the child abuse and neglect problem.

Despite this definitional challenge, data are available with which to estimate the scope, prevalence, and characteristics of child abuse and neglect across the United States. The National Child Abuse and Neglect Data System (NCANDS) is the official child abuse and neglect reporting system for cases referred to state child protection authorities. In fiscal year 2011, all states, the District of Columbia, and all territories contributed counts of the number of cases referred to child protective services, the case characteristics, and the case outcomes. Based on NCANDS data, about three-quarters of reported cases are classified as neglect, about 18 percent as physical abuse, and about 9 percent as sexual abuse (ACF, 2012). The specific rates vary among states but overall reflect the general pattern that a substantial majority of cases are neglect, with physical and sexual abuse representing much smaller groups. The characteristics of the child victims of abuse and neglect show a gender breakdown that is approximately evenly split between males and females. The highest rates of child abuse and neglect occur among the very youngest children. Perpetrators are mainly parents (81 percent), 88 percent of whom are biological parents (ACF, 2012). Somewhat more than half of perpetrators are female. These same demographic characteristics also are reflected in other research that draws its samples from national incidence studies utilizing different data sources and methodologies.

While some discrepancies exist across data sources, strong evidence indicates that sexual abuse has declined substantially in the past two decades, and the balance of evidence favors a decline in physical abuse, especially the more common and less serious forms. There is no evidence that neglect is declining overall. However, states vary significantly as to whether neglect is increasing, decreasing, or remaining constant. These disparate trends and their causes currently are not well understood. Such understanding is essential to bring clarity to the phenomena of child abuse and neglect and to identify appropriate program and policy responses.

CAUSES

Theoretical models for child abuse and neglect have progressed as the field has matured. Yet hundreds of studies have reported an association or correlation between a variety of potential risk factors and child abuse or neglect without considering these models. Drawing on the work of Brofenbrenner (1979) and Belsky (1980), who identified interrelated but embedded factors that contribute to child abuse and neglect, these risk factors can be organized into individual-level, family, and contextual factors. Contextual factors represent the broader social systems that influence parental functioning, including macrosystem factors representing the social or cultural forces that contribute to and sustain abuse or neglect.

Parental substance abuse, history of child abuse or neglect, and depression appear to have the strongest support in the literature as risk factors for child abuse and neglect. There is also a robust body of knowledge about the role of stressful environments and the impact of poverty. Other candidate risk factors that have received at least some support in the literature for an association with child abuse and neglect include children having a disability, parental psychopathology, early childbearing, low socioeconomic status, and social beliefs about discipline and corporal punishment. Acknowledging that risk factors seldom occur in isolation, some studies have shown that the presence of multiple risk factors can dramatically increase the likelihood of child abuse and neglect. It is important to acknowledge, however, that all of these factors simply describe circumstances surrounding elevated risk, but that none of these individual or contextual factors has been shown to "cause" child abuse and neglect. There is also a relative lack of understanding of why certain factors result in abuse or neglect in some situations but not others. Further, the complex interaction among multiple risk factors, especially in conjunction with protective factors and resilience, is not clearly understood.

The field's limited knowledge of causal pathways is due mainly to the fact that research in child abuse and neglect has utilized primarily correlational designs and analyses, relying heavily on cross-sectional studies and retrospective self-reports. Research in the field needs to include models that test causal pathways using rigorous research designs and analyses. This work would ideally involve longitudinal studies starting before the birth of the target children to permit better controlled studies of who does and does not commit child abuse and neglect and under what cultural, social, and individual circumstances. Animal model studies can provide insight on issues difficult to address in human studies.

CONSEQUENCES

Abuse and neglect appear to influence the course of development by altering many elements of biological and psychological development; in other words, childhood abuse and neglect have a profound and often lasting impact that can encompass psychological and physical health, neurobiological development, relational skills, and risk behaviors. The timing of the abuse or neglect and its chronicity clearly matter for outcomes. In particular, the more often children experience abuse or neglect, the worse are the outcomes.

Across human and nonhuman primate studies, perturbations to the hypothalamic-pituitary-adrenal (HPA) "stress" system often are associated with abuse and neglect and with a range of mental and physical health problems. Abused and neglected children also show behavioral and emotional difficulties that are consistent with effects on the amygdala, a structure in the brain that is critically involved in emotion and associated with internalizing of problems, heightened anxiety, emotional reactivity, and deficits in emotional processing. A number of studies suggest that abuse and neglect are associated with functional changes in the prefrontal cortex and associated brain regions, often affecting inhibitory control. Specifically, children who experience abuse and neglect appear especially at risk for deficits in executive functioning that affect behavioral regulation. Abuse and neglect also increase children's risk for experiencing academic problems.

The impact of abuse and neglect on relational skills likely operates at least partially through disorganized attachment to the caregiver, which in turn can be predictive of long-term problems. As a result of abusive or neglectful responses from caregivers, children are at risk for failing to develop effective strategies for regulating emotions in interactions with others. Further, abused and neglected children, like children with a history of institutional care, have problematic peer relations at disproportionately high rates. Similarly, abuse and neglect have been associated with dissociation among preschool- and elementary-aged children, as well as among adults.

Long-term outcomes among adolescents and adults with a history of abuse and neglect include higher rates of alcohol abuse and alcoholism, as well as elevated rates of posttraumatic stress disorder, compared with those without a history of abuse and neglect. Additionally, experiences of abuse and neglect in childhood have a large effect on suicide attempts in adolescence and adulthood. Moreover, children who experience abuse and neglect are more likely to engage in sexual activity at earlier ages than comparison groups. Childhood sexual abuse especially has been associated with heightened risks for a range of adverse outcomes related to sexual risk-taking behaviors.

Regarding impacts on physical health outcomes, at their most extreme, abuse and neglect are associated with stunted growth. The rate of untreated illness and infection is high among abused and neglected children, as has been found consistently among children living with their birth parents, children placed in foster care, and adults years after their experience of abuse or neglect. In various studies, different forms of abuse and neglect also have been linked with increased body mass index and increased rates of obesity in childhood, adolescence, and adulthood.

THE CHILD WELFARE SYSTEM

Each year, more than 3 million referrals for child abuse and neglect are received that involve around 6 million individual children. Contrary to popular belief, most investigated reports of child abuse and neglect do not result in out-of-home placement; only about 20 percent of investigated cases lead to the removal of a child from his or her home. The risk of placement and length of stay in out-of-home care can vary considerably based on such factors as a child's age and the family's race, socioeconomic status, and state of residence. Family-based care—specifically regular foster family care and relative (kinship) care—has been emphasized as the preferred option for the placement of an abused or neglected child. There has also been a policy impetus to limit the number of placements per child. The clinical literature documents that instability in placement has negative effects on children with respect to insecure attachment, psychopathology, and other problematic outcomes.

Since 1993, policy, practice, and program initiatives to improve the public child welfare system—the institution charged with providing society's response to suspected cases of child abuse and neglect formally reported to authorities—have received significant attention. The child welfare system provides four main sets of services: child protection investigation, family-centered services and supports, foster care, and adoption.

Beyond specific federal legislation that has paved the way for practice reforms, states and localities have adopted a number of system-level reforms that at their outset most likely were intended to improve child and family outcomes. These reforms have included differential response, privatization of child welfare services, models of parent and family engagement, and the implementation of practice models. The strongest evidence to date is on the effects of differential response.

Differential response systems have been implemented in 21 states, the District of Columbia, and four tribes to offer multiple pathways for addressing the needs of children and families referred to child welfare services. In its simplest form, differential response entails screening child abuse and neglect reports and, based on level of risk and other criteria, referring cases to either an assessment or a traditional investigation pathway. Results of some evaluations indicate a positive impact of this approach with regard to maintenance of child safety, fewer removals from home, increased access to services, and family satisfaction.

The child welfare system currently faces systemic concerns relating to a lack of organizational capacity to carry out some of the many promising practice and intervention models that are being developed. Barriers to sufficient organizational capacity include issues related to reduced funding; high caseloads; staff who are poorly trained, especially in addressing the social and emotional needs of the children who come in contact with the child protection services system; limited staff supervision; and a culture that does not necessarily support autonomy, quality practice, and critical thinking. Although certain organizational change strategies have been found to be evidence based and effective for improving workforce retention in child welfare, more research is needed in this area, especially research linking practice outcomes and workforce issues. Research also is needed to examine effective strategies for bringing to bear the interdisciplinary knowledge necessary to carry out all the diverse functions of a child welfare agency. And child welfare agencies need to employ more effective quality improvement strategies.

EFFECTIVE INTERVENTIONS AND SERVICE DELIVERY SYSTEMS

Since the 1993 NRC report was issued, significant advances have occurred in the development, evaluation, and dissemination of model programs for preventing or treating various forms of child abuse and neglect. In addition to the public child protection and child welfare systems found in all communities, a variety of treatment programs targeting victims and perpetrators of child abuse and neglect are offered through various mental health and social service agencies. Many communities also have access to primary and secondary prevention services designed to reduce the risk for child abuse or neglect among families experiencing difficulties. Among this growing array of service options, there is strong evidence for the efficacy of an increasing number of interventions.

In the treatment domain, trauma-focused cognitive behavioral therapy, a brief structured program based on well-established theory and treatment elements, has been tested extensively and found to be effective with children affected by abuse and other traumatic experiences. Equally important has been the successful application of a number of well-established parent management training programs to children and families involved in the child welfare system. Again, these are programs with well-established theory and large bodies of knowledge.

In terms of prevention services, strategies such as early home visiting targeting pregnant women and parents with newborns are well researched and have demonstrated meaningful improvements in mitigating the factors commonly associated with an elevated risk for poor parenting, including abuse and neglect. Promising prevention models also have been identified in other areas, including public awareness campaigns, parenting education programs, and professional practice reforms. In contrast to the reality in 1993, policy makers and practitioners have a much stronger pool of program candidates on which to draw in both remediating the impacts of abuse and neglect and reducing its incidence.

Research suggests that a degree of reciprocity exists between service models and their host agencies. In some instances, the rigor and quality of these innovations may alter the standards of practice throughout an agency, thereby improving the overall service delivery process and enhancing participant outcomes. In other cases, organizations that provide little incentive for staff to adopt new ideas or that reduce the dosage or duration of evidence-based models to accommodate their limited resources contribute to poor implementation and reduced impacts. Maximizing the impact of evidence-based models and proven approaches will require more explicit attention to the organizational strengths and weaknesses of those agencies in which such models and approaches are embedded and to how these factors impact service implementation.

While research carried out since 1993 has generated much knowledge that can inform programs and policies, some notable gaps remain. These include understanding of the underlying reasons why some individuals and families fail to benefit from treatment and prevention programs; of how evidence-based practices and interventions are implemented, replicated, and sustained; of which service attributes are most essential to achieving the desired impacts and for whom; and of costs for training and supervision, data monitoring, and monitoring of service delivery. Research also is lacking on the question of system reform and the infrastructure required to institutionalize and support such reform. Little research exists that can inform how best to improve interventions and agency performance in the areas of workforce development, data management, and system integration. While some preliminary research has been conducted in the area of system integration, it remains unclear which strategies are most effective in building a collaborative culture and a set of working relationships across public institutions and between these institutions and the community-based agencies that constitute the child abuse and neglect response system.

RESEARCH INFRASTRUCTURE

To be productive, high-quality scientific research requires a sophisticated infrastructure. This is particularly true for research that requires multiple fields, disciplines, methodologies, and levels of analysis to fully address key questions. Research on child abuse and neglect is especially complex, involving diverse independent service systems, multiple professions, ethical issues that are particularly complicated, and levels of outcome analysis ranging from the individual child to national statistics. Moreover, the building of a national research infrastructure designed to adequately address the problem of child abuse and neglect will require a dedicated and trained cadre of researchers with expertise that spans the many domains associated with research in this field and the supports necessary to sustain high-quality, methodologically sound research endeavors. Moreover, the ability of the research to achieve the goal of informing quality programming and policies will be limited if the research fails to address the complex role of culture and context in the causes, consequences, prevention, and treatment of child abuse and neglect, particularly given the increasing heterogeneity of U.S. families.

Research on child abuse and neglect entails a number of challenges. As noted, the problem cuts across a wide range of domains, such as child welfare, medicine, child development, and public health. Services must be evaluated in multiple areas, such as treatment, prevention, and policy. Moreover, children and families receiving services related to child abuse and neglect often are eligible to receive services from other systems, and diversity in the type, timing, and intensity of these additional services can be difficult to account for in research on the effects of child abuse and neglect interventions. Services designed to respond to the problem of child abuse and neglect also are provided through the many systems that interact with abused and neglected children and their families, and these systems often act independently of one another, with little or no coordination. Finally, coordination of research in the field and opportunities for support have been fragmented and generally insufficient to develop and sustain the capacity for a national child abuse and neglect research enterprise.

The formation of child abuse and neglect research centers presents an important opportunity to develop and sustain a volume of high-quality interdisciplinary research on child abuse and neglect. University-affiliated child abuse and neglect research centers also provide opportunities to train and support a new generation of researchers to ensure the growth of the field.

POLICY

Since the 1993 NRC report was issued, numerous changes have been made to federal and state laws and policies designed to impact the incidence, reporting, and negative health and economic consequences of child abuse and neglect. At its core, the debate around the development of laws and policies to help prevent child abuse and neglect involves questions of public value. It also involves trade-offs entailed in laws and policies between public benefit and private interests. Research evaluating laws and policies on child abuse and neglect can make it possible to anticipate and respond to predictable problems that may occur as a result of their implementation. Research helps address questions whose answers are critical to implementing child protection laws and policies effectively.

The research design needed to evaluate laws and policies is not always the same as the design one would use for the evaluation of child abuse and neglect practice interventions. Although some laws and policies can be evaluated by random assignment (e.g., studying the differential response approach discussed above), random assignment cannot be used if it would differentially affect the legal rights of citizens, if it would subject citizens to unequal treatment under the law, or if it would place children in jeopardy. Furthermore, simply studying the incidence of child abuse and neglect in the aggregate (such as at the state or national level) is unlikely to aid in determining and attributing potential causes.

Another difficulty in evaluating laws and policies related to child abuse and neglect is that adherence to a law, such as one on mandatory reporting, often is predicated on public knowledge, understanding, and support, which frequently vary across practitioner disciplines, as well as within and among states. Finally, much of the evolution in child abuse and neglect law and policy over the last few decades has consisted of incremental changes to existing legislation (such as CAPTA). In these cases, what is needed is research on the implementation and augmentation of the law or policy rather than the core law or policy itself.

Given these complexities in conducting analyses of child abuse and neglect laws and policies and the fact that the laws and policies vary by state, it is not surprising that little research has been done in this area. A number of federal laws set national standards for confronting child abuse and neglect issues; however, many standards are either further elucidated by or completely derived from state legislation. Research on changes in both state and federal laws and policies has been extremely limited.

The heterogeneity of state laws on child abuse and neglect can be viewed as offering the opportunity for a natural experiment. State variations in such areas as mandated reporters, definitions of abuse and neglect, and the range of penalties provide a myriad of opportunities to examine the impact of policy change. New methods, such as propensity scoring and difference-within-difference analyses, can be powerful tools for examining policy-relevant questions.

RECOMMENDATIONS

The committee formulated a set of recommendations around four pertinent areas, focused on the development of a coordinated research enterprise in child abuse and neglect that is relevant to the programs, policies, and practices that influence children and their caregivers. The four areas are (1) development of a national strategic research plan that is focused on priority topics identified by the committee and that delineates implementation and accountability steps across federal agencies (Recommendations 1-3), (2) creation of a national surveillance system (Recommendation 4), (3) development of the structures necessary to train cohorts of high-quality researchers to conduct child abuse and neglect research (Recommendations 5-7), and (4) creation of mechanisms for conducting policy-relevant research (Recommendations 8-9).

A National Strategic Research Plan

Recommendation 1: Federal agencies, in partnership with private foundations and academic institutions, should implement a research agenda designed to advance knowledge and understanding of the causes and consequences of child abuse and neglect, as well as the identification and implementation of effective services for its treatment and prevention. The research priorities listed in Figure S-1 should be considered in this agenda.

Recommendation 2: The Federal Interagency Work Group on Child Abuse and Neglect, under the auspices of the assistant secretary of the Administration for Children and Families, should develop a strategic plan that details a business plan, an implementation strategy, and de-

partmental accountability for the advancement of a national research agenda on child abuse and neglect.

Recommendation 3: The assistant secretary of the Administration for Children and Families should convene senior-level leadership of all federal agencies with a stake in child abuse and neglect research to discuss and assign accountability for the implementation of a strategic plan to advance a national research agenda on child abuse and neglect.

Causes and Consequences

- Improve understanding of the separate and synergistic consequences of different forms of child abuse and neglect.
- Initiate high-quality longitudinal studies of child abuse and neglect.
- Target innovative research on the causes of child abuse and neglect.
- Improve understanding of the behavioral and neurobiological mechanisms that mediate the association between child abuse and neglect and its sequelae.

Services in Complex Systems and Policy

- Explore highly effective delivery systems.
- Develop and test new programs for underserved children and families.
- Identify the best means of replicating effective interventions and services with fidelity.
- Identify the most effective ways to implement and sustain evidence-based programs in real-world settings.
- Investigate the longitudinal impacts of prevention.
- Encourage research designed to provide a better understanding of trends in the incidence of child abuse and neglect.
- Evaluate the impact of laws and policies that address prevention and intervention systems and services for child abuse and neglect at the federal, state, and local levels.

Disentangle the role of cultural processes, social stratification influences, ecological variations, and immigrant/acculturation status.

Apply multidisciplinary, multimethod, and multisector approaches.

Leverage and build upon the existing knowledge base of child abuse and neglect research and related fields, as well as research definitions, designs, and opportunities.

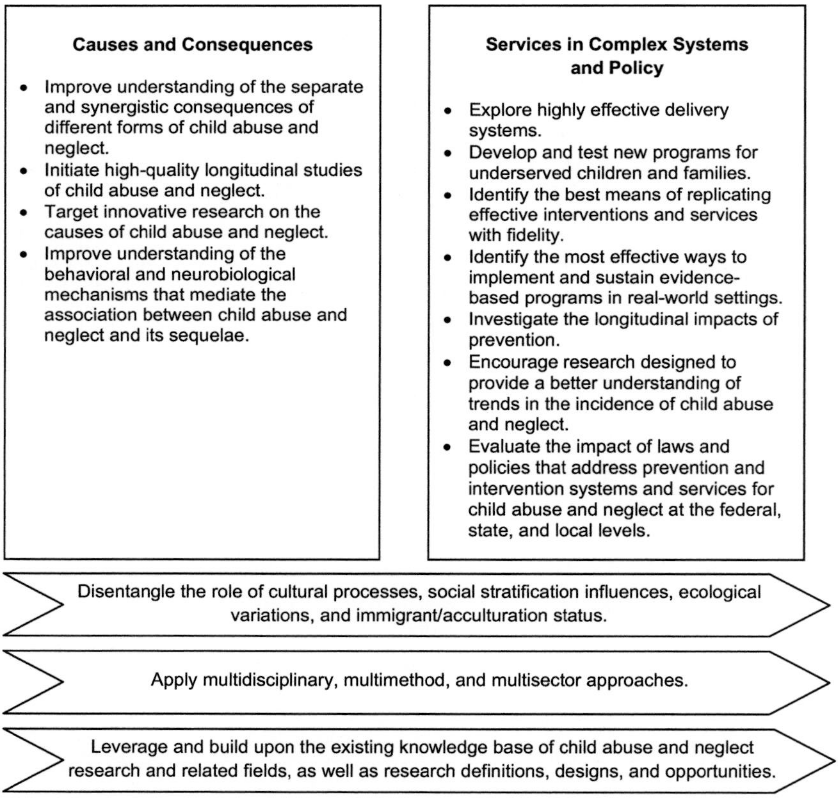

FIGURE S-1 Research priorities in child abuse and neglect.

A National Surveillance System

Recommendation 4: The Centers for Disease Control and Prevention, in partnership with the Federal Interagency Work Group on Child Abuse and Neglect, should develop and sustain a national surveillance system for child abuse and neglect that links data across multiple systems and sources.

Training of Researchers

Recommendation 5: Federal agencies, in partnership with private foundations and academic institutions, should invest in developing and sustaining a cadre of researchers who can examine issues of child abuse and neglect across multiple disciplines.

Recommendation 6: Federal agencies, in partnership with private foundations and academic institutions, should provide funding for new multidisciplinary education and research centers on child abuse and neglect in geographically diverse locations across the United States.

Recommendation 7: The National Institutes of Health should develop a new child maltreatment, trauma, and violence study section under the Risk, Prevention, and Health Behavior Integrated Review Group.

Mechanisms for Conducting Policy-Relevant Research

Recommendation 8: To ensure accountability and effectiveness and to encourage evidence-based policy making, Congress should include support in all new legislation related to child abuse and neglect, such as reauthorizations of the Child Abuse Prevention and Treatment Act, for evaluation of the impact of new child abuse and neglect laws and policies and require a review of the findings in reauthorization discussions.

Recommendation 9: To ensure accountability and effectiveness, to support evidence-based policy making, and to allow for exploration of the differential impact of various state laws and policies, state legislatures should include support in all new legislation related to child abuse and neglect for evaluation of the impact of new child abuse and neglect laws and policies and require a review of the findings in reauthorization discussions.

REFERENCES

ACF (Administration for Children and Families). 2012. *Child maltreatment, 2011 report.* Washington, DC: U.S. Deparment of Health and Human Services, ACF. http://www.acf.hhs.gov/sites/default/files/cb/cm11.pdf (accessed December 3, 2013).

Belsky, J. 1980. Child maltreatment: An ecological integration. *American Psychologist* 35(4): 320-335.

Bronfenbrenner, U. 1979. *The ecology of human development: Experiments by nature and design.* Cambridge, MA: Harvard University Press.

IOM (Institute of Medicine) and NRC (National Research Council). 2012. *Child maltreatment research, policy, and practice for the next decade: Workshop summary.* Washington, DC: The National Academies Press.

NRC. 1993. *Understanding child abuse and neglect.* Washington, DC: National Academy Press.

1

Introduction

The 1993 National Research Council (NRC) report *Understanding Child Abuse and Neglect* notes that "Child maltreatment is a devastating social problem in American society" (NRC, 1993, p. 1). The committee responsible for the present report, armed with research findings gleaned during the past 20 years, regards child abuse and neglect not just as a social problem but as a serious public health issue. Researchers have found that child abuse and neglect affects not only children but also the adults they become. Its effects cascade throughout the life course, with costly consequences for individuals, families, and society. These effects are seen in all aspects of human functioning, including physical and mental health, as well as important areas such as education, work, and social relationships. Furthermore, rigorous examinations of risk and protective factors for child abuse and neglect at the individual, contextual, and macrosystem levels have led to more effective strategies for prevention and treatment.

This public health problem requires swift and effective action. The committee's deliberations led to recommendations for responding to the problem of child abuse and neglect while remaining realistic about the nature of feasible actions in these challenging political and economic times. The intent is to capitalize on existing opportunities whenever possible while advocating for new actions when they are needed.

The committee also believes that the existing body of research creates enormous opportunities for research going forward; the nation is poised to take full advantage of a developing science of child abuse and neglect. In particular, the results of studies of the consequences of child abuse and neglect, integrating biological with behavioral and social context research, as well as studies and controlled prevention trials that integrate basic findings with services research, now provide a solid base for moving forward with more sophisticated and systematic research designs to address important unanswered questions. New knowledge and better research tools can yield a better understanding of the causes of child abuse and neglect, as well as the most effective ways to prevent and treat it.

At the same time, however, the existing research and service system infrastructures are inadequate for taking full advantage of this new knowledge. The committee hopes that this gap will narrow as researchers in diverse domains collaborate to elucidate the underlying causes and consequences of child abuse and neglect, as those implementing promising interventions learn how best to take evidence-based models to scale with fidelity, and as policies are examined more rigorously for their ability to improve outcomes and create a coordinated and efficient system of care.

THE 1993 REPORT

Two decades ago, the Administration on Children, Youth and Families (ACYF) within the U.S. Department of Health and Human Services asked the National Academy of Sciences to conduct a study of research needs in the area of child abuse and neglect. That study resulted in the 1993 NRC report, which synthesizes the research on child abuse and neglect and, adopting a child-oriented developmental and ecological perspective, outlines 17 research priorities in an agenda that addresses 4 objectives:

1. clarify the nature and scope of child maltreatment;
2. provide an understanding of the origins and consequences of child maltreatment to improve the quality of future policy and program efforts;
3. provide empirical information about the strengths and limitations of existing interventions while guiding the development of more effective interventions; and
4. develop a science policy for child maltreatment research that recognizes the importance of national leadership, human and financial resources, instrumentation, and appropriate institutional arrangements.

TRENDS SINCE 1993

Since the 1993 report, research on child abuse and neglect has expanded, and understanding of the consequences and other aspects of child abuse and neglect for the children involved, their families, and society has advanced significantly. During that same period, rates of reported physical and sexual abuse (but not neglect) have declined substantially, for reasons not fully understood. On the other hand, reports of psychological and emotional abuse have risen.

Child abuse and neglect nonetheless remains a pervasive, persistent, and pernicious problem in the United States. Each year more than 3 million referrals for child abuse and neglect are received that involve around 6 million children, although most of these reports are not substantiated. In fiscal year 2011, the latest year for which data are available, state child protective services agencies encountered 676,569 children, or about 9.1 of every 1,000 children, who were found to be victims of child abuse and neglect, including physical abuse, sexual abuse, psychological abuse, and medical and other types of neglect. More than one-quarter had been victimized previously. Of these 676,569 children, 1,545 died as a result of the abuse or neglect they suffered—most younger than 4 years old (ACF, 2012). Yet these figures are underestimates because of underreporting (GAO, 2011). For example, the estimate of the rate of child abuse and neglect by caretakers in 2005-2006 derived from the most recent National Incidence Study of Child Abuse and Neglect, a sample survey, was 17.1 of every 1,000 children (totaling more than 1.25 million children), and many more were determined to be at risk (Sedlak et al., 2010). This uncertainty as to the extent of child abuse and neglect hampers understanding of its causes and consequences, as well as effective prevention and treatment interventions.

Research conducted since 1993 has made clear that child abuse and neglect has much broader and longer-lasting effects than bruises and broken bones or other acute physical and psychological trauma. As noted above, child abuse and neglect can have long-term impacts on its victims, their families, and society. Children's experiences of these long-term consequences vary significantly, depending on the severity, chronicity, and timing of abuse or neglect, as well as the protective factors present in their lives. Nevertheless, abused and neglected children are more prone to experience mental health conditions such as posttraumatic stress disorder and depression, alcoholism and drug abuse, behavioral problems, criminal behavior and violence, certain chronic diseases, and diminished economic well-being.

Society is also affected. Each year, cases of abuse or neglect may impose a cumulative cost to society of $80.3 billion—$33.3 billion in direct costs (e.g., hospitalization, childhood mental health care costs, child welfare system costs, law enforcement costs) and $46.9 billion in indirect costs (e.g., special education, early intervention, adult homelessness, adult mental and physical health care, juvenile and adult criminal justice costs, lost work productivity) (Gelles and Perlman, 2012). An analysis by the Centers for Disease Control and Prevention found that the average lifetime cost of a case of nonfatal child abuse and neglect is $210,012 in 2010 dollars, most of this total ($144,360) due to loss of productivity but also encompassing the costs of child and adult health care, child welfare, criminal justice, and special education (Fang et al., 2012). The average lifetime cost of a case of fatal child abuse and neglect is $1.27 million, due mainly to loss of productivity. These costs are comparable to those of other major health problems, such as stroke and type 2 diabetes, issues that garner far more research funding and public attention.

THE CURRENT STUDY

In 2012, ACYF requested that the National Academies update the 1993 NRC report. ACYF asked that the updated report "provide recommendations for allocating existing research funds and also suggest funding mechanisms and topic areas to which new resources could be allocated or enhanced resources could be redirected." Box 1-1 contains the complete statement of task for this study.

BOX 1-1
Statement of Task

Building on Phase 1, an ad hoc committee will conduct a full study that will culminate in an updated version of the 1993 NRC publication entitled *Understanding Child Abuse and Neglect*. Similar to the 1993 report, the updated report resulting from this study will provide recommendations for allocating existing research funds and also suggest funding mechanisms and topic areas to which new resources could be allocated or enhanced resources could be redirected. To this end, the committee will

- build on the review of literature and findings from the evaluation of research on child abuse and neglect;
- identify research that provides knowledge relevant to the programmatic, research, and policy fields; and
- recommend research priorities for the next decade, including new areas of research that should be funded by public and private agencies and suggestions regarding fields that are no longer a priority for funding.

It is expected that the committee will give special consideration to the following key topics: preventing child maltreatment and promoting well-being; intervention and evidence-based practices; implementation and dissemination; strategies aimed at community, society, place-based, or system-level changes; parent, family, and community engagement; biological and neurobiological research on child maltreatment; culturally relevant and meaningful practice; and future directions for child maltreatment research methods and measurement.

STUDY APPROACH

The Institute of Medicine of the National Academies appointed a committee with expertise in relevant areas—child development and pediatrics, psychology and psychiatry, social work and implementation science, sociology, and policy and legal studies—to conduct this study. The chair and one committee member had been the chair and a member, respectively, of the 1993 study committee, which provided for continuity. The committee commissioned a number of background papers that reviewed research results and research infrastructure needs in key areas of child abuse and neglect research. It held four face-to-face meetings, including two public sessions, as well as many whole-committee and subcommittee conference calls, to review the literature; discuss current understanding of the extent, causes, and consequences of child abuse and neglect, the effectiveness of intervention programs, and the impact of public policies; and discuss the draft report chapters and reach consensus on findings, conclusions, and recommendations.

Evidence

In constructing the evidence base for this report, the committee looked back nearly 20 years to assess the state of research on child abuse and neglect. Doing so involved a conscious decision to privilege the peer-reviewed literature across a variety of disciplines (e.g., social-cultural science, developmental science, neuroscience, prevention and intervention science, epidemiology) and multiple dimensions of child abuse and neglect, including etiology, consequences, prevention, and intervention, as well as ethics, service delivery, and policy. The committee considered the most rigorous evidence drawn from a variety of study designs and methods, including mixed-methods, experimental, observational, prospective, retrospective, descriptive, longitudinal, epidemiological, meta-analysis, and cost-effectiveness studies.

The committee built on a literature review conducted as part of a workshop exploring major research advances since publication of the 1993 report (IOM and NRC, 2012). That initial literature review yielded a brief updated summary of selected research literature, reports, and grey literature on the topics covered in the original report (NRC, 1993). Relevant studies were selected through a search of several scientific databases and were augmented by additional research conducted by other agencies and organizations (see IOM and NRC, 2012, for more detailed information).

The committee expanded on the 2012 literature review and critically examined publications derived from a literature database search, supplemented by the committee's knowledge of relevant work in the field. The review strategy began with a keyword search of electronic citation databases, followed by a review of the literature gleaned from published research syntheses, academic books, and peer-reviewed journals (i.e., *Child Abuse and Neglect, Child Maltreatment, Children and Youth Services Review, Child Welfare, Protecting Children*); websites of research, nonprofit, and policy organizations (including evidence-based clearinghouses); professional conference proceedings; and other grey literature. Literature on child abuse and neglect in the United States was the primary focus; however, the committee also considered key studies from other countries. While the committee's approach did not represent a systematic review of the evidence, it did provide a body of research well suited to guide an understanding of critical issues and formulation of the recommendations presented in this report.

Definitions

As described in Chapter 2, definitions of child abuse and neglect can vary considerably as legal definitions differ across states, and researchers apply diverse standards in determining whether abuse or neglect has occurred. A basic yet important definition of child abuse and neglect is contained in Section 3 of the Child Abuse Prevention and Treatment Act (CAPTA)[1]:

> At a minimum, any recent act or set of acts or failure to act on the part of a parent or caretaker, which results in death, serious physical or emotional harm, sexual abuse or exploitation, or an act or failure to act, which presents an imminent risk of serious harm.

While this federal definition sets a minimum standard for legal definitions, each state has developed its own definitions of child abuse and neglect. Child abuse and neglect are usually represented by four major categories: physical abuse, neglect, sexual abuse, and emotional (or psychological) abuse. Table 1-1 presents examples of acts that are considered to represent each of these four types of abuse and neglect, as compiled by the Child Welfare Information Gateway.

The examples listed in Table 1-1 are drawn from state definitions of child abuse and neglect; however, they are not representative of any specific state. There is considerable variation across jurisdictions with regard to statutory descriptions of which acts constitute abuse or neglect. In addition, child abuse and neglect are defined in many contexts outside of legal and child protection system venues, research being the most notably germane to this report. Many studies identify cases of abuse and neglect through the use of survey instruments. Across these studies is found much variation

---

[1] 42 U.S.C. § 5101 note.

TABLE 1-1 Examples of Acts of Child Abuse and Neglect

Physical Abuse	Nonaccidental physical injury (ranging from minor bruises to severe fractures or death) as a result of punching, beating, kicking, biting, shaking, throwing, stabbing, choking, hitting (with a hand, stick, strap, or other object), burning, or otherwise harming a child, that is inflicted by a parent, caregiver, or other person who has responsibility for the child. Such injury is considered abuse regardless of whether the caregiver intended to hurt the child. Physical discipline, such as spanking or paddling, is not considered abuse as long as it is reasonable and causes no bodily injury to the child.
Neglect	The failure of a parent, guardian, or other caregiver to provide for a child's basic needs. Neglect may be • physical (e.g., failure to provide necessary food or shelter, or lack of appropriate supervision); • medical (e.g., failure to provide necessary medical or mental health treatment); • educational (e.g., failure to educate a child or attend to special education needs); or • emotional (e.g., inattention to a child's emotional needs, failure to provide psychological care, or permitting the child to use alcohol or other drugs). These situations do not always mean a child is neglected. Sometimes cultural values, the standards of care in the community, and poverty may be contributing factors, indicating the family is in need of information or assistance. When a family fails to use information and resources, and the child's health or safety is at risk, then child welfare intervention may be required.
Sexual Abuse	Includes activities by a parent or caregiver such as fondling a child's genitals, penetration, incest, rape, sodomy, indecent exposure, and exploitation through prostitution or the production of pornographic materials. Appearing in the definition of abuse and neglect itself, sexual abuse is further defined by the Child Abuse Prevention and Treatment Act (CAPTA) as "the employment, use, persuasion, inducement, enticement, or coercion of any child to engage in, or assist any other person to engage in, any sexually explicit conduct or simulation of such conduct for the purpose of producing a visual depiction of such conduct; or the rape, and in cases of caretaker or inter-familial relationships, statutory rape, molestation, prostitution, or other form of sexual exploitation of children, or incest with children."

continued

TABLE 1-1 Continued

Emotional (or Psychological) Abuse	A pattern of behavior that impairs a child's emotional development or sense of self-worth. This may include constant criticism, threats, or rejection, as well as withholding love, support, or guidance. Emotional abuse is often difficult to prove, and therefore, child protective services may not be able to intervene without evidence of harm or mental injury to the child.

SOURCE: Adapted from CWIG, 2008.

in the types of questions asked of respondents and the types of responses that indicate instances of abuse or neglect. While some standards have been developed, definitions of child abuse and neglect in this context are often tailored to the needs of specific studies.

Given this definitional landscape, which is discussed further in Chapter 2, the committee made two significant determinations with regard to definitions of child abuse and neglect for the purposes of this report. First, the scope of the discussion in this report is limited to actions (or inaction) of parents or caretakers, to the exclusion of extrafamilial abuse. This scope is reflective of the minimum definitional standard prescribed by CAPTA. Although individual jurisdictions may expand their definitions of abuse to include actions by extrafamilial parties, the CAPTA minimum standard is the most universally relevant to legal and child protection systems across the United States, as well as the data drawn from such sources for research purposes. Restricting the scope of this report to parent or caregiver actors also allowed the committee to conduct a more focused evaluation of the causes and consequences of abuse and neglect, as well as the delivery of prevention and treatment services, within the context of family and home. It is important to note that while this scope applies to the organization and content of the report, some of the studies discussed in the following chapters draw samples from jurisdictions that include instances of extrafamilial abuse in their definitions.

Second, the report does not specify a particular set of circumstances that would define whether or not an instance of child abuse or neglect has occurred. In addition to the need to review many studies that incorporate samples based on differing characterizations of acts of child abuse and neglect, there is insufficient evidence with which to determine the single most reliable, effective, and appropriate definitional approach. As studies are presented throughout the report, methodological limitations identified by the committee are described where applicable.

RESEARCH ADVANCES IN CHILD ABUSE AND NEGLECT

As noted above, research conducted in the past 20 years has revealed child abuse and neglect to be a serious public health problem, but it has also revealed that rates of physical and sexual abuse of children (although not neglect) appear to have declined. Credited with the possible declines are some policy and practice reforms that include more aggressive prosecution of offenders, especially in the area of child sexual abuse; more effective treatment programs for victims of child abuse and neglect; and increased investments in prevention programs, especially for new parents. Yet contradictions and inconsistencies in the data demand more analysis.

Publications on child abuse and neglect increased more than threefold over the past two decades. Among the key areas seeing significant advances are (1) research on the consequences of child abuse and neglect, demonstrating that its effects are severe, long-lasting, and cumulative over adulthood; (2) research demonstrating effects on the brain and other biological systems, as well as on behavior and psychosocial outcomes; and (3) rigorous treatment and prevention research demonstrating the effectiveness of interventions.

Despite these advances, however, the research evidence also underscores how much remains unknown. More specific research designs and incorporation of core questions into studies examining factors that impact parental capacity and child development are needed to enable greater understanding and more effective prevention of child abuse and neglect. Also needed is a better understanding of the remarkable declines in reported child abuse, why children have differential sensitivity to abuse of similar severity, and how different types of abuse impact a child's developmental trajectory.

Needed as well are improved theories and research that can make it possible to disentangle the multiple causes and consequences of child abuse and neglect. The complexity of child abuse and neglect requires a systems approach, employing integrated, cross-disciplinary thinking, and research methods that can support better-specified model testing. Among specific improvements needed are refined theoretical models and research designs representing the relevant disciplines and ecological levels with appropriate specification of effects; multiple measures and methods for tracking core constructs, including neurological and other biological measures such as genetic and epigenetic factors; longitudinal research designs with which to assess the sequences of events that lead to abusive and neglectful behaviors and to identify treatment and prevention interventions that can protect against the intergenerational transfer of abuse and neglect; appropriate statistical analyses that differentiate effects at various ecological levels; appropriate statistical control to create more rigorous experimental opportunities when randomized controlled trials are infeasible for evaluating interventions; and designs that account for overlapping variance due to children's being nested within multiple layers of systems. Simpler designs and analyses can still play a role, especially when descriptive studies are needed to generate hypotheses. And essential for any study is clarity of the question being examined, preferably with a hypothesis that can be tested; the appropriate research design and statistical analysis can then be identified.

While some longitudinal studies on child abuse and neglect do exist, including the Longitudinal Studies in Child Abuse (LONGSCAN) and National Survey of Child and Adolescent Well-Being (NSCAW), additional longitudinal, prospective studies are needed. An example of the kind of study required is the Fragile Families and Child Wellbeing Study, which is following a cohort of nearly 5,000 children born in large U.S. cities between 1998 and 2000, with an oversample of 75 percent children born to unmarried parents (for further information, see www.fragilefamilies.princeton.edu). This longitudinal study (now producing the sixth wave of data on children and their families 15 years after the original data collection) has examined many questions related to the nature of the sample, including child abuse and neglect (e.g., Guterman et al., 2009; Lee et al., 2008; Whitaker et al., 2007). The study employs embedded variables, such as children and parents within families, including all the variations that currently occur in families, and many types of data, from neighborhood characteristics to biological measures.

Importantly, this study serves as an example for the rigor of data analysis. A recent working paper by McLanahan and colleagues (2012) carefully reviews the literature on the causal effects of father absence to examine how study design impacts findings. The authors conclude that studies with more rigorous designs have found negative effects of father absence on child well-being, but with smaller effect sizes than have been found with standard cross-sectional designs. These conclusions demonstrate the importance of designing rigorous studies to examine complex questions such as those relating to child abuse and neglect. The Fragile Families study can provide a great deal of information on child abuse and neglect, and a similarly rigorous study designed to examine the many important questions concerning child abuse and neglect could do much more.

Both practice and policy research require similar improvements. Future research efforts need to address the impacts of service integration and the additive effects of conducting multiple interventions that simultaneously address the problem at the individual and community levels. While strengthening the response to child abuse and neglect will require continued rigorous prevention and treatment research on the efficacy of promising interventions, equally important is examining how such efforts can be replicated with quality and consistency. Finally, research is needed to understand the role and impacts of a more integrated, systemic response to child abuse and neglect with respect to participant outcomes and system performance. A better understanding also is needed of the utility and potential limitations of employing a singular focus on evidence-based decision making to guide policy and practice.

A SYSTEMS FRAMEWORK FOR CHILD ABUSE AND NEGLECT

Research advances in child abuse and neglect make clear that attaining a better understanding of the problem and mounting an effective response will require a systems perspective (e.g., Senge and Sterman, 1992). The public health problem of child abuse and neglect encompasses many embedded systems that are engaged both positively and negatively in creating, sustaining, and responding to the problem. Such systems include individual development, family systems, social relationship systems, and service systems from the local to the national level, among others. All of these systems and factors within them involve complex interdependencies, such that efforts to solve one aspect of the problem may reveal or even create problems at other levels.

Systems thinking has been adopted in the child protection field both in the United States and globally (e.g., Wulczyn et al., 2010). As Wulczyn and colleagues note, the systems approach fits well with the major theoretical model in the field of child development—that of Bronfenbrenner (1979). From any perspective, children can be considered in terms of the nested or embedded and interacting structures (e.g., families, communities) that affect them. Conversely, considering any child-related issue without taking such a perspective will be an incomplete exercise. From the perspective of the child protection system, all of the systems that work with children are highly entangled and must work in concert to achieve effective results (Wulczyn et al., 2010). Figure 1-1 depicts the interplay among the actors, contexts, and components of child protection systems.

Policy and program failures typically are considered to be system failures (Petersen, 2006). They often involve a given system's establishing unsustainable ends or goals, or the use of approaches that fail to achieve the intended results and may have unintended consequences that may be worse than the initial problem. The common system failures (e.g., Senge and Sterman, 1992; Sterman, 2002) include misspecified ends, unintended consequences, drifting goals, underinvestment in capacity, and delays in delivering results.

An underlying problem that can contribute to all of these types of system failure is incomplete analysis of opportunities and challenges at the initial stage. To be effective, change efforts and the policies designed to sustain them must include a rigorous analysis of system dynamics. For example, the usefulness of systems analysis has been demonstrated in

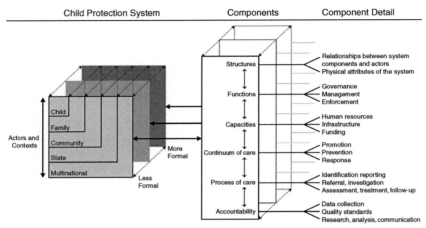

FIGURE 1-1 Child protection systems: actors, contexts, and components.
SOURCE: Wulczyn et al., 2010 (reprinted with the permission of the paper authors).

multiple successful applications to business challenges (e.g., Ford, 1990; Harris, 1999; Jones and Cooper, 1980), as well as in current efforts to apply systems analysis to the child protection system (e.g., Wulczyn et al., 2010). Systems analysis helps reveal mental models held by participants, including beliefs, assumptions, and presumed knowledge. This allows all participants in a change effort to recognize and take responsibility for their mental models and to account for them in the design of the change effort. In addition, systems analysis includes identification of potential barriers or challenges to implementation so that approaches to overcome them can be anticipated. Finally, the systems analysis approach views all solutions identified by the process as interim, systematically building feedback into the implementation of a change effort. By intentionally seeking, generating, and learning from feedback over time, participants in change efforts will improve their understanding of the system and efforts to improve it, and will see concomitant improvements in the efforts' results.

The complexity of child abuse and neglect makes the problem difficult to address in the absence of a full understanding of the diverse and multi-level systems that impact its incidence, consequences, and social response. By contrast, sustained and thoughtful systems thinking can lead to rigorous research designs that can advance knowledge and program or service implementation in meaningful ways. Such research can progress from addressing symptoms to focusing increasingly on core causes and solutions that draw more effectively on the strengths of multiple actors and domains.

Prevention of child abuse and neglect is a complex problem that can be solved only if many societal systems and the people within them cooperate to play positive roles (Wulczyn et al., 2010). As with all complex societal problems, child abuse and neglect has no single cause; therefore, tackling the problem strategically at multiple levels is the only way to make a substantial impact on the problem.

THE UNIQUE ROLE OF SOCIAL AND ECONOMIC STRATIFICATION

In the 1993 NRC report, issues concerning the influence of sociocultural factors on child abuse and neglect are addressed only marginally and, in truth, somewhat superficially. What is more, that report often implies that the racial and socioeconomic dimensions of abuse and neglect represent "cultural" effects. This misnomer distorts understanding of those social, economic, and cultural factors that influence the prevalence, mechanisms, processes, and outcomes of child abuse and neglect. The present report proposes several new conceptual and empirical directions for addressing these themes in future research on child abuse and neglect. Unfortunately, they are not well covered in existing research in the field, so the review of the literature presented herein generally is missing these perspectives.

The committee emphasizes the importance of adopting a critical stratification lens in considering and writing about the impact of social and economic factors on child abuse and neglect. *Stratification* involves the rank ordering of people based on their social and economic traits (Keister and Southgate, 2012). Based on this rank ordering, people have unequal access to resources and are differentially exposed to certain behaviors, processes, and circumstances (e.g., discrimination) that influence the nature, power, vulnerability, privilege, and protection of children who are abused, those who abuse them, and those who are charged with preventing and intervening in abuse situations. This lens therefore makes it possible to consider the various domains of stratification—race, skin color, ethnicity, class (social and economic), gender, sexual orientation, immigration status—and how the inequalities that ensue because of rank ordering in these domains impact child abuse and neglect. In addition, this lens enables intersectionality to be infused into the discourse; thus, how the multiple strata occupied by an individual (e.g., a poor dark-skinned Latino female) collectively influence the lived experiences of child abuse and child neglect for all involved can be discussed and differentiated (Burton et al., 2010; Dill and Zambrana, 2009). Finally, attention to stratification issues points to the need to consider how *place* matters relative to child abuse and neglect. Stratification processes create inequalities in physical and environmental locations that differentially shape certain behaviors and outcomes. Researchers in the field need to consider whether differences in the prevalence and nature of child abuse and neglect are observed in certain urban, suburban, rural, and regional areas of the United States and how those differences are related to population, institutional, and political inequalities.

Also important is avoiding the error of equating domains of stratification with the attributes and practices of culture. Culture is distinct from stratification. It is not necessarily circumscribed by the same mechanisms and processes as, for example, racial stratification; it encompasses but is larger than stratification issues. In Geertz's classic work *The Interpretation of Culture*, culture is defined as "an historically transmitted pattern of meanings embodied in symbols, a system of inherited conceptions expressed in symbolic forms by means of which men communicate, perpetuate, and develop their knowledge about and attitudes toward life" (Geertz, 1973, p. 89). And as Swidler notes, "seeing culture as meaning embodied in symbols focuses attention on such phenomena as beliefs, ritual practices, art forms, and ceremonies, and on informal cultural practices such as language gossip, stories, and rituals of daily life" (Swidler, 2001, p. 12). Thus, a fundamental component of culture is the social processes by which these symbols, attitudes, and modes of behavior are shared, reified, and sanctioned within families and communities. A focus on culture then directs attention to different types of questions, such as how certain religions and other collectives (not necessarily defined by race) value children, adopt harsh parenting styles, or execute certain moral codes/beliefs in the contexts in which they reside.

Attention to these issues will contribute to achieving the goal for research on child abuse and neglect of having sufficient specificity so that understanding of the problem's causes and consequences, as well as programs or services to address it, will be focused rather than overly general. Research conducted to date is informative about risk factors but not about how or why more risk factors lead to worse results, or which risk factors are more important than others and for which types of abuse or neglect. For example, poverty is a risk factor, yet many poor children are not abused or neglected. Which poor children are abused and why? The committee believes attention to these issues of social and economic stratification will yield increased understanding and more effective responses to the problem.

CONCLUSION

Significant progress has been made in efforts to understand child abuse and neglect; to document its devastating and lifelong impacts on both its victims and society; and to develop, test, and replicate evidence-based treatment and prevention strategies. Today, strong evidence demonstrates that child abuse and neglect is a public health issue in terms of both its immediate impact on child development and well-being and its impact on long-term productivity.

Research advances in child abuse and neglect underscore the importance of viewing the problem as a systemic challenge. The interdependency of myriad factors operating at multiple levels and in multiple domains complicates understanding of the causes and consequences of child abuse and neglect and challenges the ability to design, implement, and sustain effective responses. Building on the gains realized in the past 20 years will require a research paradigm and infrastructure capable of capturing this complexity.

ORGANIZATION OF THE REPORT

This report is organized into nine chapters. Between this introductory chapter and the final chapter, which contains the committee's recommendations, are seven chapters that review the state of knowledge and contain the committee's findings and conclusions related to important aspects of child abuse and neglect research. In these chapters, major research findings are summarized at the end of major sections, and each chapter ends with overall conclusions. The aspects of child abuse and neglect addressed are the extent of the problem (Chapter 2); research on its causes (Chapter 3); research on its consequences (Chapter 4); an overview of the child welfare system, which constitutes society's primary vehicle for identifying and responding to formal reports of child abuse and neglect (Chapter 5); research on the implementation and impacts of prevention and treatment programs (Chapter 6); an overview of the infrastructure for child abuse and neglect research (Chapter 7); and research on relevant public policies (Chapter 8). The recommendations presented in Chapter 9 are based on the findings and conclusions in these chapters, as well as the supporting discussion.

REFERENCES

ACF (Administration for Children and Families). 2012. *Child maltreatment, 2011 report.* Washington, DC: U.S. Department of Health and Human Services, ACF.

Bronfenbrenner, U. 1979. *The ecology of human development: Experiments by nature and design.* Cambridge, MA: Harvard University Press.

Burton, L. M., E. Bonilla-Silva, V. Ray, R. Buckelew, and E. H. Freeman. 2010. Critical race theories, colorism, and the decade's research on families of color. *Journal of Marriage and Family* 72(3):440-459.

CWIG (Child Welfare Information Gateway). 2008. *What is child abuse and neglect?* Washington, DC: U.S. Department of Health and Human Services, Children's Bureau.

Dill, B. T., and R. E. Zambrana. 2009. *Emerging intersections: Race, class, and gender in theory, policy, and practice.* New Brunswick, NJ: Rutgers University Press.

Fang, X., D. S. Brown, C. S. Florence, and J. A. Mercya. 2012. The economic burden of child maltreatment in the United States and implications for prevention. *Child Abuse & Neglect* 36:156-165.

Ford, J. D. 1990. *Tension, communication, and change in organizations.* Columbus: Ohio State University, College of Business.

GAO (Government Accountability Office). 2011. *Child maltreatment: Strengthening national data on child fatalities could aid in prevention.* Washington, DC: GAO.

Geertz, C. 1973. *The interpretation of cultures.* New York: Basic Books.

Gelles, R. J., and S. Perlman. 2012. *Estimated annual cost of child abuse and neglect.* Chicago, IL: Prevent Child Abuse America.

Guterman, N. B., Y. Lee, S. J. Lee, J. Waldfogel, and P. J. Rathouz. 2009. Fathers and maternal risk for physical child abuse. *Child Maltreatment* 14(3):277-290.

Harris, B. 1999. Pipeline inventory: The missing factor in organizational expense management. *National Productivity Review* 18(3):33-38.

IOM (Institute of Medicine) and NRC (National Research Council). 2012. *Child maltreatment research, policy, and practice for the next decade: Workshop summary.* Washington, DC: The National Academies Press.

Jones, A. N., and C. L. Cooper. 1980. *Combating managerial obsolescence.* Westport, CT: Greenwood Press.

Keister, L. A., and D. E. Southgate. 2012. *Inequality: A contemporary approach to race, class, and gender.* New York: Cambridge University Press.

Lee, S. J., N. B. Guterman, and Y. Lee. 2008. Risk factors for paternal physical child abuse. *Child Abuse & Neglect* 32(9):846-858.

McLanahan, S., L. Tach, and D. Schneider. 2012. *The causal effects of father absence.* Princeton, NJ: Bendheim-Thoman Center for Research on Child Wellbeing.

NRC (National Research Council). 1993. *Understanding child abuse and neglect.* Washington, DC: National Academy Press.

Petersen, A. 2006. Conducting policy-relevant developmental psychopathology research. *International Journal of Behavioral Development* 30(1):39-46.

Sedlak, A. J., J. Mettenburg, M. Basena, I. Petta, K. McPherson, A. Greene, and S. Li. 2010. *Fourth National Incidence Study of Children Abuse and Neglect (NIS-4): Report to Congress.* Washington, DC: U.S. Department of Health and Human Services, Administration for Children and Families.

Senge, P. M., and J. D. Sterman. 1992. Systems thinking and organizational learning: Acting locally and thinking globally in the organization of the future. *European Journal of Operational Research* 59(1):137-150.

Sterman, J. D. 2002. All models are wrong: Reflections on becoming a systems scientist. *System Dynamics Review* 18(4):501-531.

Swidler, A. 2001. *Talk of love: How culture matters.* Chicago, IL: University of Chicago Press.

Whitaker, R. C., S. M. Phillips, S. M. Orzol, and H. L. Burdette. 2007. The association between maltreatment and obesity among preschool children. *Child Abuse & Neglect* 31(11-12):1187-1199.

Wulczyn, F., D. Daro, J. Fluke, S. Feldman, C. Glodek, and K. Lifanda. 2010. *Adapting a systems approach to child protection: Key concepts and considerations.* New York: United Nations Children's Fund.

2

Describing the Problem

Child abuse and neglect is well established as an important societal concern with significant ramifications for the affected children, their families, and society at large (see Chapter 4). A critical step in devising effective responses is reasonable agreement on the definition of the problem and its scope. Yet achieving clarity in the area of child abuse and neglect has been an ongoing challenge. Legal definitions vary across states; researchers apply diverse standards in determining incidence and prevalence rates in clinical and population-based studies; and substantial obstacles hamper learning about the experiences of children, especially young children, with caregiver-inflicted abuse or neglect. As a result, definitions of the characteristics of the problem and determinations of its scope will differ depending on the data source used for analysis. This challenge was articulated in the 1993 National Research Council (NRC) report (NRC, 1993) and continues to impede a full understanding of the nature of the child abuse and neglect problem. The purpose of this chapter is to describe briefly what is known about the problem from current data sources and to highlight issues that remain problematic, as well as identify areas in which advances have been made. The chapter addresses, in turn, definitions of child abuse and neglect, incidence rates and the problem of underreporting, trends in the incidence of child abuse and neglect, and how cases are determined by medical and mental health professionals and the legal system. The final section presents conclusions.

DEFINITIONS

A key definition of child abuse and neglect is contained in Section 3 of the Child Abuse Prevention and Treatment Act (CAPTA)[1]:

> At a minimum, any recent act or set of acts or failure to act on the part of a parent or caretaker, which results in death, serious physical or emotional harm, sexual abuse or exploitation, or an act or failure to act, which presents an imminent risk of serious harm.

This definition is especially important because it is enshrined in federal legislation. To be eligible to receive funding under Section 106[2] of the act, states must, at a minimum, include the conduct described in Section 3 in their state child abuse and neglect authorizing legislation. All 50 states, as well as American Samoa, the Commonwealth of Puerto Rico, the Commonwealth of the Northern Mariana Islands, the District of Columbia, Guam, and the Virgin Islands, have mandatory child abuse and neglect reporting laws that define the terms slightly differently for their jurisdiction and lay out the requirements for mandatory reporting (CWIG, 2011). Federal law defines child abuse and neglect and identifies reporting requirements on tribal lands[3] (see CWIG, 2012b, for further information) and on military installations[4] (see Military OneSource, n.d., for further information); in some circumstances, state laws on child abuse and neglect reporting also apply to tribal lands and military installations. The Victims of Child Abuse Act[5] (also see Chapter 8) lays out requirements for reporting child abuse that occurs on federal lands and in federal facilities.

The National Child Abuse and Neglect Data System (NCANDS) is the official government data source to which all states must contribute information about child abuse and neglect reports. To collect data on reported and confirmed cases of child abuse and neglect uniformly from all states, NCANDS provides the following somewhat more comprehensive definition of child abuse and neglect:

> An act or failure to act by a parent, caregiver, or other person as defined under State law that results in physical abuse, neglect, medical neglect, sexual abuse, emotional abuse, or an act or failure to act which presents an imminent risk of harm to a child. (ACF, 2012)

Many states, reflecting the words "at a minimum" in CAPTA, have more expansive definitions of the conduct that legally constitutes child

---

[1]42 U.S.C. § 5101 note.
[2]42 U.S.C. § 52016a.
[3]25 U.S.C. § 3202 and 18 U.S.C. § 1169.
[4]10 U.S.C. § 1787.
[5]42 U.S.C. § 13001, et seq.

abuse and neglect for purposes of mandatory reporting. In some states, for example, only conduct by current caregivers is defined as reportable child abuse and neglect; in other states, the conduct must be reported regardless of the perpetrator's relationship to the child. Pennsylvania, for example, considers only acts of abuse as reportable acts of maltreatment and uses a different mechanism for capturing neglect. CAPTA permits states to limit reporting to "recent" acts, but most states have no time limit on when the conduct occurred for the mandatory reporting requirement to be invoked. A summary of the differences in states' child abuse and neglect reporting laws is available (CWIG, 2011).

How child abuse and child neglect are defined and who is obligated to report them are subject to changes in awareness or level of concern about possible abuse- and neglect-related hazards faced by children. It is common for a specific case, especially one involving an egregious situation not addressed by extant law, to prompt advocacy for legislative change (Gainsborough, 2010). Newly identified problem areas, changes in societal consensus about child protection, and revelations that certain groups of professionals are not included in mandatory reporting laws are typical scenarios for bringing about statutory reforms. In 2012, 107 bills addressing child abuse and neglect reporting were introduced in 30 states and the District of Columbia (NCSL, 2012). For example, a number of states expanded mandatory reporting to apply to university employees in response to the Penn State Sandusky scandal.

In some cases, such changes have unintended consequences. An example is the occasional inclusion of exposure to domestic violence as a statutorily specified form of reportable child abuse and neglect, a result of increasing awareness of the association between domestic violence and child abuse and neglect and concern for the welfare of children exposed to this violence, so that affected children would receive protection and services. The Minnesota state legislature instituted such a change in 1999. The result was a dramatic increase in the number of referrals, emanating mainly from law enforcement officials who responded to reports of domestic violence and, as mandated, reported the family to child protective services. Parents, primarily mothers, who themselves were victims of domestic violence thus became the subjects of neglect reports based on their alleged failure to protect their children from exposure to the violence. This was not the intent of the legislation, and the provision was quickly rescinded (Edleson et al., 2006).

Child abuse and neglect laws are for the most part concerned with parental behaviors of omission or commission that place children in jeopardy. Acts of omission usually are characterized as neglect. They include failing to provide adequate supervision; not protecting children from known dangers; and not providing for basic needs, such as proper medical care, adequate food and clothing, safe/hygienic shelter, and school attendance. Child neglect reports may also be made in some states if a child is born affected by illegal drug or alcohol abuse by the mother or if a child is living where drugs are being manufactured and/or distributed.

Child abuse, on the other hand, refers to acts of commission by a caregiver. Physical abuse encompasses physical assaults that exceed permitted corporal punishment. States may define explicitly the types of behavior that fall in this category. In some cases for example, the age of the child may determine whether a behavior is acceptable discipline (e.g., slapping an infant versus an older child across the face). Sexual abuse generally includes the range of sexual behaviors that are defined by criminal statutes, including sexual exposure, sexual touching, rape, and sexual exploitation. Emotionally abusive behaviors include threatening, terrorizing, or deliberately frightening a child; rejecting, ridiculing, shaming, or humiliating behaviors; extreme isolating or restricting behaviors; and corruption or encouraging involvement in illegal behaviors. However, of the 48 states that mention emotional abuse in law, only Delaware identifies specific emotionally abusive caregiver behaviors; most states define emotional abuse by its impact on the child's mental health (CWIG, 2011). Because the involvement of the child protection system focuses on caregivers, cases of abuse committed by non-family members or siblings may be classified as neglect. In those cases, it is the presumed or alleged failure of the caregiver to protect the child that drives the designation. For example, the majority of sexual abuse and a notable proportion of serious physical abuse cases involve non-family members as perpetrators (Finkelhor and Dziuba-Leatherman, 1994). Instances of abuse committed by a non-family member, a sibling, or another person regularly present in the household are classified as neglect if it is determined that the caregiver failed to protect the child victim from that individual.

As noted, child abuse and neglect laws also vary in how mandated reporters are defined. Some states define all adult citizens as mandated reporters, but most specify certain groups of professionals and others who work with children (CWIG, 2012a). State laws usually exempt from a reporting obligation priests acting in the role of receiving confession; states vary, however, as to whether reporting is required of priests or pastors acting in other capacities. Regardless of the groups specified, anyone not listed as a mandated reporter can still make a report. Both mandated reporters and others are legally protected for good faith reports, while mandated reporters who fail to report may be prosecuted for that failure. No evidence-based research has assessed whether the breadth of inclusion in mandatory reporting laws makes a difference in rates of reporting, although it may affect substantiation rates (McElroy, 2012; also see the discussion of mandatory reporting laws in Chapter 8).

Some acts of child abuse and neglect are also crimes. The specific statutory definitions and names of those crimes vary by state, but in general, criminal statutes cover the same acts in all states. Sexual abuse is always a crime; most cases are classified as felonies. Physical abuse is a crime unless the behavior falls within the discipline exception for corporal punishment. Most cases of physical abuse are likely to be classified as misdemeanors unless a child is seriously injured or dies. A minority of neglect cases involve criminal conduct. When the failure to supervise, protect, or provide care for a child rises to a certain level of negligent treatment, it may meet the criteria for violation of criminal codes (e.g., child endangerment or criminal neglect) and can be prosecuted. Just because child abuse and neglect falls within the statutory definition of a crime, however, does not mean it will be fully investigated by law enforcement and prosecuted. Law enforcement investigations and prosecutions tend to focus on sexual abuse and on serious physical abuse and very serious neglect that have resulted in a child's experiencing physical harm or death (e.g., starvation, inflicted medical trauma).

As with state laws, child abuse and neglect is defined in various ways for research purposes. The National Incidence Study (NIS)-4 (Sedlak et al., 2010a) applies two definitional standards: a harm standard and an endangerment standard. The harm standard is restricted to cases in which children have been harmed by child abuse and neglect, whereas the endangerment standard encompasses children who have not yet been harmed under certain circumstances. The numbers vary depending on which definition is used (NIS-4 harm standard = 1.25 million children; endangerment standard = 3 million children). Under both standards, alleged instances of abuse or neglect are classified according to eight major categories. Table 2-1 lists actions or failures to act that are representative of each type of abuse or neglect and, for the purposes of this chapter, provides examples of how these forms of maltreatment can be defined in a research setting.

A widely used method of defining child abuse and neglect in research is the classification scheme developed by Barnett and colleagues (1993). Many studies focused specifically on child abuse and neglect use these definitions rather than the officially reported labels (e.g., English et al., 2005). The Centers for Disease Control and Prevention (CDC) also has recommended a set of uniform definitions for public health purposes to allow for monitoring of incidence over time and detection of trends (Leeb et al., 2008). Notably, both the classification scheme developed by Barnett and colleagues and the CDC recommendations are designed for analysis of existing information from public sources, primarily child protective services case records.

Slack and colleagues (2003) note that research definitions developed for analysis of child protective services case records may not be applicable to survey research. They argue that these definitions may capture risk factors associated with the detection of child abuse and neglect rather than risk factors associated with the commission of child abuse and neglect. They

TABLE 2-1 National Incidence Study (NIS)-4 Abuse and Neglect Classifications

Sexual Abuse	• Intrusion sex without force • Intrusion sex involving use of force • Child's prostitution or involvement in pornography with intrusion • Molestation with genital contact • Exposure/voyeurism • Providing sexually explicit materials • Child's involvement in pornography without intrusion • Failure to supervise the child's voluntary sexual activity • Attempted/threatened sexual abuse with physical contact • Other/unknown sexual abuse
Physical Abuse	• Shake, throw, purposefully drop • Hit with hand • Hit with object • Push, grab, drag, pull • Punch, kick • Other physical abuse
Emotional Abuse	• Close confinement: tying/binding • Close confinement: other • Verbal assaults and emotional abuse • Threats of sexual abuse (without contact) • Threats of other maltreatment • Terrorizing the child • Administering unprescribed substances • Other/unknown abuse
Physical Neglect	• Refusal to allow or provide needed care for a diagnosed condition or impairment • Unwarranted delay in seeking or failure to seek needed care • Refusal of custody/abandonment • Other refusal of custody • Illegal transfer of custody • Other or unspecified custody-related maltreatment—unstable custody arrangements • Inadequate supervision • Inadequate nutrition • Inadequate personal hygiene • Inadequate clothing • Inadequate shelter • Other/unspecified disregard of child's physical needs and physical safety

TABLE 2-1 Continued

Educational Neglect	• Permitted chronic truancy • Other truancy • Failure to register or enroll • Other refusal to allow or provide needed attention to a diagnosed educational need
Emotional Neglect	• Inadequate nurturance/affection • Domestic violence • Knowingly permitting drug/alcohol abuse • Knowingly permitting other maladaptive behavior • Refusal to allow or provide needed care for a diagnosed emotional or behavioral impairment/problem • Failure to seek needed care for an emotional or behavioral impairment/problem • Overprotectiveness • Inadequate structure • Inappropriately advanced expectations • Exposure to maladaptive behaviors and environments • Other inattention to developmental/emotional needs
Other Maltreatment	• Lack of preventive health care • General neglect—other/unspecified neglect allegations • Custody/child support problems • Behavior control/family conflict issues • Parent problem • General maltreatment—unspecified/other
Not Codable by Any NIS Standard	• Involuntary neglect • Chemically dependent newborns • Nonmaltreatment cases

SOURCE: Sedlak et al., 2010a.

have built on the framework created by Barnett and colleagues (1993) to develop a set of research definitions for neglect that they intend for use in survey research.

Likewise, other investigators develop their own study-specific designations. These definitions vary in comprehensiveness and behavioral specificity. For example, a study not focused specifically on child abuse and neglect but interested in it as one of many independent variables may use a single general question to get at the construct.

Finding: Child abuse and neglect are defined differently for different purposes. Legal definitions at the state level are properly subject to the legislative process. In research, however, the variability in definitions compromises learning the true scope and characteristics of the problem, understanding trends over time, and determining the relationship between child abuse and neglect and various outcomes.

Finding: State laws vary in what groups are specified as mandated reporters of child abuse and neglect. No evidence-based research has assessed whether the breadth of inclusion in mandatory reporting laws makes a difference in rates of reporting, although it may affect substantiation rates.

INCIDENCE RATES AND THE PROBLEM OF UNDERREPORTING

Determining the true incidence of child abuse and neglect is problematic for the same reason encountered in attempting to quantify any social problem: discrepancies between actual rates and the number of cases reported to authorities. It is well established that most crimes (the exception being homicide) are not reported (Langton et al., 2012). Data on the incidence of child abuse and neglect are derived from three primary sources: NCANDS, the official reporting system for cases of child abuse and neglect referred to state child protective services; two U.S. government surveys—the Uniform Crime Reporting (UCR) system, administered by the Federal Bureau of Investigation (FBI), and the National Crime Victimization Survey (NCVS), administered by the Bureau of Justice Statistics (BJS) to a large representative sample of U.S. citizens aged 12 and older; and the NIS, a study conducted every decade by the Department of Health and Human Services on a nationally representative sample that captures both cases of abuse and neglect reported to child protective services and unreported cases identified by professionals working with children.

National Child Abuse and Neglect Data System

Each state receiving a federal Basic State Grant for child abuse and neglect prevention and treatment programs is required to submit data annually to NCANDS.[6] In fiscal year (FY) 2011, all states, the District of Columbia, and all territories contributed to NCANDS counts of the number of cases referred to child protective services, the number accepted for investigation, the number substantiated, the case characteristics, and the case outcomes. As previously noted, the definitions of child abuse and neglect used by child protective services vary by state, as do reporting requirements. Because NCANDS collects information from child protective services case files in each state, the data reflect inconsistencies in state-level definitions of

---

[6]42 U.S.C. § 5106a(d).

types of maltreatment, reporting requirements, and procedures for responding to reports of child abuse and neglect.

NCANDS reports are issued annually. According to the FY 2011 NCANDS report (ACF, 2012), there were 3.4 million referrals involving 6.2 million children; some of the children were the subject of more than one referral. Nationally, more than three-quarters of these cases are classified as neglect, 18 percent as physical abuse, and 9 percent as sexual abuse. The specific rates vary among states but overall reflect the general pattern that a substantial majority of cases are neglect, with physical and sexual abuse representing much smaller groups.

Based on NCANDS, victims of child abuse and neglect are approximately evenly divided between males and females. The highest rates of child abuse and neglect occur among the very youngest children (see Table 2-2). Perpetrators are mainly parents (81 percent) and among parents are primarily biological parents (88 percent), which reflects the legal definition for reportable cases. Somewhat more than half of perpetrators are female (ACF, 2012). These demographic characteristics are also reflected in other data sources, such as the NIS-4 (Sedlak et al., 2010a).

In FY 2011, NCANDS reported 1,545 child fatalities resulting from abuse and neglect. Again, young children were at greatest risk: 80 percent of victims were less than 4 years old. Deaths were higher among boys than girls. About 70 percent of the fatalities are associated with neglect and nearly half are attributed to physical abuse, either exclusively or in combination. A Government Accountability Office (GAO, 2011) report notes that the NCANDS method relies only on cases reported to child protective services for these figures. The report states that not all child fatalities due to abuse and neglect are known to the child welfare system, suggesting that the actual figure is likely higher, although it acknowledges the difficulty of obtaining an accurate count.

An important limitation of NCANDS is that it does not capture accurate rates of child abuse and neglect among American Indian children. Only states submit information to NCANDS; there are no mechanisms for tribal child welfare systems to submit data to the system. American Indian and Alaska Native families and children whose cases are reported to and investigated by state child protection authorities and who self-identify as American Indian or Alaska Native are included in NCANDS. Children served by tribal child welfare systems, the Bureau of Indian Affairs, or the Indian Health Service are not. Thus, "it is estimated that 40 percent of all cases of child abuse and neglect among American Indian and Alaska Native children are not reported to NCANDS" (Cross and Simmons, 2008, p. 3; also see Earle and Cross, 2001). NCANDS is further limited in its ability to reveal the levels of abuse and neglect suffered by American Indian and Alaska Native children by the fact that state or county employees, rather than

TABLE 2-2 Child Maltreatment Cases/Victims, Rates per Thousand Population Ages 0-17,[a] by Various Characteristics, 2002-2011

Characteristic	2002	2003	2004	2005	2006	2007	2008	2009	2010	2011
Total	12.3	12.4	12.0	12.1	12.1	10.6	10.3	9.3	9.3	9.1
Gender										
Male	11.6	11.6	11.2	11.3	11.4	9.9	9.7	8.8	8.7	8.7
Female	13.1	13.1	12.6	12.7	12.7	11.1	10.8	9.7	9.7	9.6
Age										
0-3	16.0	16.4	16.1	16.5	16.8	14.9	14.7	13.6	13.7	14.3
4-7	13.7	13.8	13.4	13.5	13.5	11.5	11.0	9.7	9.7	9.9
8-11	11.9	11.7	10.9	10.9	10.8	9.5	9.2	8.1	8.0	7.7
12-15	10.6	10.7	9.3	10.2	10.2	8.7	8.4	7.6	7.3	7.0
16-17	6.0	5.9	6.1	6.2	6.3	5.4	5.5	5.1	5.0	4.8
Race and Hispanic Origin of Victim[b]										
Non-Hispanic white	10.7	11.0	10.7	10.8	10.7	8.3	7.9	7.8	8.1	7.9
Non-Hispanic black	20.2	20.4	19.9	19.5	19.8	15.4	15.4	15.1	14.7	14.3
Hispanic	9.5	9.9	10.4	10.7	10.8	9.2	9.0	8.7	8.6	8.6
Non-Hispanic American Indian or Alaska Native	21.7	21.3	15.5	16.5	15.9	12.4	12.6	11.5	11.3	11.4
Non-Hispanic Asian	—	2.7	2.9	2.5	2.5	2.2	2.2	2.0	1.9	1.7
Non-Hispanic Pacific Islander	—	21.4	17.6	16.1	14.3	11.5	10.7	11.3	9.8	8.5
Multiple races	12.4	12.8	14.6	15.0	15.4	11.8	12.4	12.4	10.0	10.1

Type of Maltreatment[c]										
Neglect	7.2	7.5	7.4	6.3	6.4	6.2	7.4	8.1	7.1	7.2
Physical abuse	2.3	2.3	2.1	1.7	1.6	1.1	1.7	1.8	1.6	1.6
Sexual abuse	1.2	1.2	1.2	0.9	0.9	0.8	1.0	1.0	0.8	0.8
Psychological or emotional abuse	0.8	0.6	0.9	0.7	0.7	0.4	0.8	0.8	0.7	0.8
Medical neglect	0.3	0.3	0.3	0.2	0.2	0.1	0.2	0.3	0.2	0.2
Other	3.3	3.7	3.2	1.5	1.5	0.4	0.9	—	—	0.9

[a]Includes "substantiated" cases, in which investigation results in a disposition concluding that the allegation of maltreatment or risk of maltreatment was supported or founded according to state law or policy—the highest level of finding by a state agency. Also includes cases designated "indicated" or "reason to suspect," which are those not substantiated by investigation but for which there is reason to suspect that the child may have been maltreated or was at risk of maltreatment. Not all states distinguish between substantiated and indicated dispositions. All data for 2009 and later represent "unique" cases—children who have experienced at least one instance of substantiated or indicated maltreatment (see definition above), with duplicate cases removed.

[b]Estimates for specific racial groups have been revised to reflect the new Office of Management and Budget race definitions and include only those who are identified with a single race. Hispanics may be of any race.

[c]A child may be a victim of multiple types of maltreatment and is counted once for each type (2007, when children were counted once only, was an exception).

SOURCES: CDC, 2003; Children's Bureau, 1995-2011, reprinted with permission from Child Trends (2013).

tribal workers, collect the data reported to NCANDS. Therefore, not only does NCANDS lack data on many cases that occur on tribal lands, but the data it does include may be flawed because non-Native workers unfamiliar with American Indian or Alaska Native culture often are tasked with making determinations of abuse or neglect in such settings (Fox, 2004).

U.S. Government Surveys

The U.S. government uses the two surveys noted above to learn about crime rates. The UCR covers crimes reported to police, whereas the NCVS is a household survey of a large representative sample of individuals aged 12 and older that asks about both reported and unreported crimes. Self-reported rates of crime victimization frequently are several times the rates of official reports, with the discrepancies being especially high for sexual assault.

The ability of such surveys to capture cases accurately hinges, in part, on how the question is asked. Using official terminology or labels for acts of child abuse and neglect requires respondents to label their own experiences as abusive or neglectful. In some cases, respondents may not know the official definitions or exactly what they encompass. For example, many children and adults may consider hitting a child with a belt appropriate corporal punishment. In other cases, the victim may be reluctant to define what happened as abusive. For example, evidence suggests that labeling acts as intentionally abusive is associated with increased distress in children (Kolko et al., 2002).

These labeling considerations are particularly acute in cases of sexual assault. Asking a single question—such as "Have you ever been raped?"—yields far fewer responses than a series of behaviorally specific questions about acts that meet the legal definition of sexual abuse and rape. For example, rates of endorsement of child sexual abuse in self-report research vary substantially based on how the question is posed. A meta-analysis of studies that used self-report surveys to examine childhood sexual abuse experiences around the world found that differences in the way sexual abuse was defined and the specific questions asked produced dramatically different rates of sexual abuse prevalence (Stoltenborgh et al., 2011).

In addition to these survey design issues, the point in time and circumstances under which respondents provide information about child abuse and neglect are crucial. Surveys of adults about their childhood experiences may yield very different rates than surveys of children. For example, population-based telephone interviews of youth aged 10 and older provide extensive information about self-reported victimization and exposure to violence (Finkelhor, 2009; Kilpatrick and Saunders, 1995). However, the rates of intrafamilial sexual and physical abuse reported in these studies are relatively low compared with the rates reported among adult samples when asked their childhood abuse experiences. Children may be less likely to report intrafamilial crimes when they are still children and are living at home.

Another method of learning about child abuse and neglect is asking adults about their behavior toward their children. Surveys using the Conflict Tactics Scale can provide a picture of self-reported corporal punishment and parental acts that would meet legal criteria for child physical abuse (Straus and Stewart, 1999; Straus et al., 1998; Theodore et al., 2005). This method has the obvious limitation, however, that even when responding to anonymous surveys, parents may underreport socially undesirable or illegal acts.

Discrepancies between official reports and child and adult self-reports can be in either direction. Children or adults may not define their experiences as child abuse and neglect because they do not know better or believe the conduct was deserved or acceptable, or because of the distress associated with reporting that caregivers are behaving abusively toward them. Adults may not define their own behavior as abusive or neglectful because of fears of being reported, social undesirability, or shame about the conduct. On the other hand, substantial evidence shows that careful and detailed questioning of children about their experiences produces substantially higher rates than official reports. For example, computer-assisted interviews were used to obtain self-reports of abuse and neglect from a sample of youth aged 12-13 enrolled in a prospective study of high-risk and abused children (Everson et al., 2008). This method yielded rates that were four to six times higher than those in the official child protective services records. At the same time, close to half of adolescents in the sample with confirmed child protective services reports failed to note that experience in the interview.

The National Incidence Study

The NIS is a congressionally mandated report on the incidence of child abuse and neglect that has been issued periodically since 1974 (OPRE, 2009). It estimates national rates of reported and unreported child abuse and neglect based on a representative sample of counties. The study uses official data and also collects information from "sentinels" representing community professionals who may encounter child abuse and neglect victims during the course of their work. The methodology of the NIS is explicitly designed to uncover child abuse and neglect that may not have been reported to authorities but was identified by professionals. The most recent report, issued in 2010, is based on data collected in 2005-2006 (Sedlak et al., 2010a). As noted above, the NIS defines child abuse and neglect differently from federal and state law, applying both a harm and an endangerment standard. All cases sampled in the study—both those identified by child protective services agencies and those reported by sentinels—are evaluated to determine whether they meet the definitional standards of the NIS for physical abuse, sexual abuse, emotional abuse, physical neglect, emotional neglect, and educational neglect. The NIS considers only abuse and neglect perpetrated or permitted by a parent or caregiver, aligning its definitions with those of child protective services.

The primary investigators of the NIS-4 note that findings of differential incidence rates for abuse and neglect of black and white children are limited by the range of risk factors available for analysis in multifactor risk models, which exclude such key elements as neighborhood characteristics, social isolation, substance use, and mental illness (Sedlak et al., 2010b). Likewise, many children's records lacked information on socioeconomic status, and the socioeconomic status measures used classified black and white children differently, limiting the utility of the data for examining socioeconomic status as a risk factor for child abuse and neglect.

Reasons for Underreporting

It is well known that not all child abuse and neglect cases come to the attention of authorities at the time they happen. Retrospective reports from adults abused or neglected as children reveal that most cases are not reported to anyone, and fewer still are reported and investigated by child protection workers or law enforcement officials (e.g., Finkelhor, 1994; MacMillan et al., 2003). Adults abused or neglected as children give a variety of explanations for why they did not tell anyone or make an official report, including not realizing that what was happening was wrong, illegal, or a form of child abuse and having fears or concerns about what would happen if they reported the experience or attempted to seek help.

Child abuse and neglect can sometimes be identified without a child's making a statement about it. Examples include certain types of injuries or medical conditions that are noticed by others or become known to a medical provider. Some types of neglect can also be detected through observable behaviors, such as young children found wandering the streets or coming to school unclean or very disheveled. But detection of many cases of physical abuse and neglect and almost all cases of sexual abuse depends largely on children making statements and adults acting on those statements. The statements may be made spontaneously or may be in response to adult inquiries about behaviors, circumstances, or injuries observed in the children. Once abuse or neglect has been detected, many variables can affect whether adults take action, including personal attitudes and beliefs about what will happen as a result of reporting, the relationship of the adult to the child or the caregiver who may have committed the abuse or neglect, the certainty of the concern about maltreatment, and understanding of the child abuse reporting laws (Alvarez et al., 2004; Khan et al., 2005; Sedlak et al., 2010a).

Therefore, official reports do not capture all instances in which child abuse and neglect is suspected or even is detected and acted upon. For example, adults in a child's life may learn about child abuse and neglect and take informal actions on behalf of the child without necessarily reporting to authorities. Although citizens are protected if they make a good faith report of suspected child abuse or neglect, there are many reasons why they might be hesitant about or deterred from making an official report even if strong evidence or suspicion exists. For example, they may fear retaliation or rejection by the abuser or negative consequences for the child or family. Indeed, despite the fact that relatives, neighbors, and friends are most likely to observe or hear about child abuse or neglect because of their proximity and involvement in children's lives, they account for only a minority (18 percent) of reporters of cases to child protective services (ACF, 2012).

Professionals account for the other three-fifths of child abuse and neglect reports, with teachers (16 percent), law enforcement officials (17 percent), and social service providers (11 percent) making the majority of these reports (ACF, 2012). However, mandated reporters do not always make a report when they suspect child abuse or neglect. Among mandated reporters involved as sentinels in the NIS-4, a significant percentage have had suspicion and not made a report. Professionals identify a variety of reasons for not reporting their suspicions (Sedlak et al., 2010a). The most common reasons given are concerns that intervention by child protective services will be more harmful than helpful and the professionals' belief that they can do a better job of addressing the suspected child abuse or neglect on their own without involving the authorities. Rates of reporting also may vary by profession and relationship with the family. In one state survey of pediatricians, only 10 percent had ever not reported a suspected case of abuse or neglect; the most common reason given was not feeling that the evidence for suspicion was strong enough or believing that the case could be better handled by the physician or family without the involvement of child protective services (Theodore and Runyan, 2006). For mental health providers, the dilemma may be more acute. For example, Steinberg and colleagues (1997) found that among psychologists who had made a report to child protective services, 27 percent stated that their client ended the therapy relationship because of the child abuse report.

In addition to the concerns of professionals about the consequences of reporting for themselves and their practice, a lack of clarity exists as to what constitutes reasonable suspicion as defined by the law. There is little dispute about suspicion when the basis for concern is clear-cut (e.g., the child makes a credible statement about being sexually abused or has hand print bruises on the cheek). In many cases, however, the information available to the reporter is vague, inconclusive, or only suggestive. Is it neglect when a child comes to school in dirty clothes and smelling bad? How young a child can be left alone at home? What if a child says, "I am afraid to go home"? If a child is engaging in highly sexualized behavior, is that indicative of abuse? There is a substantial gray area that is open to interpretation with respect to whether a statement or behavior meets criteria for triggering a legally mandated report of child abuse and neglect. A lack of consensus exists even among expert child abuse doctors. Levi and Crowell (2011) found no agreement among experts on how high child abuse and neglect would have to be on the list of differential diagnoses and how certain the provider would have to be that child abuse and neglect accounted for the child's presentation to meet the reporting criterion of reasonable suspicion.

On the other hand, only about 60 percent of referrals to child protection authorities are accepted and screened in for some type of official response (ACF, 2012). Cases may be screened out because they do not meet the legal criteria for child abuse and neglect or state standards for accepting cases, or because information about the case is insufficient to enable completing a report. Among states, screen-in rates range from a low of 25 percent to a high of virtually all referrals (ACF, 2012). Thus citizens and professionals likely recognize many situations in which they suspect child abuse and neglect, but their suspicions do not meet the threshold of concern required by local statute to justify an investigation.

Disproportionality

Concerns have been raised about possible racial and ethnic bias in child abuse and neglect reporting and investigations because African American and American Indian children are referred to child protective services at higher rates than their representation in the population, whereas Asian American and Latino children are referred at lower rates. A recent study used a birth cohort methodology and linked vital statistics and child abuse report records for young children (Putnam-Hornstein, 2011). Prior child abuse reports were associated with an almost sixfold increase in the probability of intentional death and double the rate of unintentional fatal injury; the rates were higher for African American and American Indian children and lower for Asian American and Latino children relative to the general population. In other words, the racial/ethnic patterns of injury and death mirror the child abuse and neglect reporting rates by racial and ethnic group. Moreover, the overall underrepresentation of Latino children in referrals to the child welfare system masks significant differences between the experiences of Latino children of U.S.-born mothers and Latino children of foreign-born mothers, both in rates of referral (Putnam-Hornstein et al., 2013) and in type of abuse or neglect (Dettlaff and Johnson, 2011).

Authoritative commentators (Drake et al., 2011; Putnam-Hornstein, 2012; Putnam-Hornstein et al., 2013) agree that there are real group differences in the rates of child abuse and neglect and conclude that these differences reflect the higher burden of social ills borne by some groups. As Putnam-Hornstein concludes: "The findings suggest that the overrepresentation of black and Native American children in the child welfare system may be a manifestation of historical and contemporary racial inequities that place these minority children at a disproportionate risk of maltreatment" (2012, p. 171).

Disproportionality extends beyond referrals. Miller (2011) examined disproportionality in Washington state at both the referral point and key decisions points after cases had been screened in (e.g., risk rating, placement, length of time in care). As with other states, disproportional rates of referral were seen. When disproportionality from the point of referral was examined, virtually no differences were found among whites, Asians, and Latinos following case entry into the child welfare system. After case receipt, rates of disproportionality were reduced for African American families at most decision points, with the largest discrepancy remaining in length of time in care. For American Indian cases, the disproportionality continued at every decision point following case acceptance. These results suggest that the observed disproportionality may have a variety of causes, some that reflect larger social forces and others that may be more reflective of professional assumptions and local practices. Disproportionality is discussed further in Chapter 5 of this report.

Finding: According to NCANDS data from FY 2011, there were 3.4 million child abuse and neglect referrals involving 6.2 million children. Nationally, more than three-quarters of these cases are classified as neglect, 18 percent as physical abuse, and 9 percent as sexual abuse. The highest rates of child abuse and neglect occur among young children, specifically those less than 3 years old.

Finding: Tribal child welfare systems, the Bureau of Indian Affairs, and the Indian Health Service do not report to NCANDS and are therefore not included in the datasets, thus limiting the ability to determine levels of abuse and neglect among many American Indian and Alaska Native populations. Moreover, non-Native workers report on cases of child abuse and neglect without familiarity with or consideration of the culture in these communities.

Finding: Difficulties arise in determining rates of child abuse and neglect. When researchers attempt to identify instances of child abuse and neglect through survey instruments, results can vary based on the types of questions asked and the point in time and circumstances under which respondents provide the information. Conducting retrospective surveys of childhood experiences, asking children about recent experiences, and surveying parents about their behaviors toward children all can yield different results.

Finding: African American and American Indian children are referred to child protective services at disproportionate rates relative to their representation in the general population.

INCIDENCE TRENDS

Questions about whether child abuse and neglect are increasing, decreasing, or being detected and reported more often have become prominent in recent years. At the time of the 1993 NRC report, there was a general consensus that child abuse and neglect was underreported. Since that time, substantial changes have occurred in the social climate with regard to awareness of child abuse and neglect, attitudes toward reporting it, and the availability of programs and services for children and families affected by it. These developments have explicitly been intended to increase reporting of child abuse and neglect by victims, the general public, and professionals. However, establishing whether changes in official reporting represent true changes in incidence is complicated by the limitations of the reporting systems discussed above, as well as the difficulties inherent in ascertaining rates of events that happen to children, many of whom are very young, and that occur mainly in the private context of family life. As revealed by the review below, discrepancies exist in some areas and considerable ambiguity in others regarding the conclusions to be drawn from the available trend data, suggesting outstanding questions that would benefit from more systematic empirical analyses of these trends over time.

Sexual abuse has shown the largest decline in reported rates. NCANDS reports a decline of 62 percent since 1992 (Finkelhor and Jones, 2012). The sharpest declines occurred during the late 1990s, but the downward trajectory has continued, with a 3 percent decline being reported between 2009 and 2010. This same pattern is demonstrated in the NIS-4, issued in 2010, which reported a 47 percent decline from the mid-1990s through 2005, when the data for that report were collected (Finkelhor and Jones, 2012).

Additional information on trends in sexual abuse is derived from surveys of youth. The NCVS documents a 68 percent decrease in reported and unreported sexual assault or rape of 12- to 17-year-olds between 1993 and 2010 (White and Lauritsen, 2012). In a national survey on sexual and reproductive activity, young women (aged 15-24) reported a 39 percent decline in sexual experiences with a partner 3 or more years older before the age of 15 (Finkelhor and Jones, 2012). This survey follows the same pattern as NCANDS, with the declines being steepest in the 1990s and tapering off although still continuing in the 2000s. Finkelhor and colleagues (2010b) compare results from the National Survey of Children Exposed to Violence (NatSCEV) in 2003 and 2008 and find that reports of sexual assault declined from 3.3 percent of all children aged 2-17 in 2003 to 2.0 percent of children in 2008. In contrast, the National Survey of Adolescents (NSA), a survey of a large nationally representative sample of youth, found no decline in self-reported sexual assault between 1995 and 2005 (Finkelhor and Jones, 2012).

The trend data are more ambiguous with respect to physical abuse. NCANDS reports a decline of 56 percent in physical abuse reports from the early 1990s through 2010 (Finkelhor et al., 2010a). The decrease for physical abuse began somewhat later than that for sexual abuse but has followed the same slope, with steep declines in the late 1990s that tapered off by 2009. Likewise, the NIS-4 reported a 29 percent drop in endangerment-standard physical abuse starting in the early 1990s (Finkelhor and Jones, 2012).

Survey results produce a somewhat different picture. The NCVS reports a 69 percent decline in aggravated physical assaults on children (aged 12-17) from 1993 through 2008; however, these events are mainly peer and sibling assaults rather than physical abuse by parents (Finkelhor and Jones, 2012). Zolotor and colleagues (2011) compared results from a 2002 survey of parents in North Carolina (Carolina Survey of Abuse in the Family Environment) using the Parent-Child Conflict Tactics Scale with the findings of a Gallup survey completed in 1995 and the results of two National Family Violence Surveys, conducted in 1975 and 1985, that used the same scale. The results show a decline in parental reports of physical abuse. On the other hand, neither the NatSCEV nor the NSA found significant declines in youth-reported physical abuse by caregivers (Finkelhor and Jones, 2012).

Another source of data on physical abuse is admissions to a hospital for abuse-related injury. Physical abuse encompasses a broad range of acts. The most common is striking a child such that bruising results—ranging from relatively minor, temporary, and localized marks caused by pinching or slapping to significant marks caused by whipping or hitting with an object that may leave scars. These types of injuries do not typically entail admission to a hospital or even require medical care. On the other hand, a relatively small percentage of physical abuse cases involve injuries, such as fractures, burns, blunt trauma, and abusive head trauma (formerly known as shaken baby syndrome), that require medical care and possibly hospitalization (Zolotor and Shanahan, 2011). Approximately 1.4 percent of physical abuse cases are estimated to result in hospitalization (Leventhal et al., 2012).

A number of studies have investigated changes in rates of admission for head injuries resulting from child physical abuse—the most common reason for child abuse-related hospital admission. Leventhal and Gaither (2012) found a small but concerning increase in the rate of serious injuries as documented in coding on medical records in a series of children's hospitals (from 6.1 to 6.4/100,000) from 1997 to 2009. Additional studies, attempting to show an association between economic indicators and child abuse, similarly have found increases in rates of injuries coded as child abuse occurring during the 2000s (Berger and Waldfogel, 2011; Berger et al., 2011; Wood et al., 2012). A national study conducted in Taiwan also found a significant increase from 1996 to 2007, but only for infants and largely accounted for by changes in coding practices since 2003 (Chiang et al., 2012).

Neglect reports show the most mixed trends picture. NCANDS neglect reports declined by 10 percent between 1990 and 2010 (Finkelhor et al., 2010a), but there was significant variability across states. From 1992 to 2010, for example, fluctuations ranged from a 90 percent decline in neglect in Vermont to a 189 percent increase in Michigan. These dramatic state variations are not mirrored in the sexual and physical abuse rates, which declined across almost all states over the same period. The NIS-4 found no decline in neglect cases (Sedlak et al., 2010a). Self-report survey data are not available for neglect to permit comparisons over time. In part, this is due to the fact that retrospective self-report surveys are poorly suited to gathering information about neglect involving very young children, which is the most frequent form of child abuse and neglect.

Child maltreatment–related fatalities include deaths caused by both physical abuse and neglect, with a majority being attributed to neglect. NCANDS reports an increase of 46 percent in abuse- and neglect-related fatalities between 1993 and 2007 (Finkelhor and Jones, 2012). In contrast, homicide rates for children fell by 43 percent during the same period, with a 26 percent decline for the youngest children (aged 0-5) (Finkelhor and Jones, 2012); between 1980 and 2008, 63 percent of murdered children aged 0-5 were killed by a parent (Cooper and Smith, 2011). It is unclear to what extent cases officially reported by law enforcement as homicides correspond to cases included in the NCANDS child abuse and neglect dataset, most of which, as noted, are attributed to neglect.

Trends in child abuse and neglect occur in the larger context of rates of crime and violence in the United States. The consensus is that crime has decreased substantially, although there are some year-to-year fluctuations and pockets where these results are not seen. Both official reports as reflected in the UCR and population-based counts of reported and unreported crime as determined by the NCVS reveal declines in virtually all crime categories since the mid-1990s (FBI, 2010; Truman and Planty, 2012). These declines extend to sexual assault and domestic violence, crimes that share characteristics of child sexual and physical abuse and often involve people in close interpersonal relationships or family members. As with child abuse and neglect, extensive efforts have been undertaken to change the social climate around these crimes, encourage reporting, and expand service availability. The NCVS shows a 68 percent decline in the number of children aged 17 and younger living in households in which someone aged 12 and older was the victim of sexual assault or violent crime between 1993 and 2010 (Truman and Smith, 2012).

In sum, trends are inconsistent across types of child abuse and neglect, and in the case of neglect are inconsistent across states. Sexual abuse reporting appears to indicate a clear decline that is not reflected in only a single data source. Although most sexual abuse is not committed by immediate family members, the declines here appear to extend equally to family and nonfamily sexual assaults. It is worth noting that the declines in child sexual abuse began about the same time as general declines in crime and have followed a similar slope. Physical abuse presents a more complicated picture, with some official sources showing overall declines and several surveys not showing declines. Although physical assaults in general (e.g., nonfamily assault, bullying) appear to be down, it is not clear that these trends extend to intrafamilial physical abuse.

Increases in child abuse-related hospital admissions are especially concerning because these data represent the most severe assaults, even though they make up a very small subgroup of child abuse cases. There are several possible explanations for these increases. First, they may represent actual increases in serious injury. Several studies have directly examined the correlation between the increases in identified cases and larger economic forces (Berger and Waldfogel, 2011; Berger et al., 2011; Wood et al., 2012). Berger and colleagues (2011) hypothesize an association between the economic recession and rising rates of child abuse-related injury, citing increases in child abuse and neglect reports from the prerecession to the recession period. However, they find no association with local unemployment rates. Wood and colleagues (2012) link data on child abuse-related hospital admissions to mortgage delinquency, foreclosures, and unemployment rates between 2000 and 2009. They find increases in admission rates to be correlated with mortgage foreclosure and delinquency rates but not with unemployment rates. Another possibility is that the increases reflect greater awareness and willingness of health care providers to label injuries as child abuse. The increases coincide with the advent of growing use of hospital diagnostic and billing codes that specify child abuse as the injury cause and a period when a child abuse subspecialty was created in pediatrics. These changes may have contributed to greater willingness to identify child abuse as the cause of injury in official records. Now that abusive head trauma is being captured more accurately in administrative data, it could potentially account for a decline in other forms of head injury (Leventhal and Gaither, 2012). It is also possible that caregivers who inflict severe injuries have more severe psychopathology or are otherwise different from the typical child abuser, and are therefore less amenable to the influences associated with general societal changes and less likely to accept offers of voluntary assistance.

The lack of a significant decline in child neglect and the large jurisdictional variations in this area remain the least understood. The past two decades have seen a growing emphasis on encouraging recognition of neglect as its deleterious effects have increasingly been documented. Awareness campaigns have been undertaken to encourage reporting of neglect, and in some cases its definition has been expanded to incorporate a variety of risky circumstances and conditions. For example, the relationship of parental substance abuse to child abuse and neglect has received widespread attention. These forces may have contributed to increased reporting of a broader spectrum of neglect cases. Greater awareness and expanded definitions may have offset any declines in reports of traditionally defined neglect.

Poverty often is considered a major contributor to neglect, yet there is little empirical support for a strong relationship between changes in indicators of poverty and neglect reporting rates. For example, there was a great deal of concern that welfare reform, especially the timelines for receiving Temporary Assistance for Needy Families (TANF), would produce an increase in cases of neglect as parents were forced off income support. However, no significant change in neglect rates was seen during this period. And as mentioned, two separate investigations failed to find a relationship between unemployment rates and child abuse and neglect reports.

A better understanding is needed of whether and why rates of physical and sexual abuse are declining while no change in neglect is being observed. Criminologists have focused on understanding the substantial declines in crime rates as well as the occasional fluctuations or stubborn persistence of high crime rates in a few areas. Multiple commentators have examined possible causes and explanations (Finkelhor et al., 2010b; Levitt, 2004; Oppel, 2011; Zimring, 2008, 2011). Other fields, such as medicine, would certainly have devoted extensive scientific inquiry to understanding an epidemiological phenomenon as significant and inconsistent across different forms of the same problem area. Yet there has been no similar focus in the field of child abuse and neglect. Attention to the topic has been limited to a few investigators who have repeatedly reported on trends (e.g., Finkelhor and Jones, 2012) and to targeted examinations of specific subareas, such as hospital admissions (e.g., Chiang et al., 2012; Leventhal and Gaither, 2012). A greater focus on understanding the fluctuations in child abuse reporting data and other indicators of child injury both nationally and within specific communities and populations could have important implications for the design and targeting of intervention and prevention efforts.

Finding: Strong evidence indicates that sexual abuse has declined substantially in the past two decades; the balance of evidence favors a decline in physical abuse, especially its more common and less serious forms. There is no evidence that neglect is declining overall; however, states vary significantly as to whether neglect is increasing, decreasing, or remaining constant. These disparate trends have important implications for understanding the nature of child abuse and neglect and the forces that potentially affect its trends. Social policy endeavors are hampered when insufficient attention is paid to understanding the various aspects of the problem.

Finding: Understanding is incomplete with respect to whether and why rates of physical and sexual abuse are declining while no change in neglect is being observed. Research on these trends has received inadequate attention given their important implications for intervention and prevention efforts.

DETERMINATION OF CHILD ABUSE AND NEGLECT

This section reviews the various methods of determining whether child abuse and neglect has occurred. The basis for the determination can range from a citizen's or family member's simply believing what a child says about being abused or neglected or being convinced by something observed, to a medical examination and diagnosis or the formation of a professional opinion, to the results of administrative or legal procedures. The process for making a determination by medical and mental health professionals is established by professional standards of practice, whereas legal standards of investigative practice, rules of evidence, and burdens of proof govern how legal determinations are made.

Determination by Medical and Mental Health Professionals

Medical determination or diagnosis is relevant in a small but very high-stakes minority of child abuse and neglect cases. A medical opinion is the only way to determine whether certain physical injuries—especially very serious injuries such as head injuries, fractures, and burns—are the result of child abuse and neglect in children who are too young to provide a verbal account of how the injury occurred. In certain cases involving children old enough to say what happened, a medical opinion may be necessary to distinguish accidental from nonaccidental injuries when the children's or parents' accounts are discrepant. In some neglect cases, such as those entailing malnutrition or failure to thrive, a medical opinion may be an essential component of the investigative process.

Taking a medical history is standard practice when medical professionals conduct a medical examination. In situations involving child abuse and neglect, especially when sexual abuse is suspected or the cause of an injury is in dispute, the child's history may be the primary basis for a medical professional's opinion or diagnosis. In such cases, although medical professionals may have specialized expertise in interviewing children, they, like other professionals and ordinary citizens, have no special ability to distinguish true from false or mistaken statements. However, statements made to a health care provider may be admissible in legal proceedings as an exception to the hearsay rule.

Overall, within the child abuse medical subspecialty, substantial consensus exists regarding the diagnostic criteria for forming a medical opinion about whether injuries or medical conditions are attributable to child abuse and neglect. However, there have been high-profile controversies about medical opinions in some child abuse cases. For example, questions have been raised about certain medical diagnoses, such as shaken baby syndrome, which as noted, is now called abusive head trauma. In some cases, child abuse experts have concluded that intentional injury has occurred, but other medical professionals have attributed the injuries to causes such as brittle bones or vitamin deficiencies. In large part, such conflicting opinions are due to the adversarial nature of the U.S. legal system. Opposing experts provide testimony to contradict a child abuse and neglect allegation and opine that alternative medical explanations account for the injuries, often, it has been argued, invoking scientifically unsupported assertions (Chadwick et al., 1998). Although there have been some salient scientific developments in terms of the causes of injuries, in most cases these disputes do not reflect significant scientific uncertainties.

Outstanding questions do remain about the types of tests and procedures that are most appropriate for making a determination of child abuse and neglect. For example, radiographic skeletal survey is the standard procedure for detecting clinically unsuspected fractures in possible child abuse victims since a certain percentage of children will have occult fractures. Standards for additional tests and their timing have not been definitively established. Absent consensus standards, practice shows considerable variability.

Other presentations for which a medical opinion is absolutely necessary include complex conditions such as Munchausen syndrome by proxy, or medical child abuse (Davis and Sibert, 1996; Fisher and Mitchell, 1995; Roesler and Jenny, 2008). While this condition is very rare (0.5/100,000 children), the potential consequences to children are extreme and severe (McClure et al., 1996). Parents repeatedly take their children to medical providers, often many different ones, with reports of multiple and sometimes extremely serious symptoms or conditions. In some cases, the child has or had a legitimate underlying condition, and the parents have extreme anxiety and repeatedly seek out additional tests and procedures or exaggerate symptoms. In other cases, parents fabricate or cause the medical symptoms to obtain psychological gratification from the attention they receive in the role of concerned parent. Making a determination of medical child abuse in these cases is fraught with complications and frequently cannot occur until the child has suffered significant harm or endured unnecessary tests, procedures, and even surgeries. Suspicion does not even arise until the pattern of visits, procedures, and contacts with multiple providers emerges. Child abuse doctors face a daunting task in challenging the opinions and practices of other medical providers who may have been mistaken, but genuinely believed the child had a serious medical condition.

In sexual abuse cases, although medical assessment is the standard of care, medical diagnosis is relevant in only a small subset of cases. Physical signs or symptoms, such as genital changes or injuries, sexually transmitted diseases, pregnancy, or the presence of seminal fluids or sperm, are present in only about 4 percent of cases; the vast majority of children medically evaluated for sexual abuse have normal exams (Heger et al., 2002). Even when there are genital findings, most are nonspecific and cannot be linked conclusively to sexual assault (Heger et al., 2002). Cases with definitive medical evidence, such as the presence of semen or pregnancy, are exceedingly rare. Standards for making a medical determination of sexual abuse have been published (Kellogg and Committee on Child Abuse and Neglect, 2005).

There are two important reasons beyond medical diagnosis why medical assessment of children who may have been or report being sexually abused is the standard of care. One purpose is to allay the child's and parents' worries about the potential physical effects of sexual contact. A visit with a medical provider creates a nonstigmatizing opportunity for support and validation, psychoeducation about the impact of sexual abuse, and encouragement to engage in available treatment services. The second is that citizens, judges, and juries assume that medical findings will be present in sexual abuse cases, even though this frequently is not the case. Child protection and criminal legal professionals believe it is often necessary to have a medical exam and expert medical testimony primarily to counter this widespread misconception.

Mental health professionals may be asked by parents or other professionals to provide a professional opinion as to whether a child was abused. Most such requests involve concern about sexual abuse. A diagnosis is not made because sexual abuse is an event, not a medical or psychiatric condition. In many cases, the mental health professional's opinion is sought in a forensic context when a report has been made to authorities or a legal action has been initiated, and the opinion is expected to help guide legal decision making or provide the basis for expert testimony in a legal proceeding. In other cases, however, the opinion is sought to determine whether to initiate reporting or other legal actions.

Typically in these situations, mental health providers consider a range of information, including what the child says in an interview, what the child has told others, the circumstances of the discovery of abuse concerns, results of medical examinations, and the emotional and behavioral functioning of the child based on a psychosocial assessment or administration of a standardized checklist of tests. The degree of thoroughness and the formality of the process depend largely on the purpose the opinion will serve.

Whereas child abuse mental health professionals do bring specialized expertise, knowledge, and skills to the evaluation process, there are scientific limits on the conclusions that can be drawn about whether an event occurred based on psychosocial assessment. No psychological profile has sufficient specificity to permit conclusions about an event as the cause of a presentation (APA, 2013). In addition, the emotional and behavioral consequences of child abuse and neglect are varied and nonspecific (see Chapter 4). Conditions typically associated with child abuse and neglect, such as posttraumatic stress, anxiety, depression, and behavioral problems, are common mental health problems for children and have many other causes. The only behavioral problem that has a specific and significant relationship with child abuse and neglect is inappropriate sexual behavior. However, the majority of sexually abused children do not have sexual behavior problems, and there are other potential causes for sexual behavior in children (Friedrich, 1993; Friedrich and Trane, 2002; Friedrich et al., 1998, 2003).

To a large extent, professional opinions on child abuse and neglect rely heavily on determinations about the credibility of children's statements. There is no reason to believe that children cannot give reliable and accurate information about events or that they are prone to making false complaints about abuse (Brown et al., 2007; Cederborg et al., 2008; Lamb et al., 2007; Lyon, 1999). On the other hand, it is well established that memory, especially in young children, is susceptible to error and distortion, and that children can form false beliefs that they have experienced events (Cederborg et al., 2008; Lyon, 1999). It turns out that the characteristics of true and untrue statements have many commonalities; some true statements are not very credible, and some untrue statements are highly detailed and convincing. Mechanisms devised for rating child reports about abuse and neglect and classifying them as accurate or inaccurate have not proven reliable (Hershkowitz et al., 2007). In other words, professionals have no special ability to detect truthfulness, nor is there a scientifically reliable method for doing so. This is why courts generally do not permit professionals to opine about the credibility of witnesses, but reserve that function for the fact finder (Myers, 2012).

Standards have been established for conducting forensic assessments for purposes of providing an opinion about possible sexual abuse (e.g., Kuehnle and Connell, 2009; Sparta and Koocher, 2006). The standards cover the assessment process, interviewing approaches, the proper use of psychosocial information, and limits on the accuracy of opinions based largely on statements that cannot be verified and behaviors that are non-specific. Unfortunately, the types of cases for which such assessments are sought are those that are most ambiguous and complex, such as when children are unable or unwilling to give a clear and credible history, they are very young, they have not made statements, their statements are vague or inconsistent, or they suffer from emotional and behavioral problems that affect their credibility.

Mental health professionals routinely form opinions on the basic truth of reports about historical events that are potentially relevant in explaining why clients present with emotional and behavioral problems. Mental health providers commonly inquire about a range of past events, such as child abuse and neglect; other forms of trauma; events and experiences such as divorce, family moves, and experiences at school or with peers; illness and hospitalization; and other relevant life experiences. This information is integrated with information derived from clinical observation and the results of assessment measures with respect to symptoms and behaviors. Except for what providers observe directly in session, nearly all the information that serves as the basis for an opinion about events and mental health problems is derived from self-reports. Reliance on self-reports, including reports of child abuse and neglect, is therefore a cornerstone of standard clinical practice.

Determination by the Legal System

Legal Investigations

Before a child abuse and neglect case arrives before a legal fact finder (judge or jury), an arm of the government investigates the case. Child protective services and law enforcement conduct the investigations that serve as the basis for the state's actions regarding dependency or prosecution. In many cases, the parents or defendants come to an agreement with the government, and no actual fact-finding hearing takes place. If it does, the official legal determination is made by civil or criminal court.

Child protective services usually is responsible for investigating civil dependency cases; such cases are screened in by the child welfare system, and they fall under the jurisdiction of the juvenile court. Given that the greatest number of reported cases involve neglect, and most do not involve criminal conduct, the child protective services investigation is the only process applied to making a determination about child abuse and neglect in the majority of cases. Caseworkers make home visits and observe the safety and hygiene status of the household; inspect bruises and injuries; and conduct interviews with children (when appropriate), caregivers, reporters, and others who may have relevant information (such as relatives, teachers, and health care providers). They then draw conclusions about whether the information and evidence thus obtained meet the legal standards for child abuse and neglect.

Law enforcement officials investigate crimes. They generally engage in the same activities as child welfare system caseworkers (e.g., interviewing victims and witnesses, examining home conditions); they may also collect evidence from crime scenes, undertake forensic analyses, and interrogate suspects. In many jurisdictions, child protective services and law enforcement officials conduct joint investigations (Cross et al., 2005).

A key activity in many child abuse and neglect dependency and criminal investigations, especially in cases involving sexual abuse and some involving physical abuse, is interviewing the child. Interviewing methods most likely to lead to accurate and complete reports have been extensively investigated (e.g., Cronch et al., 2006; Lamb et al., 2009; Larsson and Lamb, 2009; Saywitz et al., 2002). The protocol of the National Institute for Child Health and Development (NICHD) is the approach that has been the most researched in real-life settings and in laboratory analogue experiments, and serves as the model for the current standard of practice (Lamb et al., 2007). Other extant models, none of which has undergone the same level of empirical evaluation, share almost all the same procedures and practices as the NICHD protocol (Anderson et al., 2010).

Legal Determinations

A legal determination of child abuse and neglect is based on the weighing of admissible evidence that is collected following the accepted procedures for the specific legal arena. The common law legal system in the United States is adversarial and is based on principles that protect the due process rights of those who are accused and risk loss of liberty, access to their children, or assets. The legal contexts vary by whether they are criminal or civil, the intended outcomes of the case, and the standard of proof that applies.

The two primary legal systems that make determinations about child abuse and neglect are the child protection system and the criminal justice system (Myers, 2012). The child protection system carries out an administrative and civil justice process that involves the state's seeking to intervene in families, often but not always to assume temporary custody of children (e.g., establishing child abuse or neglect and then obtaining authority of the court for the child's placement) or in a small fraction of cases to terminate parental rights. In these court cases (often called dependency cases), the standard of proof typically is more probable than not; in a case involving termination of parental rights, a higher standard of clear and convincing evidence has been set by the U.S. Supreme Court. The goals of the criminal justice system are to hold lawbreakers accountable and punish them, to bring justice for victims, and to protect the community. The standard of proof here is the highest (beyond a reasonable doubt) because the case involves the government's restricting an adult's liberty, including the possibility of incarceration. Child abuse and neglect also may be addressed in family court custody matters when it is alleged by one parent seeking to restrict the other parent's access to the child. In addition, civil tort actions may be brought in which a child, or someone on his/her behalf, sues a caregiver, the government, or another entity for negligence, seeking monetary damages.

The large majority of both civil and criminal proceedings regarding child abuse and neglect do not progress to a formal fact-finding hearing or a trial. In many child protection cases, usually those not requiring a court order to remove a child from home against parental wishes, no formal legal process is even initiated; the family agrees to a voluntary service plan that is overseen by the state. Even when a dependency petition is filed in court, in the large majority of cases the parent reaches an agreement or case settlement regarding dependency, often without admitting to having committed an act of child abuse and neglect. On the criminal side, charges are not filed in many cases, even when prosecutors may believe a crime occurred, because of difficulties entailed in proving the case and in meeting the legal standard of proof of beyond a reasonable doubt. In the majority of cases when charges are filed, the accused pleads guilty to the crime or to a lesser crime.

Substantiation

The child protection system's classification of a child abuse and neglect case as substantiated is an administrative procedure for making a formal recorded determination about the validity of a child abuse and neglect report. In most states, the result of an investigation of a report is classified as substantiated or unsubstantiated, although some states use other terminology (e.g., founded/unfounded) to describe the investigative outcome. In 2011, approximately 19 percent of screened-in cases were substantiated, or "indicated" (ACF, 2012). Substantiation can be legally disputed because the consequences of a substantiated report can be significant for caregivers (e.g., job loss or being barred from certain professions or by certain employers) (CWIG, 2013; McCarthy et al., 2005).

No formal conclusion about whether child abuse and neglect occurred is recorded in cases that are referred for an alternative response (sometimes called a family assessment or differential response) and not formally investigated (CWIG, 2013). In 2011, about 10 percent of all cases reported to NCANDS received an alternative response (ACF, 2012), but that percentage is increasing. As of 2011, 17 states were implementing differential response at some level, and 6 states planned to implement it in the near future.

Rates of substantiation vary dramatically across states (ACF, 2012), and there is little consensus on what accounts for this variation. Overall, every method used to determine the accuracy of child abuse and neglect allegations has weaknesses and cannot be considered definitive. To some extent, this does not matter as long as the victims are safe and receive needed services. For example, most crimes will not be reported or prosecuted or result in conviction of the perpetrator; however, crime victims will still have access to many services designed to help them recover from the effects of the crime, and most can take at least some steps toward protecting themselves from the perpetrator. Although child abuse victims are dependent on caregivers for future protection, many parents can and do take steps to protect their children from known perpetrators or correct their own neglectful or abusive behavior. In terms of access to needed services, what happens officially in a case is unrelated to receipt of services in the child welfare system. The National Survey of Child and Adolescent Well-Being, a large longitudinal study of a nationally representative sample of cases reported to child protective services, produced illustrative results. Comparisons of cases that were closed or kept open, or were substantiated or not, revealed no difference in key variables related to services or outcomes (Hussey et al., 2005; Kohl et al., 2009).

The difficulty of ascertaining the validity of cases using official reporting or procedural outcomes may have more of an effect on research and interpretation of findings than on the lives of children who enter the child welfare system. For example, Kohl and colleagues (2009) argue that if substantiation does not discriminate true from untrue cases of child abuse and neglect, it is not a meaningful or accurate way of learning about the characteristics of actual abuse and neglect and its relationships to outcomes since the comparison group of unsubstantiated cases will contain many true cases. Therefore, child abuse research may benefit if consensus is achieved not only on definitions, but also on the meaning of different classification mechanisms for child abuse and neglect reports.

Finding: Significant advances have been made in dealing with children who may have been abused and neglected when they come in contact with medical, mental health, or social services professionals. It has become more common for these professionals to screen children routinely for abuse and other traumatic experiences. The children's accounts are generally accepted, at least for purposes of meeting the "reasonable suspicion" standard for making a child abuse report, except when there is significant evidence for coercion or contamination of their statements. Children who are suspected of being abused are commonly referred for specialized assessment, as well as clinical and support services.

Finding: Overall, substantial improvements have been achieved in the assessment and investigative procedures for determining whether child abuse and neglect has occurred since the 1993 NRC report was issued. Widely accepted standards for proper interviewing have been adopted by child protective services, law enforcement officials, and forensic evaluators and are well known even among general health, mental health, and other professionals (Lamb et al., 2007).

Finding: Rates of substantiation of child abuse and neglect allegations by child protective services vary dramatically across states, and there is little consensus on what accounts for this variation. Overall, every method of determining the accuracy of child abuse and neglect allegations has weaknesses, and no method can be considered definitive. This limits the substantiation classification as a meaningful way to learn about the characteristics of actual abuse and neglect and their relationships to outcomes.

CONCLUSIONS

Child abuse and neglect is a pervasive societal problem, with recent NCANDS data indicating that 3.4 million child abuse and neglect referrals involving 6.2 million children were made in a single year across the United States and its territories. As will be discussed in Chapter 4, these incidents of child abuse and neglect entail a substantial risk for deleterious consequences that can hinder child development and lead to problems that persist across the life course.

Cases of child abuse and neglect are referred to child protective services based on mandatory reports by professionals such as teachers, law enforcement officials, social service providers, and physicians, as well as good-faith reports by citizens. Not all cases of child abuse and neglect are reported, and standards for reasonable suspicion of abuse and neglect are not always clear-cut. Therefore, official reports do not capture all cases in which child abuse and neglect is suspected or even is detected and acted upon. For research purposes, then, sole reliance on referral data from child protective services cannot capture the full scope of child abuse and neglect. Incorporating data from additional sources is necessary to determine the true incidence of the problem.

In addition, child abuse and neglect are defined differently for the varying purposes for which related information is collected, confounding attempts to portray the scope of the problem accurately or examine the surrounding circumstances. Results across studies based on surveys also may vary according to the survey methodology employed. Movement toward a reasonable degree of standardization in these areas is therefore needed.

Difficulties in ascertaining the scope of child abuse and neglect have contributed to uncertainties regarding whether the incidence of the problem is increasing or decreasing or cases are being detected and reported more frequently. Available trend data provide strong evidence that sexual abuse has declined substantially in the past two decades; the balance of evidence favors a decline in physical abuse, especially its more common and less serious forms. There is no evidence that neglect is declining overall. However, states vary significantly as to whether neglect is increasing, decreasing, or remaining constant. Discrepancies and ambiguity across analyses of different data sources highlight a need for more systematic empirical analyses of these trends over time. Research is needed to learn more about trends in child abuse and neglect and the variables that may account for decreases in the incidence of the problem or the lack thereof.

REFERENCES

ACF (Administration for Children and Families). 2012. *Child maltreatment, 2011 report.* Washington, DC: U.S. Department of Health and Human Services, ACF.

Alvarez, K. M., M. C. Kenny, B. Donohue, and K. M. Carpin. 2004. Why are professionals failing to initiate mandated reports of child maltreatment, and are there any empirically based training programs to assist professionals in the reporting process? *Aggression and Violent Behavior* 9(5):563-578.

Anderson, J., J. Ellefson, J. Lashley, A. Lukas Miller, S. Olinger, A. Russell, J. Stauffer, and J. Weigman. 2010. Cornerhouse forensic interviewing protocol: RATAC. *Thomas M. Cooley Journal of Practical and Clinical Law* 12:193-331.

APA (American Psychiatric Association). 2013. *DSM-5 diagnostic and statistical manual of mental disorders,* 5th ed. Arlington, VA: APA.

Barnett, D., J. T. Manly, and D. Cicchetti. 1993. Defining child maltreatment: The interface between policy and research. *Child Abuse, Child Development, and Social Policy* 8:7-73.

Berger, L. M., and J. Waldfogel. 2011. *Economic determinants and consequences of child maltreatment.* OECD social, employment and migration working papers, no. 111. Paris, France: OECD Publishing.

Berger, R. P., J. B. Fromkin, H. Stutz, K. Makoroff, P. V. Scribano, K. Feldman, L. C. Tu, and A. Fabio. 2011. Abusive head trauma during a time of increased unemployment: A multicenter analysis. *Pediatrics* 128(4):637-643.

Brown, D. A., M. E. Pipe, C. Lewis, M. E. Lamb, and Y. Orbach. 2007. Supportive or suggestive: Do human figure drawings help 5- to 7-year old children to report touch? *Journal of Consulting and Clinical Psychology* 75(1):33-42.

CDC (Centers for Disease Control and Prevention). 2003. *2000 and 2001 population estimates for calculating vital rates.* http://www.cdc.gov/nchs/about/major/dvs/popbridge/popbridge.htm (accessed November 14, 2013).

Cederborg, A. C., D. La Rooy, and M. E. Lamb. 2008. Repeated interviews with children who have intellectual disabilities. *Journal of Applied Research in Intellectual Disabilities* 21(2):103-113.

Chadwick, D. L., R. H. Kirschner, R. M. Reece, L. R. Ricci, R. Alexander, M. Amaya, J. A. Bays, K. Bechtel, R. Beltran-Coker, C. D. Berkowitz, S. D. Blatt, A. S. Botash, J. Brown, M. Carrasco, C. Christian, P. Clyne, D. L. Coury, J. Crawford, N. Cunningham, M. D. DeBellis, C. Derauf, J. de Triquet, B. P. Dreyer, H. Dubowitz, K. W. Feldman, M. A. Finkel, E. G. Flaherty, L. Frasier, L. Gari, J. Glick, P. Grant, G. Fortin, S. Halpert, R. A. Hicks, D. Huyer, C. Jenny, M. Joffe, S. W. Kairys, K. M. Kaplan, M. Kaufhold, K. J. Kemper, E. J. Krane, H. Krous, M. Lorand, J. McCann, M. Mian, K. Moran, L. M. Osborn, V. Palusci, M. A. Radkowski, M. E. Rimsza, D. Runyan, M. Ryan, M. D. Sadof, C. Schubert, R. Sege, R. A. Shapiro, B. Siegel, A. Sirotnak, W. Smith, R. Socolar, D. Soter, S. P. Starling, C. Stashwick, R. D. Steiner, J. Stirling, N. Sugar, T. Truman, D. Turkewitz, C. Wang, J. M. Whitworth, and J. A. Zenel. 1998. Shaken baby syndrome—a forensic pediatric response. *Pediatrics* 101(2):321-323.

Chiang, W. L., Y. T. Huang, J. Y. Feng, and T. H. Lu. 2012. Incidence of hospitalization due to child maltreatment in Taiwan, 1996-2007: A nationwide population-based study. *Child Abuse & Neglect* 36(2):135-141.

Child Trends. 2013. *Child maltreatment: Indicators on children and youth.* Bethesda, MD: Child Trends DataBank.

Children's Bureau. 1995-2011. *Child maltreatment.* http://www.acf.hhs.gov/programs/cb/research-data-technology/statistics-research/child-maltreatment (accessed December 3, 2013).

Cooper, A., and E. L. Smith. 2011. *Homicide trends in the United States, 1980-2008.* Washington, DC: U.S. Department of Justice.

Cronch, L. E., J. L. Viljoen, and D. J. Hansen. 2006. Forensic interviewing in child sexual abuse cases: Current techniques and future directions. *Aggression and Violent Behavior* 11(3):195-207.

Cross, T. L., and D. Simmons. 2008. *Child abuse and neglect and American Indians. Overview and policy briefing.* Portland, OR: National Indian Child Welfare Association.

Cross, T. P., D. Finkelhor, and R. Ormrod. 2005. Police involvement in child protective services investigations: Literature review and secondary data analysis. *Child Maltreatment* 10(3):224-244.

CWIG (Child Welfare Information Gateway). 2011. *Definitions of child abuse and neglect.* Washington, DC: U.S. Department of Health and Human Services, Children's Bureau.

CWIG. 2012a. *Mandatory reporters of child abuse and neglect.* Washington, DC: U.S. Department of Health and Human Services, Children's Bureau.

CWIG. 2012b. *Tribal-state relations.* Washington, DC: U.S. Department of Health and Human Services, Children's Bureau.

CWIG. 2013. *How the child welfare system works.* Washington, DC: U.S. Department of Health and Human Services, Children's Bureau.

Davis, P. M., and J. R. Sibert. 1996. Munchausen syndrome by proxy or factitious illness spectrum disorder of childhood. *Archives of Disease in Childhood* 74(3):274-275.

Dettlaff, A. J., and M. A. Johnson. 2011. Child maltreatment dynamics among immigrant and U.S. born Latino children: Findings from the National Survey of Child and Adolescent Well-Being (NSCAW). *Children and Youth Services Review* 33(6):936-944.

Drake, B., J. M. Jolley, P. Lanier, J. Fluke, R. P. Barth, and M. Jonson-Reid. 2011. Racial bias in child protection? A comparison of competing explanations using national data. *Pediatrics* 127(3):471-478.

Earle, K., and A. C. Cross. 2001. *Child abuse and neglect among American Indian/Alaska Native children: An analysis of existing data.* Seattle, WA: Casey Family Programs and National Indian Child Welfare Association.

Edleson, J. L., J. Gassman-Pines, and M. B. Hill. 2006. Defining child exposure to domestic violence as neglect: Minnesota's difficult experience. *Social Work* 51(2):167-174.

English, D. J., R. Thompson, J. C. Graham, and E. C. Briggs. 2005. Toward a definition of neglect in young children. *Child Maltreatment* 10(2):190-206.

Everson, M. D., J. B. Smith, J. M. Hussey, D. English, A. J. Litrownik, H. Dubowitz, R. Thompson, E. D. Knight, and D. K. Runyan. 2008. Concordance between adolescent reports of childhood abuse and child protective service determinations in an at-risk sample of young adolescents. *Child Maltreatment* 13(1):14-26.

FBI (Federal Bureau of Investigation). 2010. *Table 1: Crime in the United States by volume and rate per 100,000 inhabitants, 1991-2010.* Washington, DC: U.S. Department of Justice.

Finkelhor, D. 1994. Current information on the scope and nature of child sexual abuse. *The Future of Children* 4(2):31-53.

Finkelhor, D. 2009. The prevention of childhood sexual abuse. *Future Child* 19(2):169-194.

Finkelhor, D., and J. Dziuba-Leatherman. 1994. Children as victims of violence: A national survey. *Pediatrics* 94(4):413-420.

Finkelhor, D., and L. Jones. 2012. *Have sexual abuse and physical abuse declined since the 1990s?* Durham: University of New Hampshire, Crimes Against Children Research Center.

Finkelhor, D., L. Jones, and A. Shattuck. 2010a. *Updated trends in child maltreatment, 2010.* Durham: University of New Hampshire, Crimes Against Children Research Center.

Finkelhor, D., H. Turner, R. Ormrod, and S. L. Hamby. 2010b. Trends in childhood violence and abuse exposure: Evidence from 2 national surveys. *Archives of Pediatrics & Adolescent Medicine* 164(3):238-242.

Fisher, G. C., and I. Mitchell. 1995. Is Munchausen-syndrome by proxy really a syndrome? *Archives of Disease in Childhood* 72(6):530-534.

Fox, K. 2004. Are they really neglected? A look at worker perceptions of neglect through the eyes of a national data system. *First Peoples Child and Family Review* 1(1):73-82.

Friedrich, W. N. 1993. Sexual victimization and sexual-behavior in children: A review of recent literature. *Child Abuse & Neglect* 17(1):59-66.

Friedrich, W. N., and S. T. Trane. 2002. Sexual behavior in children across multiple settings—commentary. *Child Abuse & Neglect* 26(3):243-245.

Friedrich, W. N., J. Fisher, D. Broughton, M. Houston, and C. R. Shafran. 1998. Normative sexual behavior in children: A contemporary sample. *Pediatrics* 101(4):E9.

Friedrich, W. N., W. H. Davies, E. Feher, and J. Wright. 2003. Sexual behavior problems in preteen children—developmental, ecological, and behavioral correlates. *Sexually Coercive Behavior: Understanding and Management* 989:95-104.

Gainsborough, J. F. 2010. *Scandalous politics: Child welfare policy in the states (American governance and public policy series).* Washington, DC: Georgetown University Press.

GAO (Government Accountability Office). 2011. *Child maltreatment: Strengthening national data on child fatalities could aid in prevention.* Washington, DC: GAO.

Heger, A., L. Ticson, O. Velasquez, and R. Bernier. 2002. Children referred for possible sexual abuse: Medical findings in 2,384 children. *Child Abuse & Neglect* 26(6-7):645-659.

Hershkowitz, I., S. Fisher, M. E. Lamb, and D. Horowitz. 2007. Improving credibility assessment in child sexual abuse allegations: The role of the NICHD investigative interview protocol. *Child Abuse & Neglect* 31(2):99-110.

Hussey, J. M., J. M. Marshall, D. J. English, E. D. Knight, A. S. Lau, H. Dubowitz, and J. B. Kotch. 2005. Defining maltreatment according to substantiation: Distinction without a difference? *Child Abuse & Neglect* 29(5):479-452.

Kellogg, N., and Committee on Child Abuse and Neglect. 2005. The evaluation of sexual abuse in children. *Pediatrics* 116(2):506-512.

Khan, A., D. H. Rubin, and G. Winnik. 2005. Evaluation of the mandatory child abuse course for physicians: Do we need to repeat it? *Public Health* 119(7):626-631.

Kilpatrick, D. G., and B. E. Saunders. 1995. *National survey of adolescents in the United States, 1995.* ICPSR 2833. Washington, DC: U.S. Department of Justice.

Kohl, P. L., M. Jonson-Reid, and B. Drake. 2009. Time to leave substantiation behind: Findings from a national probability study. *Child Maltreatment* 14(1):17-26.

Kolko, D. J., E. J. Brown, and L. Berliner. 2002. Children's perceptions of their abusive experience: Measurement and preliminary findings. *Child Maltreatment* 7(1):41-53.

Kuehnle, K., and M. Connell. 2009. *The evaluation of child sexual abuse allegations: A comprehensive guide to assessment and testimony.* Hoboken, NJ: John Wiley & Sons, Inc.

Lamb, M. E., Y. Orbach, I. Hershkowitz, P. W. Esplin, and D. Horowitz. 2007. A structured forensic interview protocol improves the quality and informativeness of investigative interviews with children: A review of research using the NICHD investigative interview protocol. *Child Abuse & Neglect* 31(11-12):1201-1231.

Lamb, M. E., Y. Orbach, K. J. Sternberg, J. Aldridge, S. Pearson, H. L. Stewart, P. W. Esplin, and L. Bowler. 2009. Use of a structured investigative protocol enhances the quality of investigative interviews with alleged victims of child sexual abuse in Britain. *Applied Cognitive Psychology* 23(4):449-467.

Langton, L., M. Berzofsky, C. P. Krebs, and H. Smiley-McDonald. 2012. *Victimizations not reported to the police, 2006-2010.* Washington, DC: U.S. Department of Justice, Office of Justice Programs, Bureau of Justice Statistics.

Larsson, A. S., and M. E. Lamb. 2009. Making the most of information-gathering interviews with children. *Infant and Child Development* 18(1):1-16.

Leeb, R. T., L. J. Paulozzi, C. Melanson, T. R. Simon, and I. Arias. 2008. *Child maltreatment surveillance: Uniform definitions for public health and recommended data elements.* Atlanta, GA: CDC, National Centers for Injury Prevention and Control.

Leventhal, J. M., and J. R. Gaither. 2012. Incidence of serious injuries due to physical abuse in the United States: 1997-2009. *Pediatrics* 130(5):1-6.

Leventhal, J. M., K. D. Martin, and J. R. Gaither. 2012. Using us data to estimate the incidence of serious physical abuse in children. *Pediatrics* 129(3):458-464.

Levi, B. H., and K. Crowell. 2011. Child abuse experts disagree about the threshold for mandated reporting. *Clinical Pediatrics* 50(4):321-329.

Levitt, S. D. 2004. Understanding why crime fell in the 1990's: For factors that explain the decline in six that do not. *Journal of Economic Perspectives* 18(1):163-190.

Lyon, T. D. 1999. The new wave in children's suggestibility research: A critique. *Cornell Law Review* 84(4):1004-1087.

MacMillan, H. L., E. Jamieson, and C. A. Walsh. 2003. Reported contact with child protection services among those reporting child physical and sexual abuse: Results from a community survey. *Child Abuse and Neglect* 27(12):1397-1408.

McCarthy, J., A. Marshall, J. Collins, G. Arganza, K. Deserly, and J. Milon. 2005. *A family's guide to the child welfare system*. Washington, DC: National Technical Assistance Center for Children's Mental Health.

McClure, R. J., P. M. Davis, S. R. Meadow, and J. R. Sibert. 1996. Epidemiology of Munchausen syndrome by proxy, non-accidental poisoning, and non-accidental suffocation. *Archives of Disease in Childhood* 75(1):57-61.

McElroy, R. 2012. *Analysis of state laws regarding mandated reporting of child maltreatment with appendix*. Washington, DC: State Policy Advocacy and Reform Center.

Military OneSource. n.d. *Legislation*. http://www.militaryonesource.mil/abuse/service-providers?content_id=267333 (accessed July 15, 2013).

Miller, M. 2011. *Family team decision making: Does it reduce racial disproportionality in Washington's child welfare system?* Olympia: Washington State Institute for Public Policy.

Myers, J. E. B. 2012. "Nobody's perfect"—partial disagreement with Herman, Faust, Bridges, and Ahern. *Journal of Child Sexual Abuse* 21(2):203-209.

NCSL (National Council of State Legislatures). 2012. *Mandatory reporting of child abuse and neglect: 2012 introduced state legislation*. http://www.ncsl.org/issues-research/human-services/2012-child-abuse-mandatory-reporting-bills.aspx (accessed February 11, 2013).

NRC (National Research Council). 1993. *Understanding child abuse and neglect*. Washington, DC: National Academy Press.

Oppel, R. A. 2011. Steady decline in major crime baffles experts. *New York Times*, May 23.

OPRE (Office of Planning Research and Evaluation). 2009. *National Incidence Study of Child Abuse and Neglect (NIS-4), 2004-2009*. http://www.acf.hhs.gov/programs/opre/research/project/national-incidence-study-of-child-abuse-and-neglect-nis-4-2004-2009 (accessed April 22, 2013).

Putnam-Hornstein, E. 2011. Report of maltreatment as a risk factor for injury death: A prospective birth cohort study. *Child Maltreatment* 16(3):163-174.

Putnam-Hornstein, E. 2012. Preventable injury deaths: A population-based proxy of child maltreatment risk in California. *Public Health Reports* 127(2):163-172.

Putnam-Hornstein, E., B. Needell, B. King, and M. Johnson-Motoyama. 2013. Racial and ethnic disparities: A population-based examination of risk factors for involvement with child protective services. *Child Abuse & Neglect* 37(1):33-46.

Roesler, T. A., and C. Jenny. 2008. *Medical child abuse: Beyond Munchausen syndrome by proxy*. Elk Grove, IL: AAP Press.

Saywitz, K. J., G. S. Goodman, and T. D. Lyon. 2002. Interviewing children in and out of court. In *The ASPAC handbook on child maltreatment*, edited by J. E. Myers, L. Berliner, J. Briere, C. T. Hendrix, C. Jenny, and T. A. Reid. Thousand Oaks, CA: Sage Publications, Inc. Pp. 349-378.

Sedlak, A. J., J. Mettenburg, M. Basena, I. Petta, K. McPherson, A. Greene, and S. Li. 2010a. *Fourth National Incidence Study of Children Abuse and Neglect (NIS-4): Report to Congress*. Washington, DC: U.S. Department of Health and Human Services, ACF.

Sedlak, A. J., K. McPeherson, and B. Das. 2010b. *Supplementary analyses of race differences in child maltreatment rates in the NIS-4*. Rockville, MD: Westat, Inc.

Slack, K. S., J. Holl, L. Altenbernd, M. McDaniel, and A. B. Stevens. 2003. Improving the measurement of child neglect for survey research: Issues and recommendations. *Child Maltreatment* 8(2):98-111.

Sparta, S. N., and G. P. Koocher, eds. 2006. *Forensic mental health assessment of children and adolescents*. New York: Oxford University Press.

Steinberg, K. L., M. Levine, and H. J. Doueck. 1997. Effects of legally mandated child-abuse reports on the therapeutic relationship: A survey of psychotherapists. *American Journal of Orthopsychiatry* 67(1):112-122.

Stoltenborgh, M., M. H. van Ijzendoorn, E. M. Euser, and M. J. Bakermans-Kranenburg. 2011. A global perspective on child sexual abuse: Meta-analysis of prevalence around the world. *Child Maltreatment* 16(2):79-101.

Straus, M. A., and J. H. Stewart. 1999. Corporal punishment by American parents: National data on prevalence, chronicity, severity, and duration, in relation to child and family characteristics. *Clinical Child and Family Psychology Review* 2(2):55-70.

Straus, M. A., S. L. Hamby, D. Finkelhor, D. W. Moore, and D. Runyan. 1998. Identification of child maltreatment with the parent-child conflict tactics scales: Development and psychometric data for a national sample of American parents. *Child Abuse & Neglect: The International Journal* 22(4):249-270.

Theodore, A. D., and D. K. Runyan. 2006. A survey of pediatricians' attitudes and experiences with court in cases of child maltreatment. *Child Abuse & Neglect* 30(12):1353-1363.

Theodore, A. D., J. J. Chang, D. K. Runyan, W. M. Hunter, S. I. Bangdiwala, and R. Agans. 2005. Epidemiologic features of the physical and sexual maltreatment of children in the Carolinas. *Pediatrics* 115(3):e331-e337.

Truman, J. L., and M. Planty. 2012. *Criminal victimization, 2011*. Washington, DC: Bureau of Justice Statistics.

Truman, J. L., and E. L. Smith. 2012. *Prevalence of violent crime among households with children, 1993-2010*. Washington, DC: Bureau of Justice Statistics.

White, N., and J. L. Lauritsen. 2012. *Violent crime agains youth, 1994-2010*. Washington, DC: U.S. Department of Justice, Office of Justice Programs, Bureau of Justice Statistics.

Wood, J. N., S. P. Medina, C. Feudtner, X. Luan, R. Localio, E. S. Fieldston, and D. M. Rubin. 2012. Local macroeconomic trends and hospital admissions for child abuse, 2000-2009. *Pediatrics* 130(2):e358-e364.

Zimring, F. E. 2008. *The great American crime decline*. New York: Oxford University Press.

Zimring, F. E. 2011. How New York beat crime. *Scientific American* 305:74-79.

Zolotor, A. J., and M. Shanahan. 2011. Epidemiology of physical abuse. In *Child abuse and neglect: Diagnosis, treatment and evidence*, edited by C. Jenny. St. Louis, MO: Saunders. Pp. 10-15.

Zolotor, A. J., A. D. Theodore, D. K. Runyan, J. J. Chang, and A. L. Laskey. 2011. Corporal punishment and physical abuse: Population-based trends for three-to-11-year-old children in the United States. *Child Abuse Review* 20(1):57-66.

3

Causality

As the field of child abuse and neglect has progressed, theoretical models have become more complex (e.g., Belsky, 1993; Cicchetti and Lynch, 1993; Cicchetti and Toth, 1998; Cicchetti and Valentino, 2006), and the number of studies has increased dramatically. Most have reported an association or correlation between a variety of potential risk factors and child abuse and neglect, contributing to the description of the problem, but few have investigated causes. This chapter reviews the literature on the candidate explanatory factors for child abuse and neglect and considers whether it is appropriate to draw causal inferences regarding these associations. Major challenges to the field are discussed, and the committee suggests that research needs to move beyond correlational designs and analyses to test causal models.

In contrast to other areas covered in the 1993 National Research Council (NRC) report, relatively little progress has been made in understanding the causes of child abuse and neglect. Risk factors for child abuse and neglect, which have been identified by research based on nonexperimental and correlational studies, provide valuable information to practitioners working directly with abused and neglected children, as well as policy makers and researchers seeking to launch inquiries into new areas of investigation. For example, the extensive research on risk factors has been applied in the creation of valuable risk assessment tools used by many child welfare agencies to predict whether children are at low, medium, or high risk for reoccurrence of abuse or neglect based on individual case characteristics (see Chapter 5). Yet while the existing research on risk factors can help in predicting abuse or neglect for the purposes of identifying individuals and populations in need of prevention and treatment efforts, it cannot explain why these factors result in abuse and neglect in certain situations but not in others. This limits the guidance that the research can provide for the creation and implementation of effective policies and programs. To design more effective prevention and treatment policies and interventions, therefore, a better understanding of the causal mechanisms of child abuse and neglect is required.

ESTABLISHING A CAUSAL CONNECTION

Muehrer and Koretz (1992) argue that a theoretical framework explaining the mechanisms and processes leading to certain outcomes provides the groundwork for the development and implementation of interventions that are preventive in nature. They stress the importance of identifying "factors that may play a causal, not simply correlational, role in the development of targeted outcomes" (p. 10). According to Blalock (1964), the noted methodologist and statistician, "the fact that causal inferences are made with considerable risk of error does not, of course, mean that they should not be made at all" (p. 5). Similarly, the committee believes it is important to advance the field with respect to determining the causes of child abuse and neglect.

According to formal tests of causal models, at least four conditions must be met to support the causal influence of hypothesized risk factors. First, one must demonstrate that a logical relationship exists. Second, one must demonstrate that an empirical association exists. Third, one must demonstrate that the correct temporal sequence exists. And finally, one must demonstrate that the relationship is not spurious, or due to some other characteristic or variable(s) (Hill, 1965; Schuck and Widom, 2001).

The vast majority of the existing literature on risk factors for child abuse and neglect provides a logical justification for the relationship, and numerous studies report an empirical association. Determining whether these studies meet the third criterion—demonstration of the correct temporal sequence—is more difficult and complex. One of the major problems with studies using retrospective measures of child abuse and neglect is that the temporal ordering of risk factors and abuse and neglect cannot be established reliably. Although a few prospective longitudinal studies exist (e.g., Dixon et al., 2005; Pears and Capaldi, 2001), most studies rely on cross-sectional designs, with information being collected at one point in time. Although one might assume that the temporal relationships are correct when asking parents whether they were abused as a child and at the same time asking whether they abuse their own children, memories are faulty, and questions have been raised about the validity and reliability of such measures (Gale et al., 1988; Henry et al., 1994; Ross, 1989; Squire, 1989;

White et al., 2007; Williams, 1994). According to Offer and colleagues (2000, p. 736), what one remembers depends on many factors, including "length of time since the event; frequency of the event; level of emotionality caused by the event; personal interpretation of and value placed on the event; and present expectations, needs, and beliefs" (see also Hardt and Rutter, 2004).

The fourth criterion (lack of spuriousness) has been addressed infrequently. To establish that a relationship is causal rather than spurious, one must control for variables that serve either theoretically or empirically as common covariates. Because many individual, family, and neighborhood risk factors that increase the likelihood of child abuse and neglect are also associated with other outcomes (Korbin, 1980; Leung and Carter, 1983; Widom et al., 1995), a causal relationship between those factors and child abuse and neglect becomes more credible if the relationship persists despite controls for these important covariates. At present, it is difficult to determine the nature of the association between risk factors and the perpetration of child abuse and neglect (Schuck and Widom, 2001).

Prospective longitudinal designs, ideally beginning before the birth of the child, provide an opportunity to determine the correct temporal order of risk factors and child abuse and neglect, to adjust for social and individual confounding factors as they occur, and to minimize reliance on recall and the selection of participants on the basis of outcomes (Gilbert et al., 2009). Animal analogue studies also provide an opportunity to examine these relationships systematically, but questions will remain about the extent to which findings can be generalized and the extent to which the experiences of abuse and neglect in animal models are representative of abuse and neglect in humans. Longitudinal ethnographic study designs may also offer additional perspectives on how certain life-course and everyday experiences shape child abuse and neglect (Burton et al., 2009). Ethnographies may be particularly helpful in discerning the meaning of abuse and neglect in everyday life and how one might characterize them as "normal" attributes in the lives of those mired in social and economic inequalities and uncertainty. The following excerpt from ethnographic fieldwork is illustrative of the more nuanced understanding of child abuse and neglect experiences that such research can provide:

> The ten-year-old girl sat on an idle swing, chatting with the caseworker on the swing beside her. "How many times," the girl asked, "have you been raped?" The question came casually, as if it could merely glide into the conversation. The caseworker, "Barbara," tried to stay composed. "I said that I hadn't, and she was surprised," Barbara recalled. "I thought everybody had been," she remembered the girl saying. "Her friends talked about it in school," Barbara observed. "It's an everyday thing." (Shipler, 2004, p. 142)

CANDIDATE EXPLANATORY FACTORS FOR
CHILD ABUSE AND NEGLECT

This review is organized into individual-level, family, contextual, and macrosystem factors that have been hypothesized as risk factors for the abuse or neglect of children. The discussion draws on the work of Bronfenbrenner (1979) and Belsky (1980), who identified these interrelated and mutually embedded factors that contribute to child abuse and neglect. Contextual factors represent the broader social systems (e.g., employment, neighborhoods) that influence parental functioning, whereas macrosystem factors represent the social or cultural forces that contribute to and maintain abuse or neglect.

Individual-Level (Parental) Risk Factors

Individual-level (parental) risk factors for child abuse and neglect include a history of child abuse and neglect, or intergenerational transmission; early childbearing; and parental psychopathology.

History of Childhood Abuse and Neglect (Intergenerational Transmission)

The most pervasive assumption on the part of the public and some policy makers is that a parent's past experience of abuse or neglect during childhood increases the risk for that parent to abuse or neglect his or her own children. This notion of intergenerational transmission was the premier developmental hypothesis in the field of abuse and neglect (Garbarino and Gilliam, 1980); according to these authors, however, the alleged relationship had not really "passed scientific muster" (p. 111).

Since that time, a number of studies have found evidence to support a history of child abuse or neglect as a risk factor for perpetration of abuse or neglect. Estimates are that about one-third of individuals who were abused or neglected will abuse or neglect their own children, with the proportion ranging from 25 to 35 percent (Jackson et al., 1999; Kaufman and Zigler, 1987). These figures suggest that the majority of parents with a history of abuse or neglect do not go on to abuse or neglect their own children.

Kaufman and Zigler (1987) critically reviewed the literature related to the hypothesis of intergenerational transmission of child abuse and neglect, concluding that many studies lacked the evidence needed to support the hypothesis because of weaknesses in the representative samples, in methodology, in formal definitions, and in descriptive statistics (Kim, 2009). More than 10 years later, Ertem and colleagues (2000) systematically reviewed studies of the intergenerational transmission of child physical abuse that met two criteria: the study used information about physical abuse in two consecutive generations, and it included a comparison or nonabused group. The authors developed a scale of eight methodological standards derived from a hypothetical experimental design to examine the validity of the studies they included in their review. Among the 10 studies they reviewed, only 1 met all eight standards, 3 met more than four, and 2 met only one. Ertem and colleagues (2000) also calculated the relative risk of child abuse between the abused and nonabused parents, and found that it varied from 1.05 to 37.80 (Ertem et al., 2000; Kim, 2009).

Stith and colleagues (2009) conducted a meta-analysis of 155 studies published between 1975 and 2000 in which parents' prior experience of abuse was included. Collectively, these studies examined 39 different risk factors for child physical abuse and 22 for neglect. Stith and colleagues found that parents' experience of childhood abuse had a moderate effect size in predicting subsequent acts of physical abuse ($d = 0.44$) and a smaller, but significant, effect size in predicting neglect ($d = 0.31$). As Stith and colleagues (2009) note, the meta-analysis cannot make any claims about the causal relationship between the risk factors examined and child abuse and neglect outcomes because their review encompasses studies that explore causality among indicators in different directions, as well as studies with both cross-sectional and longitudinal designs.

Thornberry and colleagues (2012) also examined the strength of the evidence base for the intergenerational transmission of child abuse and neglect, including in their review studies of child neglect and sexual abuse in addition to child physical abuse. They identified 47 studies that they evaluated against 11 methodological criteria. While most of the studies reported support for the hypothesis that a parental history of child abuse and neglect is a risk factor for perpetration of abuse and neglect, the authors express concern about the predictive value of many of these studies because of methodological limitations. Most of the studies met fewer than half of the methodological criteria. Among the 9 studies deemed most methodologically sound, the results were mixed with regard to the intergenerational transmission hypothesis. Four of the studies generally supported the theory (Dixon et al., 2005; Egeland et al., 1988; Pears and Capaldi, 2001; Thompson, 2006), 3 provided very limited support for only one type of abuse or neglect (Berlin et al., 2011; Renner and Slack, 2006; Sidebotham et al., 2001), and 2 found no evidence of transmission of abusive or neglectful behavior (Altemeier et al., 1984; Widom, 1989). The authors conclude that the widespread acceptance of the theory of intergenerational transmission of abuse and neglect is unsupported by these studies given their substantial methodological limitations.

Despite the broad acceptance of parental experience of abuse and neglect as a risk factor for perpetration of abuse and neglect and despite some progress in research on this hypothesis, the extent to which this risk factor explains the perpetration of child abuse and neglect remains unclear. Concerns remain as to the methodological validity of the evidence on this subject. A particular challenge to this body of research is the fact that experiences of child abuse and neglect need to be measured across two generations. Yet in much of the existing literature, a history of parental abuse and neglect often is measured by asking parents to recount memories across long periods of time, lessening the validity of the results. Also, a single reporter sometimes is called upon to assess a history of abuse and neglect for both generations (parent and child) (Thornberry et al., 2012; Widom, 1989). Problematic as well is when the sample is involved in parent training programs, institutionalized, or in some other specialized setting. Given society's disapproval of various forms of family violence, this issue is of particular concern because much of the child abuse literature is based on self-reports by parents (often mothers) who are typically participants, either voluntarily or involuntarily, in groups for abusing parents (Widom, 1989).

A related issue is whether researchers should focus not on whether parents with a history of abuse directly abuse their children but on whether they consistently put them in harm's way at the hands of others. Burton and colleagues (2009), reporting findings for the Three-City Study ethnography, indicate that many of the mothers in their sample who had suffered abuse as children serially entered and exited short-term relationships with romantic partners and often "unsuspectingly" invited abusive men into their homes and the lives of their children. In this way, mothers consistently increased the risk for abuse and neglect of their children by others, as had been done to many of them as children.

Similarly, Renner and Slack (2006) examined the relationship between mothers' childhood experiences of family violence—including physical abuse, sexual abuse, neglect, and witnessing domestic violence—and child abuse and neglect reports to child protective services regarding their children. They found that women with a history of sexual or physical abuse in childhood were three times more likely to have both experiences of adulthood intimate partner violence and allegations of child abuse and neglect toward their own children than (compared with) women with no history of childhood sexual or physical abuse. In contrast, the study found no association between any form of victimization during childhood and perpetration of child abuse or neglect in adulthood in the absence of experiences of intimate partner violence. Renner and Slack (2006) conclude that the complex relationship among childhood experiences of abuse and neglect, adulthood experiences of intimate partner violence, and adulthood perpetration of child abuse and neglect warrants further study and may shed light on the mixed findings on intergenerational transmission.

Early Childbearing

Early childbearing has been linked to an increased risk for child abuse (Connelly and Straus, 1992). Compared with older mothers, for example, younger mothers are more likely to have children referred to child protective services for abuse and neglect or circumstances suggestive of child abuse and neglect (Parrish et al., 2011; Putnam-Hornstein and Needell, 2011). Brown and colleagues (1998) found that the relative youth of a mother at childbirth was a significant risk factor for physical abuse, sexual abuse, and neglect.

Using data from two waves of the National Institute of Mental Health's Epidemiologic Catchment Area Study, Chaffin and colleagues (1996) separately assessed the relative impact of potential risk factors for child physical abuse and neglect in a representative community sample. To assess risk factors for their impact on the initiation of abuse and neglect, the analysis focused on parents who did not report any abuse or neglect in the first wave of the study but reported either physical abuse or neglect in the second wave. Parental age (mothers younger than 18 at the birth of their first child) was one of only two social or demographic factors shown to have a significant effect on the onset of both physical abuse and neglect, with younger parents showing a higher likelihood to commit both.

On the other hand, Klerman (1993) notes that the increased risk of child abuse and neglect for young compared with older mothers may be due in part to socioeconomic factors, such as income, education, family size, mobility, and stress. Using demographic data on parents with indicated abuse and neglect reports in 1988 and parents with children in out-of-home care in Illinois in 1990, Massat (1995) found that adolescent parents were not overrepresented among abusing and neglecting parents or among parents with children in out-of-home care, although low maternal age was associated with a number of negative outcomes for children. As Simkins (1984, p. 45) notes: "Age happens to be correlated with a large array of other variables such as the quality of prenatal and postnatal care, the socioeconomic status of the mother, and whether there are other caretakers in addition to the teenage mother." Thus, low socioeconomic status is a risk factor for early childbearing as well as for child abuse and neglect.

Using data from the Fragile Families and Child Wellbeing Study, Lee (2009) examined the relationship between harsh parenting behaviors (self-reports that included maternal spanking) by mothers who were aged 19 or younger compared with mothers who were 26 or older at the birth of the target child. Adolescent motherhood was significantly related to harsh parenting behavior, even after controlling for demographic and maternal characteristics. It is unclear why Lee omitted mothers who were aged 20-25 at the birth of the target child and whether the study controlled for the number of other children the mother had at the time of the birth of the target child.

A different picture emerges from an inspection of national statistics on child abuse and neglect. Table 3-1 summarizes the age of the perpetrators identified in child abuse and neglect reports by state and overall. Overall, only 6 percent of substantiated cases involve perpetrators under age 20; in contrast, 18 percent of all first-time births are to women (girls) under 20. The percentage has dropped dramatically since the 1970s, when 35 percent of all first-time births were to teens. This discrepancy between research findings and national statistics suggests a need for further exploration of the complex relationship between early childbearing and perpetration of child abuse and neglect. One question is whether a substantial proportion of teen parents who are reported/confirmed for child abuse were themselves foster children. This group of teen parents might be a good target for and benefit substantially from preventive services. Nonetheless, this body of research suggests that early childbearing may be implicated as a risk factor for child abuse and neglect, but not necessarily a causal factor.

Parental Psychopathology

Early writings reflected a belief that parental psychopathology was one of the causes of child abuse and neglect (Baumrind, 1993, 1995). While maternal mental health problems have been linked to an increased risk of child abuse and neglect (Brown et al., 1998), Wolfe (1999) found that fewer than 10 percent of abusing parents had a primary psychiatric disorder that was linked to their abusive behavior. Reviewed below is the literature on several psychiatric disorders that have been implicated in the etiology of child abuse and neglect, although few of these studies meet the criteria for drawing conclusions about causality. At present, the existing evidence suggests that specific forms of psychopathology may play a role in a parent's abuse or neglect of a child.

In one of the rare longitudinal studies of risk for child abuse and neglect beginning in infancy, Kotch and colleagues (1995) recruited mothers of newborn infants with biomedical and sociodemographic risk factors from community and regional hospitals and local health departments in 42 counties of North and South Carolina. The study considers maternal psychopathology, along with other risk factors for child abuse and neglect. For every four at-risk mother and infant pairs, the next mother to deliver a normal newborn was recruited to serve as part of a comparison group, and both groups were interviewed shortly after giving birth. State central registries of child abuse and neglect were reviewed when each infant was 1 year old. Kotch and colleagues found that several characteristics of the mothers (education, depression, and whether the mother lived with her own mother at age 14) were the best predictors of an abuse or neglect report. However, they also found that the number of other dependent children in the home and receipt of Medicaid were significant predictors of abuse and neglect reports, suggesting that multiple factors must be considered in thinking about causality.

Depression Several prospective studies have reported high rates of depression in abusing and neglecting parents (Kotch et al., 1999); thus, these findings meet at least one of the important criteria (correct temporal sequence) for establishing causality. Mothers who are depressed and/or anxious are at higher risk for physically abusing their children (Brown et al., 1998). Maternal depression also has been associated with childhood neglect (Bishop and Leadbeater, 1999; Brown et al., 1998; Éthier et al., 1995). Studies have shown that mothers who experience depression may be more disparaging, pessimistic, and ill tempered and less responsive to their children's needs relative to mothers without depression (Downey and Coyne, 1990; Nolen-Hoeksema et al., 1995). Pears and Capaldi (2001) found that, in addition to a history of abuse reported by parents, disciplinary inconsistency, depression, and posttraumatic stress disorder among parents were predictive of their abuse of their male children.

In a review of the literature on this topic, Knutson and Schartz (1997) conclude that about half of the studies examined failed to support the relationship between depression and child abuse. They suggest that unexamined moderators or confounders may play a role. In addition, since most of the research on this topic is based on cross-sectional studies, the temporal order of these relationships is unknown. The link between maternal depression and child abuse may be a consequence of having engaged in abusive behavior toward a child, or depression may play a causal role in the perpetration of child abuse because depressed parents may be more likely to react to their child's misbehavior with abuse or other forms of harsh or neglectful parenting (Belsky, 1993). The findings of the few existing prospective studies provide some evidence that maternal depression may play a causal role, but further research clearly is needed.

Substance abuse Substance (alcohol and drug) abuse is thought to be a major risk factor for the perpetration (Dubowitz et al., 2011; Ondersma, 2002) and recurrence (Jonson-Reid et al., 2010) of child abuse and neglect. Chaffin and colleagues (1996) found that parents who had a substance abuse disorder at the onset of their study were more than four times as likely as parents without such a disorder to commit physical abuse and more than 2.5 times as likely to have an episode of neglect. In an analysis of administrative data on a large sample of abused and neglected children in Florida, Yampolskaya and Banks (2006) found that caregiver alcohol and

TABLE 3-1 Perpetrators Identified in Child Abuse and Neglect Reports by Age, 2010 (Unique Count)

State	6-19		20-29		30-39		40-49	
	Number	Percent	Number	Percent	Number	Percent	Number	Percent
Alabama	848	10.8	2,845	36.1	2,099	26.6	820	10.4
Alaska	82	3.8	823	38.2	690	32.0	376	17.4
Arizona	248	4.0	2,373	38.1	2,198	35.3	991	15.9
Arkansas	1,012	10.1	3,582	35.6	2,859	28.4	1,318	13.1
California	3,141	5.2	20,075	33.5	19,909	33.3	10,923	18.2
Colorado	629	7.3	3,002	35.0	2,812	32.7	1,328	15.5
Connecticut	310	3.8	2,782	34.2	2,571	31.6	1,650	20.3
Delaware	87	5.3	616	37.3	540	32.7	314	19.0
District of Columbia	62	3.1	663	32.8	674	33.3	325	16.1
Florida	1,127	3.0	14,525	39.0	12,241	32.9	6,355	17.1
Georgia*								
Hawaii	44	3.2	456	32.7	458	32.8	286	20.5
Idaho	48	3.6	515	38.6	471	35.3	239	17.9
Illinois	1,535	8.0	7,716	40.3	5,958	31.1	2,677	14.0
Indiana	1,639	9.3	6,783	38.6	5,216	29.7	2,088	11.9
Iowa	550	5.6	3,882	39.8	3,250	33.4	1,337	13.7
Kansas	205	16.9	408	33.7	333	27.5	163	13.4
Kentucky	456	3.9	4,924	42.3	3,895	33.5	1,507	13.0
Louisiana	248	4.0	2,557	41.7	2,175	35.4	805	13.1
Maine	127	4.2	1,246	41.1	944	31.1	494	16.3
Maryland	753	8.2	2,527	27.5	2,958	32.2	1,772	19.3
Massachusetts	780	3.9	6,833	34.4	6,427	32.3	3,876	19.5
Michigan	1,174	4.7	9,876	39.3	8,625	34.3	3,995	15.9
Minnesota	327	9.4	1,231	35.5	1,171	33.8	528	15.2
Mississippi	435	7.5	2,082	35.9	2,003	34.5	832	14.3
Missouri	213	4.5	1,668	35.4	1,460	31.0	762	16.2
Montana	54	5.3	384	37.8	333	32.7	132	13.0
Nebraska	181	5.7	1,310	41.2	1,011	31.8	499	15.7

Nevada	122	3.2	1,465	38.7	1,304	34.5	654	17.3
New Hampshire	65	8.8	262	35.4	225	30.4	138	18.6
New Jersey	258	3.7	2,203	31.8	2,194	31.6	1,383	19.9
New Mexico	191	4.2	1,639	36.2	1,396	30.8	539	11.9
New York	2,117	3.4	18,998	30.7	20,985	33.9	14,015	22.6
North Carolina	167	3.6	1,663	35.9	1,606	34.7	825	17.8
North Dakota	26	3.4	223	29.4	210	27.7	120	15.8
Ohio	2,566	10.1	9,292	36.4	7,008	27.5	2,993	11.7
Oklahoma	393	5.6	2,988	42.4	2,145	30.5	888	12.6
Oregon*								
Pennsylvania	447	12.4	1,011	28.1	973	27.1	714	19.8
Puerto Rico	162	2.5	1,192	18.2	1,248	19.1	579	8.9
Rhode Island	186	7.1	981	37.6	862	33.1	424	16.3
South Carolina	261	3.0	3,318	37.7	3,237	36.8	1,456	16.5
South Dakota	34	3.7	436	47.0	284	30.6	126	13.6
Tennessee	795	15.1	2,028	38.5	1,364	25.9	586	11.1
Texas	4,765	9.3	22,179	43.1	15,254	29.7	6,198	12.1
Utah	1,026	11.3	3,220	35.6	3,016	33.3	1,263	14.0
Vermont	116	21.0	152	27.5	148	26.8	75	13.6
Virginia	236	4.4	1,859	34.7	1,558	29.1	901	16.8
Washington	136	2.4	2,023	36.1	1,978	35.3	940	16.8
West Virginia	118	3.4	1,354	38.7	1,185	33.9	430	12.3
Wisconsin	286	7.4	1,154	29.8	955	24.7	451	11.7
Wyoming	26	4.8	223	40.8	182	33.3	65	11.9
Total	30,814		185,547		162,598		82,155	
Percent	6.0		36.3		31.8		16.1	
States Reporting	50		50		50		50	

continued

TABLE 3-1 Continued

State	50-59 Number	50-59 Percent	60-69 Number	60-69 Percent	70-75 Number	70-75 Percent	Unknown Number	Unknown Percent	Total Unique Perpetrators
Alabama	289	3.7	79	1.0	906	11.5	58	2.7	7,886
Alaska	94	4.4	23	1.1	11	0.5	49	0.8	2,157
Arizona	292	4.7	64	1.0	7	0.1	635	6.3	6,222
Arkansas	447	4.4	172	1.7	36	0.4	1,596	2.7	10,061
California	3,137	5.2	785	1.3	292	0.5	312	3.6	59,858
Colorado	387	4.5	99	1.2	18	0.2	219	2.7	8,587
Connecticut	473	5.8	104	1.3	29	0.4			8,138
Delaware	71	4.3	19	1.2	4	0.2			1,651
District of Columbia	115	5.7	23	1.1	2	0.1	158	7.8	2,022
Florida	2,147	5.8	601	1.6	145	0.4	71	0.2	37,212
Georgia*									
Hawaii	89	6.4	28	2.0	7	0.5	27	1.9	1,395
Idaho	44	3.3	15	1.1	3	0.2			1,335
Illinois	797	4.2	173	0.9	65	0.3	238	1.2	19,159
Indiana	655	3.7	172	1.0	67	0.4	944	5.4	17,564
Iowa	377	3.9	76	0.8	18	0.2	253	2.6	9,743
Kansas	48	4.0	19	1.6	4	0.3	32	2.6	1,212
Kentucky	468	4.0	110	0.9	45	0.4	224	1.9	11,629
Louisiana	224	3.6	75	1.2	53	0.9	1	0.0	6,138
Maine	108	3.6	28	0.9	5	0.2	83	2.7	3,035
Maryland	606	6.6	173	1.9	29	0.3	365	4.0	9,183
Massachusetts	1,085	5.5	199	1.0	59	0.3	630	3.2	19,889
Michigan	1,082	4.3	290	1.2	64	0.3	5	0.0	25,111
Minnesota	152	4.4	45	1.3	12	0.3	1	0.0	3,467
Mississippi	311	5.4	100	1.7	24	0.4	19	0.3	5,806
Missouri	270	5.7	92	2.0	22	0.5	224	4.8	4,711
Montana	43	4.2	13	1.3	3	0.3	55	5.4	1,017
Nebraska	109	3.4	33	1.0	6	0.2	31	1.0	3,180

Nevada	201	5.3	29	0.8	10	0.3			3,785
New Hampshire	32	4.3	11	1.5	2	0.3	6	0.8	741
New Jersey	374	5.4	93	1.3	385	5.6	45	0.6	6,935
New Mexico	156	3.4	37	0.8	13	0.3	559	12.3	4,530
New York	4,353	7.0	1,044	1.7	282	0.5	92	0.1	61,886
North Carolina	265	5.7	70	1.5	36	0.8	1	0.0	4,633
North Dakota	25	3.3	3	0.4					758
Ohio	956	3.7	248	1.0	2,426	9.5	151	19.9	25,494
Oklahoma	300	4.3	103	1.5	38	0.5	5	0.0	7,044
Oregon*							189	2.7	
Pennsylvania	255	7.1	117	3.3	36	1.0	44	1.2	3,597
Puerto Rico	175	2.7	48	0.7	20	0.3	3,112	47.6	6,536
Rhode Island	100	3.8	21	0.8	7	0.3	26	1.0	2,607
South Carolina	386	4.4	102	1.2	30	0.3	18	0.2	8,808
South Dakota	25	2.7	3	0.3	1	0.1	18	1.9	927
Tennessee	227	4.3	71	1.3	25	0.5	175	3.3	5,271
Texas	2,128	4.1	643	1.3	209	0.4	52	0.1	51,428
Utah	386	4.3	94	1.0	19	0.2	25	0.3	9,049
Vermont	35	6.3	12	2.2	6	1.1	8	1.4	552
Virginia	267	5.0	86	1.6	33	0.6	412	7.7	5,352
Washington	277	4.9	74	1.3	14	0.2	167	3.0	5,609
West Virginia	131	3.7	39	1.1	8	0.2	233	6.7	3,498
Wisconsin	106	2.7	24	0.6	13	0.3	881	22.8	3,870
Wyoming	22	4.0	6	1.1			22	4.0	546
Total	25,102		6,588		5,549		12,471		510,824
Percent	4.9		1.3		1.1		2.4		100.0
States Reporting	50		50		48		46		50

NOTE: Fifty states reported case-level data about perpetrators. One state did not report perpetrator data in the Child File and one state submitted an SDC file, which does not have fields for perpetrator data.

SOURCE: ACF, 2011.

substance use was related to neglect but not abuse. Using data from a lon-gitudinal study of 224 children (selected from pediatric clinics that served primarily low-income urban families) who were followed over a 10-year period, Dubowitz and colleagues (2011) found that maternal drug use was one of five risk factors that significantly predicted a subsequent report to child protective services for abuse and neglect. Mothers who indicated they had ever used drugs were 1.7 times more likely to have a child reported to child protective services for abuse and neglect than mothers who had never used drugs.

The association between substance use disorders and deviant parenting is likely complex, encompassing both short- and long-term effects of sub-stances used in addition to the context and characteristics of parents (Moss and Tarter, 1993). Moreover, a parent with a substance use disorder can cause parenting difficulties for the other parent (Ammerman et al., 1999). It is also likely that caseworkers' perceptions of caregivers' substance abuse influence their perceptions of neglect and its severity (Berger et al., 2010). Studies have found as well that parental drinking or a family history of alcoholism is a risk factor for childhood sexual and physical abuse (Miller et al., 1997; Vogeltanz et al., 1999).

Kelleher and colleagues (1994) studied the association between alco-hol and drug disorders and child abuse and neglect using a sample drawn from the National Institute of Mental Health's Epidemiologic Catchment Area Study, a representative, community-based survey. The prevalence of substance use disorders was much higher among the group of adults who reported either physical abuse or neglect of a child than among those who did not report abuse and neglect (40 percent and 16 percent, respectively), after controlling for potential confounding variables.

In sum, a number of studies have described an elevated rate of sub-stance abuse problems in parents who abuse or neglect their children, controlling for at least some moderating factors.

Antisocial personality disorder Antisocial personality disorder (ASPD) in parents has been implicated as another risk factor for child abuse or ne-glect (Belsky and Vondra, 1989). As suggested by Capaldi (Capaldi, 1992; Capaldi and Stoolmiller, 1999), antisocial behavior interferes with the de-velopment of social competence, causing a chain reaction of developmental failures in young adulthood. In the longitudinal study described earlier, Brown and colleagues (1998) examined a number of parental mental health factors to determine whether they predicted child abuse and neglect. They found that maternal sociopathy (similar to ASPD) was a significant risk factor for physical abuse, neglect, and child sexual abuse, whereas paternal psychopathology and sociopathy predicted child neglect.

Summary Several types of parental psychopathology have been examined as risk factors for child abuse and neglect. Of the forms of parental psychopathology (primarily maternal) considered thus far, the strongest evidence suggests that maternal depression and substance abuse play an important role in the perpetration of child abuse and neglect by parents. Further research is needed, however, to begin to establish whether that role is causal.

Individual-Level (Child) Characteristics

Although the potential link is controversial and difficult to assess in methodologically rigorous ways, some research has suggested that children can be at greater risk of abuse and neglect if they have a physical and/or mental disability (e.g., mental retardation, physical impairments such as deafness and blindness, serious emotional disturbance). Using data from 35 child protective services agencies selected to be representative of U.S. counties, Westat, Inc., estimated that children with disabilities were 1.7 times more likely to experience child abuse and neglect than children without disabilities (Crosse et al., 1993; Sullivan and Knutson, 2000). However, the authors point out that child protective services agencies rarely recorded disability status in a systematic manner, and agency workers' opinions, rather than diagnoses by medical or other trained professionals, were relied upon in determining the presence or absence of disabilities. In addition, because this work combined different types of disabilities (physical and mental), it is difficult to determine whether each of these characteristics increases risk.

In terms of national statistics, the National Incidence Study (NIS)-4 is the first cycle of this study to examine the relationship between the incidence of abuse and neglect and a child's disability status (ACF, 2012). The findings are complex. Under the harm standard, children with documented disabilities had significantly lower rates of physical abuse and moderate harm from abuse and neglect compared with children without disabilities, but significantly higher rates of emotional neglect and serious injury or harm. Under the endangerment standard, children with disabilities had lower rates of abuse overall and of sexual abuse, neglect, physical neglect, and emotional neglect. However, children with disabilities were more likely to be seriously injured or harmed when they experienced abuse or neglect.

Empirical studies show an association between child abuse and neglect and disabilities (Algood et al., 2011; Govindshenoy and Spencer, 2007; Jonson-Reid et al., 2004; Sullivan and Knutson, 1998, 2000; Turner et al., 2011). In an epidemiological study involving a hospital-based sample with medical record information on diagnoses, for example, Sullivan and Knutson (1998) used records from child protective services, foster care, and law enforcement to assess evidence of child abuse and neglect. Based on this large sample of maltreated and nonmaltreated children, they found that disabilities were a risk factor for maltreatment, although they also found evidence that maltreatment could be relevant in the development of some disabilities (specifically, conduct disorder). Because there were questions about the generalizability of the hospital-based sample, the authors conducted a second study to examine this issue. In this study, Sullivan and Knutson (2000) used an entire school-based population drawn from the same geographic region as the first study and used a school-based disability criterion to reflect inclusion of a broad range of disabilities (not limited to hospital definitions as in the earlier study). The authors found a strong association between disabilities and child abuse and neglect. Among children with disabilities, the abuse and neglect rate was 31 percent, compared with 9 percent among children without disabilities. Specifically, the former children were 3.76 times more likely to be victims of neglect, 3.79 times more likely to be physically abused, and 3.14 times more likely to be sexually abused than children without disabilities. Unfortunately, no data were available on the age at first diagnosis of disability, making it impossible to determine whether the disabilities occurred before or after the child abuse and neglect. Thus the authors conclude: "Because the present data do not really address questions regarding cause and effect, future maltreatment research should consider the role of disabilities as either a risk factor or an outcome" (p. 1271).

Govindshenoy and Spencer (2007) conducted a systematic review of articles published between 1966 and 2006 in the Medline, Embase, Cinahl, Cochrane Library, National Research Register, Social Sciences, and PsychInfo databases. They included articles on population-based cohort, case-control, and cross-sectional studies of children less than 18 years of age and articles describing the results of an empirical analysis of the association between child abuse and neglect and disability. Meta-analysis was not possible because of the heterogeneity of the studies and the small number of studies that met their inclusion criterion. Of the studies reviewed, two were longitudinal, one was a retrospective birth cohort study, and the others were cross-sectional surveys. Methods of ascertaining abuse and neglect and the types of disability studied varied widely. Only two studies described analyses that included potential confounders. Considering these limitations, Govindshenoy and Spencer conclude that "the evidence base for an association of disability with abuse and neglect is weak. Psychological and emotional problems, and learning difficulties appear to be associated with abuse but this association might arise because these conditions share a common aetiological pathway with abuse. There is limited evidence that physical disability predisposes to abuse" (p. 552).

Family Characteristics

Studies have examined several family characteristics as risk factors for child abuse and neglect, including family structure, deficient parenting skills, intimate partner violence, and social isolation.

Family Structure

Over the past several decades, America's families have become increasingly complex, creating a multiplicity of contexts in which child abuse and neglect may occur. Of special note is the rise in nonmarital cohabitation among romantic partners and multiple-partner fertility (Cherlin, 2010). Multiple-partner fertility involves individuals having biological children with more than one partner, frequently in the context of nonmarital romantic relationships (Burton and Hardaway, 2012; Cancian et al., 2011; Carlson and Furstenberg, 2006). These unions often are characterized by "contentious relations among adults and serial childbearing through serial repartnering, which ultimately produces fairly broad, fluid, and complex networks of multiple biological parents, 'potential' coparents, half-siblings, and kin" (Burton and Hardaway, 2012, p. 344; Harknett and Knab, 2007; Sweeney, 2010). Such networks can create considerable inequality and uncertainty in the lives of children that can result in increased risk for child abuse and neglect. For example, ethnographic studies have noted that biological parents in new relationships can divert resources meant for their biological children from previous romantic unions to the children of their new partners, essentially taking the food out of one child's mouth to give to another (Meyer and Cancian, 2011; Tach et al., 2010). Moreover, as Hall (2010) and others have suggested, such complex families with variable biological parents may open the door for the emergence of inequalities that potentially put children at risk for abuse and neglect. It also has been suggested that colorism, or discrimination based on the lightness or darkness of one's skin color, may put darker-skinned children in these networks at greater risk for abuse and neglect compared with those with fairer skin (Glenn, 2009; Herring et al., 2004; Hunter, 2007).

Other literature documents the risk of abuse and neglect for children living in single-parent households, households with nonbiological parents, and chaotic families. Several studies have found that single parents are overrepresented among perpetrators of child abuse and neglect (Brown et al., 1998; Dufour et al., 2008; Gillham et al., 1998; Sedlak et al., 2010). Using data from the National Longitudinal Survey of Youth, Berger (2004) found that families with a biological mother and nonbiological father scored poorly on the Emotional Support subscale of the Home Observation for Measurement of the Environment, indicating that such parents may invest less than biological mother and father pairs in creating sufficient caregiving environments. Furthermore, using data from the Fragile Families and Child Wellbeing Study, Berger and colleagues (2009) found that children living in single-mother families and families with a nonbiological cohabitating father had higher rates of involvement with child protective services than children in families with biological father and mother pairs.

According to the most recent statistics from the NIS-4 (Sedlak et al., 2010), children living with their married biological parents had the lowest rates of abuse and neglect, whereas children living with a single parent who had a cohabiting partner in the household had the highest rates of abuse and neglect in all categories. "Compared to children living with married biological parents, those whose single parent had a live-in partner had more than 8 times the rate of abuse and neglect overall, over 10 times the rate of abuse, and nearly 8 times the rate of neglect" (p. 12). According to National Child Abuse and Neglect Data System (NCANDS) data, the highest rates of child sexual abuse occurred among single parents who had a cohabiting partner; children living in these households had a rate of abuse 10 times higher than that of children living with married biological parents (Sedlak et al., 2010). Finally, families in which children are abused or neglected move twice as often as nonmaltreating families from similar socioeconomic backgrounds (Eckenrode et al., 1995). In sum, although there is fairly consistent evidence that the rates of child abuse and neglect are higher in families without two biological parents, it is not clear how these alternative family structures or complex families act as causal factors in abuse and neglect.

Deficient Parenting Skills

A growing body of research explores the relationship between deficiencies in specific parenting skills and perpetration of child abuse and neglect. A number of studies have characterized parents who abuse or neglect their children as engaging in less interaction with them (Azar, 2002; Thomas and Zimmer-Gembeck, 2011; Timmer et al., 2005), being hyperresponsive to child-related stimuli (Chen et al., 2010; McCormack et al., 2009), engaging in harsher discipline (Koenig et al., 2000), having unrealistic expectations of their children (Reid et al., 1987), knowing less about child development (Burke et al., 1998; Dore and Lee, 1999), and overreporting their children's negative behaviors (Haskett et al., 1995). Compared with nonneglecting parents, neglecting parents have been shown to exhibit less empathy toward their children (Shahar, 2001) and less proficient caretaking skills (e.g., preparing food, keeping a clean home), poorer stress management, and less maternal motivation (Coohey, 1998).

Many of these studies examine differences in parental behaviors between abusing and neglecting parents and a comparison group of nonabusing and nonneglecting parents. Therefore, to be judged abusive and to be involved in these studies, these individuals had to have shown parenting behaviors that met some criteria or exceeded community standards of acceptable behavior. Thus, these descriptive findings are not surprising, but do not permit conclusions about causality. In general, these parental characteristics have been used to design interventions and treatment programs for abusing and neglecting parents on the assumption that changing these deficient parenting qualities will lead to lower rates of recurrence of child abuse and neglect. Overall, more research is needed in this area to identify the specific constructs of parenting that are most relevant to child abuse and neglect for the purposes of understanding the phenomenon, identifying at-risk families, and designing and implementing effective prevention and treatment efforts. Still, while these characteristics may be markers or risk factors for child abuse and neglect, further research is needed to determine causality.

Intimate Partner Violence

Numerous studies have reported that interparental violence and child abuse co-occur in families at a high rate (Capaldi et al., 2009; Rumm et al., 2000; Shipman et al., 1999), although studies vary on the extent of the co-occurrence reported, ranging from 18 to 67 percent (Appel and Holden, 1998; Edleson, 1999; Jouriles et al., 2008). Compared with nonabusive mothers, mothers who physically abuse their children report higher rates of victimization by intimate partner violence (Coohey and Braun, 1997). In one study of 1,232 partnered women, Zolotor and colleagues (2007) found the following odds ratios of child abuse in homes experiencing versus those not experiencing domestic violence: physical abuse, 2.7; neglect, 2.04; psychological abuse, 9.8; and sexual abuse, 4.90. As noted, Renner and Slack (2006) found no evidence for the intergenerational transmission of child abuse and neglect in the absence of adulthood experiences of intimate partner violence. Using NCANDS data in an analysis of children reported for neglect, Fox (2004) found that American Indian children were more likely than white children to come from homes where there was violence among caretakers. In another study, using National Survey of Child and Adolescent Well-Being (NSCAW) data, Dettlaff and colleagues (2009) compared Latino children of immigrants and children in native-born families in the child welfare system and found few significant differences in terms of use of excessive discipline, domestic violence, low social support, and difficulty meeting basic needs. Although both of these studies were limited to children already identified by the system, these findings suggest that further research might investigate the role of ethnic differences in the role of family violence and risk for child abuse and neglect.

Social Isolation

Social isolation has been associated with risk for abusing or neglecting children (Connelly and Straus, 1992; Coohey and Braun, 1997; Kelley et al., 1992; Kotch et al., 1997), although the evidence base on this association varies widely. Studies have reported that abusing and neglecting families lack significant social connections with their extended families, neighborhoods, and communities (Coohey, 1996, 2001; Coohey and Braun, 1997; Coulton et al., 2007). In particular, neglectful parents have been characterized as having no social networks, poor-quality marriages, and briefer relationships with their partners (Brown et al., 1998; Coohey, 1996; DePanfilis, 1996; Dubowitz, 1999). Compared with nonneglectful mothers, neglectful mothers have been found to perceive their own mothers more negatively, to have poorer relationships with their own mothers, and not to perceive their mothers as a source of emotional support (even when relying on them for money and help with child care) (Coohey, 1995).

While most of the studies reported thus far are focused on American families, Gracia and Musitu (2003) examined these issues using abusive and nonabusive families from Spanish and Colombian cultural backgrounds. In both cultures, the abusive parents reported "lower levels of community integration, participation in community social activities, and use of formal and informal organizations" compared with the nonabusive parents (p. 153). However, the families from the two cultures did not differ in the relationship between community social support and child abuse and neglect. Thus, these findings from studies in different cultural contexts regarding the role of community isolation in relation to child abuse and neglect suggest similarities to the earlier findings from studies with Anglo-Saxon families and perhaps generalizability of the phenomenon.

Summary

In sum, several characteristics of complex families, as well as deficient parenting in general, intimate partner violence, and social isolation, are associated with risk for child abuse and neglect. However, the evidence base thus far does not permit a determination of whether these factors or mechanisms play a causal role in the abuse and neglect of children.

Contextual Factors

The ecological model described earlier emphasizes that the social context within which the family lives may influence the likelihood of abuse or neglect. Several studies have examined the extent to which aspects of the broader social system (e.g., employment, neighborhood characteristics) are related to a parent's risk for becoming abusive or neglectful. The following discussion highlights studies in which the evidence is relatively strong, and also describes characteristics that place children at risk for abuse and neglect.

Poverty, Unemployment, and Low Socioeconomic Status

Poverty, unemployment, and low socioeconomic status have been reported as risk factors for child abuse and neglect (Berger, 2004; Chaffin et al., 1996; Fryer and Miyoshi, 1996; Kotch et al., 1997; Slack et al., 2003, 2004). Among all types of abuse and neglect, neglect is most strongly associated with poverty and low socioeconomic status (Brown et al., 1998; Chaffin et al., 1996; Drake and Pandey, 1996; Jones and McCurdy, 1992; Korbin et al., 1998), although there is evidence that poverty also is associated with physical abuse (Chaffin et al., 1996; Pears and Capaldi, 2001). Poverty may reduce a parent's capacity to nurture, monitor, and provide consistent parenting by contributing to the number of stressful life events experienced while also limiting available material and emotional resources. On the other hand, the potential role of poverty as a risk factor for abuse or neglect is complicated by the transmission of poverty, as a household characteristic, from one generation to the next (Behrman et al., 1990; Duncan et al., 1998; Mayer and Lopoo, 2001). Longitudinal designs that might be able to tease out the role of poverty and the associated stressors in influencing the risk for child abuse and neglect would be a worthwhile focus for future work. In addition, experimental studies evaluating the impact on child abuse and neglect of providing economic assistance to impoverished families could inform understanding of the causal role of poverty.

Neighborhood Characteristics

Characteristics of neighborhoods in which children and their families live have been associated with differences in the likelihood of child abuse and neglect (Coulton et al., 1999; Freisthler et al., 2006; Garbarino and Kostelny, 1992). For example, rates of child abuse and neglect have been associated with structural aspects of the neighborhood and community (poverty, large number of children per adult resident, population turnover, and high concentrations of single-parent families) (Coulton et al., 2007;

Drake and Pandey, 1996; Korbin et al., 1998, 2000). Lynch and Cicchetti (1998) found that rates of child abuse and neglect (particularly physical abuse) were related to levels of child-reported violence in the community and to the severity of child neglect.

Using an ecological framework and multilevel modeling, Coulton and colleagues (1999, p. 1019) examined the impact of "neighborhood structural conditions and individual risk factors for child abuse and neglect. Parents of children under the age of 18 were selected systematically from 20 randomly selected census-defined block groups with different risk profiles for child maltreatment report rates" and were administered a variety of questionnaires designed to assess characteristics of the environment and the potential for child abuse. The authors found that neighborhood poverty and child care burden affected the potential for child abuse after controlling for individual risk factors. However, they also found that the effects of neighborhood characteristics were weaker than has been reported in studies of official child abuse and neglect reports, and that there was greater variation in the potential for child abuse within than among neighborhoods.

In a subsequent paper, Coulton and colleagues (2007) review the existing literature and conclude that "only a few studies examine direct measures of parenting behaviors associated with maltreatment, and these show a weaker relationship with neighborhood disadvantage. Moreover, the processes that link neighborhood conditions to either maltreatment reports or parenting behaviors are not yet confirmed by the research literature" (p. 1117). The authors note problems with selection bias, variations in neighborhood definitions, and the failure to control for spatial influences in the existing research.

Based on concerns about the disproportionate number of racial and ethnic minority children in the child welfare system, Freisthler and colleagues (2007) examined how rates of child abuse and neglect for black, Hispanic, and white children might vary by neighborhood characteristics. Using data from 940 census tracts in California, they found that for black children, higher rates of poverty and higher density of alcohol outlets were positively associated with abuse and neglect rates, but other characteristics (population changes, population mobility, and higher percentage of black residents) were associated with lower rates. For Hispanic children, poverty, unemployment, and percentage of female-headed families were associated with increased risk for abuse and neglect. For white children, the percentages of poverty, elderly people, and Hispanic residents and the ratio of children to adults were positively associated with neighborhood rates of abuse and neglect. These findings suggest that the role of these contextual factors varies with the demographic characteristics of children and families and needs to be taken into account in future studies aimed at understanding causality.

Guterman and colleagues (2009) studied whether mothers' individual perceptions of their neighborhood social processes are related to self-reported predicted risk for physical child abuse and neglect. They examined this question using cross-sectional data from a national birth cohort sample of 3,356 mothers across 20 U.S. cities when the index child was 3 years of age. The authors used multiple-group structural equation modeling to test for differences across African American, Hispanic, and white mothers and found that perceived negative neighborhood processes had an indirect effect on the risk for physical abuse through parenting stress and personal control pathways. In contrast, however, they found that their predictor models did not differ significantly across ethnic groups. Unfortunately, because this is a cross-sectional study, the temporal relationship of these variables is unclear.

The vast majority of the literature examining the associations of neighborhood characteristics with rates and risks of child abuse and neglect has focused on national and urban samples. In contrast, Weissman and colleagues (2003, p. 1145) studied these relationships in one rural area of the United States. They analyzed "county-level data from Iowa between 1984 and 1993 for associations between county characteristics and rates of child abuse. Rates of single-parent families, divorce, and elder abuse were significantly associated with reported and substantiated child abuse ... while economic factors were not." Thus, these authors conclude that family structure is more strongly related to rates of child abuse reports and substantiation than are socioeconomic factors in this rural area.

Although limited, the findings of this body of research suggest that the role of contextual factors (as highlighted in the more complex ecological models) is important in understanding the risk for child abuse and neglect.

Macrosystem Factors

Social attitudes, such as attitudes toward violence or beliefs about discipline and corporal punishment, have been examined as risk factors for child abuse and neglect (Bower-Russa et al., 2001). One of the assumptions of an ecological perspective on child abuse and neglect is that a society's willingness to accept elevated levels of violence establishes precedence for family violence, such as physical child abuse (Belsky, 1980; Gelles, 1997). Norms within an individual's peer group and community can contribute to the likelihood that violence will be viewed as an acceptable solution to difficulties within the family (Straus et al., 1980).

In the United States, physical punishment is widely practiced and accepted, and these attitudes create an environment in which abuse and neglect may occur (Cicchetti and Lynch, 1993). However, the rate of corporal punishment has been declining since the mid-1980s (Straus and Stewart, 1999; Zolotor et al., 2011). Most schools have banned the use of physical punishment, foster care parents are not allowed to use physical discipline/ corporal punishment, and physical abuse is illegal in all 50 states (Center for Effective Discipline, 2013). On the other hand, all states allow parents to discipline their children physically (Davidson, 1997). On some level, therefore, there is a sense that physical punishment is tolerated when it is committed by a parent, but not by another person.

Coohey (2001) examined whether differences exist in the extent of familism (defined as attitudes, behaviors, and family structures operating within an extended family system) and child abuse and neglect in Latino and Anglo families. The author reports that both Latina and Anglo mothers who did not abuse or neglect their children appeared to have a higher level of familism than the abusive and neglectful mothers in both groups.

Recent work by Dunlap and colleagues (2009) uses ethnographic data to examine the "normalization of violence" that appears to characterize the childhood experiences of inner-city crack users. About half of them recalled being physically abused by their mothers or their mothers' various male partners. Those who did not report being beaten in childhood typically reported various types of physical attacks that they "deserved." Physical abuse, especially by mothers, frequently was seen as an expression of love. The authors suggest that these crack users viewed this type of abuse as a normal occurrence during their childhood and adolescence. They suggest that this type of physical discipline socialized and prepared them for the violence that would likely take place as they grew up in the inner-city environment. These findings suggest the importance of social context and, in some instances, "how much not being abused may serve as a protective factor among poor inner-city populations" (p. 16).

Complex Interaction of Multiple Risk Factors

The sections above have reviewed a large body of research focused on the impact of individual risk factors on the likelihood of perpetrating or experiencing child abuse and neglect. However, many of the risk factors that have been identified are interrelated and seldom are present in isolation from other risk factors. Some studies have shown that the presence of multiple risk factors can dramatically increase the likelihood of child abuse and neglect. In one longitudinal analysis of potential risk factors for child physical abuse, sexual abuse, and neglect, for example, Brown and colleagues (1998) collected data on abuse and neglect from both retrospective self-report surveys and official New York state records and considered a broad array of demographic, familial, child, and parenting factors as predictors of risk for child abuse and neglect. These authors found a substantial increase in the likelihood of child abuse and neglect when four or more risk factors were present. Their results also showed that the incidence of physical abuse, sexual abuse, or neglect increased from 3 percent among families with no risk factors present to 24 percent among families subject to four or more risk factors, and similar increases for each specific type of abuse or neglect. In their 18-year longitudinal study of a New Zealand birth cohort, Woodward and Fergusson (2002) found that young people reared by mothers with both alcohol/drug problems and depression tended to report higher levels of their mother's use of physical punishment and child abuse and neglect during childhood (birth to age 16).

Another example of the complex interaction of risk factors for child abuse and neglect is based on the proposition that dissociation may act as a mediator of child abuse and neglect across generations (Egeland and Susman-Stillman, 1996). Dissociation is defined as a "disruption of and/or discontinuity in the normal, subjective integration of one or more aspects of psychological functioning, including—but not limited to—memory, identity, consciousness, perception, and motor control" (Spiegel et al., 2011, p. 826). In one longitudinal study of severely sexually abused girls followed into parenthood, Kim and colleagues (2010) found that increased dissociation, together with a history of experiencing self-reported punitive parenting as a child, predicted whether a mother would parent her own children in a harsh and punitive manner. Thus, these authors hypothesize a tentative generational loop in which harsh and abusive parenting increases the risk for higher child- and adolescent-level dissociation, which in turn increases the risk for impulsive behavior and harsh parenting of offspring.

Together, these findings suggest that children being raised in families with multiple risk factors are at considerably higher risk for abuse and neglect than children not raised in such families. However, the complex interaction of multiple risk factors is not clearly understood, especially in conjunction with protective factors and resilience (discussed on p. 95), nor is it understood with respect to how children from different backgrounds in terms of culture, race, ethnicity, socioeconomic status, immigrant status, or geographic region of the country are at risk for child abuse and neglect.

Finding: Despite the broad acceptance of parental experience of abuse and neglect as a risk factor for perpetration of abuse and neglect, the extent to which this risk factor explains the perpetration of child abuse and neglect remains unclear. Major methodological concerns with the existing body of evidence on intergenerational transmission include reliance on parents' recounting of memories over a long period of time, reliance on parents' reports of abuse and neglect for both themselves and their children, and samples being drawn from specialized abuse- and neglect-related settings. Emerging research on more complex questions about intergenerational transmission may reconcile the mixed evidence on this topic.

Finding: Early childbearing has been linked to an increased risk for child abuse and neglect, although national statistics on child abuse and neglect do not reflect this relationship, suggesting that further research to understand this discrepancy is warranted. Some research suggests that low socioeconomic status is a risk factor for both early child-bearing and child abuse and neglect, while other research finds early childbearing to be significantly related to harsh parenting behavior after controlling for demographic and maternal characteristics.

Finding: Of the forms of parental (primarily maternal) psychopathology examined as risk factors for child abuse and neglect, the strongest evidence suggests that substance abuse and maternal depression play an important role in the perpetration of child abuse and neglect by parents. Further research is needed to establish whether parental depression and substance abuse play a causal role.

Finding: Research suggests that children can be at greater risk of abuse and neglect if they have a physical and/or mental disability, although this relationship is complicated and requires further research. Methodological concerns within this body of research include inconsistent definitions and procedures for establishing disability status, failure to distinguish among types of disabilities, limited knowledge about the temporal relationship between abuse and neglect and disability diagnosis, and insufficient attention to confounders.

Finding: There is fairly consistent evidence that the rates of child abuse and neglect are higher in families without two biological parents. Data from NCANDS and the NIS-4 show that children living in households with a single parent and cohabitating partner were at the highest risk of abuse and neglect compared with children in other arrangements. In addition, complex networks arising from multiple-partner fertility can create considerable inequality and uncertainty in the lives of children that can result in increased risk for abuse and neglect.

Finding: Some research suggests that deficiencies in parenting behaviors may indicate an increased risk for or serve as a marker for child abuse and neglect. More research is required to understand the relationship between specific parenting practices and child abuse and neglect.

Finding: Numerous studies have reported that interparental violence and child abuse co-occur in families at a high rate, suggesting a strong relationship between intimate partner violence and child abuse and neglect.

Finding: Findings from numerous studies, including some in diverse cultural contexts, identify social isolation as a risk factor for child abuse and neglect.

Finding: Poverty, unemployment, and low socioeconomic status have been reported as risk factors for child abuse and neglect, with neglect being most strongly associated with poverty and low socioeconomic status, followed by physical abuse.

Finding: Some structural aspects of neighborhoods and communities have been associated with rates of child abuse and neglect. Additional findings suggest that the role of contextual factors varies with the demographic characteristics of children and families, as well as with the community's location on the urban-rural continuum. Some research indicates that mothers' perceived negative neighborhood processes have an indirect effect on the risk for physical abuse through parenting stress and personal control pathways.

Finding: Important macrosystem factors that have been associated with child abuse and neglect include social attitudes about physical punishment and violence and the extent of familism among mothers.

Finding: Research suggests that children being raised in families with multiple risk factors are at considerably higher risk for abuse and neglect than children not raised in such families. However, the complex interaction of multiple risk factors is not clearly understood, especially in conjunction with protective factors and with demographic characteristics.

PROTECTIVE FACTORS

The importance of protective factors—dispositional attributes, environmental conditions, biological predispositions, and positive events that can act to mitigate risk factors (Garmezy, 1991; Masten, 2001, 2011; Masten et al., 1990)—is increasingly being recognized. Most of this research has focused on factors that enable children exposed to severe stressors to overcome the negative consequences of these experiences; relatively little is known about factors that protect at-risk children from being abused or neglected. In one of the most frequently cited studies on "breaking the cycle of abuse," Egeland and colleagues (1988) found that abused mothers who did not repeat the cycle of abuse were more likely than those who did repeat the cycle to have received emotional support from a nonabusive adult during childhood; to have participated in therapy during any period of their lives; and to have had a nonabusive and more stable, emotionally supportive, and satisfying relationship with a mate. More recently, Kotch and colleagues (1995, 1997) found that social support modified the negative impact of stressful life events on families at risk for child abuse and neglect. As Thompson (1995, p. 170) notes: "one secure, supportive social relationship may be all that is necessary to promote more adequate functioning in troubled parents." Clearly, more research is needed on protective factors that may act to prevent abuse and neglect in families at risk.

> *Finding:* Relatively little is known about factors that protect at-risk children from being abused or neglected. Some research suggests that social support, in the form of secure, supportive relationships, may play a significant role in protecting against the risk factors for child abuse and neglect. Clearly, more research is needed on protective factors that may act to prevent abuse and neglect in families at risk.

METHODOLOGICAL CHALLENGES

Since the 1993 National Research Council (NRC) report was issued, researchers in the field of child abuse and neglect have continued to face considerable methodological challenges. This chapter has reviewed several papers that identify methodological limitations of existing studies. Much of that research involves retrospective cross-sectional designs and is based on specialized, nonrepresentative samples. Method bias may arise if the same respondents, usually parents, provide information about both the parenting they received in their own childhood (or their own characteristics) and the parenting practices they use with their children. A related concern is parents' potential unwillingness to admit to engaging in poor parenting practices with their children because of social desirability issues or fear of outside intervention mandated by reporting laws. Conducting research with abused and neglected children in general is a challenging process because of difficulties in recruiting samples and in navigating ethical and legal reporting requirements. Finally, studies vary widely in the definitions and measures of child abuse and neglect used, hindering comparisons across studies. In the few studies that include "neglect," for example, definitions range from "lack of supervision" to a broader conceptualization of parental omissions, including extreme failure to provide necessary food, clothing, medical attention, and shelter.

> *Finding:* Studies of risk and protective factors for as well as causes of child abuse and neglect are limited by significant methodological challenges, including a reliance on data from retrospective cross-sectional designs with nonrepresentative samples, reports from a single responder

about two generations' experiences of abuse and neglect, responses potentially compromised by concerns about social desirability and legal reporting requirements, and a lack of consistency and clarity regarding definitions of abuse and neglect.

CONCLUSIONS

The review of the empirical literature on the causes of child abuse and neglect presented in this chapter provides some clues as to likely candidate risk factors. As risk factors, parental substance abuse, a history of child abuse and neglect, and depression appear to have the strongest support in the literature. However, it is important to acknowledge that all of these factors simply describe elevated risk, and none of them has been shown to "cause" child abuse and neglect. Indeed, the best estimates suggest that a minority of abused children will repeat the cycle with their own children. The studies reviewed also address the role of stressful environments and the impact of poverty, but it likewise is unclear whether these contextual factors "cause" child abuse and neglect. What is clear from this review is that there are a number of candidate risk factors for child abuse and neglect, but insufficient evidence to conclude that they are causal factors.

Since the 1993 NRC report was published, minimal progress has been made in understanding the causes of child abuse and neglect, particularly compared with the substantial progress made in understanding the nature of the problem and its consequences (discussed in the next chapter). Determining causality remains one of the most difficult challenges in the field. Research in the field needs to move beyond correlational designs and analyses to test causal models. Knowledge of the causes of child abuse and neglect has direct implications for the design and targeting of prevention efforts.

How do researchers investigate what causes parents or other caretakers to abuse or neglect the children in their care? In a paper on the causes of behavior, Killeen (2001) argues that understanding a phenomenon involves identifying its origin, structure, substrate, and function and representing these factors in some formal system. He cites the work of Aristotle, who described these types of explanations, referring to them as "efficient causes (triggers), formal causes (models), material causes (substrates or mechanisms), and final causes (functions)." Scholars in the field of child abuse and neglect have provided formal models of its causes (Cicchetti and Toth, 1998), and these models have been helpful in framing the prevention response. Because of the methodological challenges outlined in this chapter, however, understanding of the causes of child abuse and neglect is limited.

This chapter began with a brief discussion of four factors that are needed to establish causality. This review of the existing literature has shown that most published research makes a case for a logical relationship between a particular risk factor and the occurrence of child abuse and neglect. Risk factor studies have produced some evidence of an empirical association. Longitudinal studies would provide evidence of correct temporality, and the lack of spuriousness can be established by experimental controls. Indeed, more researchers have begun to question the strength of the evidence for some risk factors and to examine directly the role of potentially confounding factors. In some cases, these analyses have led to the conclusion that results are explained largely by the psychosocial context within which these children and families are living (Fergusson et al., 2006).

Studies of risk factors for child abuse and neglect have been conducted with methodologies heavily reliant on cross-sectional designs and retrospective self-reports, although there are some notable exceptions. The committee recognizes that not every study can be prospective and longitudinal. Correlational studies can be informative regarding causes, for example, if they use statistical controls to examine spuriousness, particularly when they show that two variables thought to be related are no longer related once one controls for a third variable. A good example is a paper that looks at the effect of male height on wages (Persico et al., 2004). No one knew why male adult height was associated with higher wages, but when the researchers controlled for height in adolescence (age 16), male adult height had no effect on wages. Thus, this was a correlational study, but it made an important contribution because it provided a better understanding of this relationship. Similar studies might be undertaken in the field of child abuse and neglect.

Nonetheless, longitudinal designs starting before the birth of the target children permit better controlled studies of who does and does not harm their children under what cultural, social, and individual circumstances. Such designs are rare in this field because they take time and are expensive. The best designs will take multiple factors into account, such as the candidate risk factors described here, and will involve large enough sample sizes to make it possible to determine what predicts abusive and neglectful behavior, under what conditions, and with which children. The work of Kotch and colleagues (1997, 1999) is an excellent example of such an approach. These designs can provide the strongest evidence for the causes of child abuse and neglect. What the field no longer needs are large population studies of "social addresses" that identify risk but not cause. There have now been many studies of this kind, and future correlational studies need to be clear about what new descriptive questions they can address or how they will analyze the data to examine whether hypothesized effects are in fact due to third variables.

The National Children's Study (NCS) provides an opportunity to engage in rigorous research to answer questions of causality. The NCS was authorized by the Children's Health Act of 2000 and is sponsored by a collaboration among four federal agencies: the National Institute of Child Health and Human Development, the National Institute of Environmental Health Sciences, the Centers for Disease Control and Prevention, and the Environmental Protection Agency. The study's objective is to recruit and follow a nationally representative sample of 100,000 children from before birth until age 21, examining the effects of the physical, chemical, and social environments on the growth, development, and health of children across the United States. The study includes attention to family dynamics, community and cultural influences, and genetics.

Ten years ago, in 2003, Barry Zuckerman, John Lutzker, and Ruth Brenner testified before the NCS steering committee to argue for the inclusion of child abuse and neglect in the study (IOM and NRC, 2012):

> To document the "natural history" of child maltreatment and to understand how environmental, child, and parent characteristics influence occurrences of child maltreatment and subsequent child development, large-scale prospective longitudinal research, such as the NCS, is required.... The ability to identify early markers of problematic parent-child interactions and factors that contribute to the likelihood of child maltreatment across different stages in children's and families' lives will provide invaluable information for the timing and delivery of cost-effective services to prevent child maltreatment.... The NCS also can provide information about the timing, dosage, and content of interventions necessary to address the consequences of child maltreatment and facilitate healthy child development through the study of interventions occurring within the sample and through using the NCS cohort as a control group in prevention and intervention research involving independent samples.

The committee urges the leadership of the NCS to include child abuse and neglect as one of its focal topics.

Studies of early neglect and deprivation with animal models, particularly rats and mice, may also offer opportunities to understand the causes of child abuse and neglect, including transgenerational processes that affect behavior (Champagne and Meaney, 2001; Champagne et al., 2003; Kaufman et al., 2000; Maestripieri, 2005; Maestripieri et al., 2006; Suomi, 1997) and the influence of substance abuse (Johns et al., 2005, 2010). No good primate analogue exists for neglect, except in the extreme case of infant abandonment. However, emerging research focused on infant physical abuse among nonhuman primates provides an opportunity not only to observe behavior and obtain biological data but also to experiment with parenting through cross-fostering (Sanchez and Pollak, 2009; Sanchez et al., 2010). Nonhuman primates also afford the advantage of a life span about one-fourth that of humans, making longitudinal studies across generations more feasible. Physical abuse of infants by mothers occurs annually at rates of 2-15 percent at the Yerkes Primate Research Center (Sanchez et al., 2010). The behaviors constituting physical abuse occur in short bouts amid otherwise more normal parenting, but when infant abuse occurs, it is severe and results in infant distress, serious injury, and occasionally death. Thus, animal analogue studies provide a way to manipulate characteristics of parents to determine whether some of the candidate risk factors identified by research in humans lead to animal versions of abuse and neglect. The findings from these animal studies will likely provide important hypotheses for processes to investigate among humans.

Research needs to examine whether there are common underlying factors that result in child abuse and neglect, or discrete behaviors have different etiologies. Are there differences or similarities in the causes of child abuse and neglect by the cultural context, sex, race, and ethnicity of parents? Some of the research described here suggests that candidate risk factors are similar across different contexts. However, relatively little attention has been paid to this issue.

Although children often experience multiple forms of abuse and/or neglect over their lifetimes, little is known about risk factors for specific types of abuse or neglect. That is, are the causes of physical abuse similar to the causes of neglect? Are the causes of sexual abuse different from those of physical abuse and neglect? Research addressing these questions will have direct implications for interventions and prevention programs. Are the causes of child abuse and neglect different in the context of multiple-problem families and communities compared with more cohesive and non-problematic families and communities? This issue is related to the concern described by Damashek and Chaffin (2012) as the "bundling" of child abuse and neglect with other life adversities. They argue that this bundling results in the inclusion of other risk factors—unmeasured or unaccountable for in research designs—that make it difficult to attribute effects to particular risk factors. This bundling also ignores one of the recommendations of the 1993 NRC report that identifies as essential "research that clarifies the common and divergent pathways in etiologies of different forms of child maltreatment for diverse populations" (p. 32).

Finally, in this chapter, the term "parental" has been used to refer to characteristics of the individual at risk for becoming abusive or neglectful. Because of the nature of laws determining who is reported and defined as an abusing and neglecting parent, however, it is the biological mother (or substitute mother) who is most often the caretaker and whose characteristics have been examined. Fortunately, recent research has begun to address the role of fathers as perpetrators of child abuse and neglect (Lee et al., 2008, 2011). In the future, particularly with the increase in fathers who remain at home, more attention should be paid to paternal characteristics that place children at risk for abuse and neglect.

REFERENCES

ACF (Administration for Children and Families). 2011. *Child maltreatment, 2010 report.* Washington, DC: U.S. Department of Health and Human Services, ACF.

ACF. 2012. *Child maltreatment, 2011 report.* Washington, DC: U.S. Department of Health and Human Services, ACF.

Algood, C. L., J. S. Hong, R. M. Gourdine, and A. B. Williams. 2011. Maltreatment of children with developmental disabilities: An ecological systems analysis. *Children and Youth Services Review* 33(7):1142-1148.

Altemeier, W. A., S. O'Connor, P. Vietze, H. Sandler, and K. Sherrod. 1984. Prediction of child abuse: A prospective study of feasibility. *Child Abuse & Neglect* 8(4):393-400.

Ammerman, R. T., D. J. Kolko, L. Kirisci, T. C. Blackson, and M. A. Dawes. 1999. Child abuse potential in parents with histories of substance use disorder. *Child Abuse & Neglect* 23(12):1225-1238.

Appel, A. E., and G. W. Holden. 1998. The co-occurrence of spouse and physical child abuse: A review and appraisal. *Journal of Family Psychology* 12(4):578-599.

Azar, S. T. 2002. Parenting and child maltreatment. In *Handbook of parenting*, Vol. 4, edited by M. H. Bornstein. Mahwah, NJ: Lawrence Erlbaum Associates. Pp. 361-388.

Baumrind, D. 1993. The average expectable environment is not good enough: A response to Scarr. *Child Development* 64(5):1299-1317.

Baumrind, D. 1995. *Child maltreatment and optimal caregiving in social contexts.* New York: Garland.

Behrman, J., P. Taubman, and R. C. Sickles. 1990. Survivor functions with covariates: Sensitivity to sample length, functional form and unobserved frailty. *Demography* 27(2):267-284.

Belsky, J. 1980. Child maltreatment: An ecological integration. *American Psychologist* 35(4): 320-335.

Belsky, J. 1993. Etiology of child maltreatment: A developmental-ecological analysis. *Psychological Bulletin* 114(3):413-434.

Belsky, J., and J. Vondra. 1989. Lessons from child abuse: The determinants of parenting. In *Child maltreatment: Theory and research on the causes and consequences of child abuse and neglect*, edited by D. Cicchetti and V. Carlson. New York: Cambridge University Press. Pp. 153-202.

Berger, L. M. 2004. Income, family structure, and child maltreatment risk. *Children and Youth Services Review* 26(8):725-748.

Berger, L. M., C. Paxson, and J. Waldfogel. 2009. Mothers, men, and child protective services involvement. *Child Maltreatment* 14(3):263-276.

Berger, L. M., K. S. Slack, J. Waldfogel, and S. K. Bruch. 2010. Caseworker-perceived caregiver substance abuse and child protective services outcomes. *Child Maltreatment* 15(3):199-210.

Berlin, L. J., K. Appleyard, and K. A. Dodge. 2011. Intergenerational continuity in child maltreatment: Mediating mechanisms and implications for prevention. *Child Development* 82(1):162-176.

Bishop, S. J., and B. J. Leadbeater. 1999. Maternal social support patterns and child maltreatment: Comparing parison of maltreating and nonmaltreating mothers. *American Journal of Orthopsychiatry* 69(2):172-181.

Blalock, H. M. 1964. *Causal inferences in nonexperimental research.* Chapel Hill: University of North Carolina Press.

Bower-Russa, M. E., J. F. Knutson, and A. Winebarger. 2001. Disciplinary history, adult disciplinary attitudes, and risk for abusive parenting. *Journal of Community Psychology* 29(3):219-240.

Bronfenbrenner, U. 1979. *The ecology of human development: Experiments by nature and design*. Cambridge, MA: Harvard University Press.

Brown, J., P. Cohen, J. G. Johnson, and S. Salzinger. 1998. A longitudinal analysis of risk factors for child maltreatment: Findings of a 17-year prospective study of officially recorded and self-reported child abuse and neglect. *Child Abuse & Neglect* 22(11):1065-1078.

Burke, J., J. Chandy, A. Dannerbeck, and J. W. Watt. 1998. The parental environment cluster model of child neglect: An integrative conceptual model. *Child Welfare* 77(4):389-405.

Burton, L. M., and C. R. Hardaway. 2012. Low-income mothers as "othermothers" to their romantic partners' children: Women's coparenting in multiple partner fertility relationships. *Family Process* 51(3):343-359.

Burton, L. M., D. Purvin, R. Garrett-Peters, G. H. Elder, and J. Z. Giele. 2009. Longitudinal ethnography: Uncovering domestic abuse in low-income women's lives. In *The craft of life course research*, edited by G. H. Elder and J. Z. Giele. New York: Guilford Press. Pp. 70-92.

Cancian, M., D. R. Meyer, and S. T. Cook. 2011. The evolution of family complexity from the perspective of nonmarital children. *Demography* 48(3):957-982.

Capaldi, D. M. 1992. Co-occurrence of conduct problems and depressive symptoms in early adolescent boys: A 2-year follow-up at grade 8. *Development and Psychopathology* 4(1):125-144.

Capaldi, D. M., and M. Stoolmiller. 1999. Co-occurrence of conduct problems and depressive symptoms in early adolescent boys: Prediction to young-adult adjustment. *Development and Psychopathology* 11(1):59-84.

Capaldi, D. M., H. K. Kim, and K. C. Pears. 2009. The association between partner violence and child maltreatment: A common conceptual framework. In *Preventing partner violence: Research and evidence-based strategies*, edited by D. J. Whitaker and J. R. Lutzker. Washington, DC: American Psychological Association. Pp. 93-111.

Carlson, M. J., and F. F. Furstenberg. 2006. The prevalence and correlates of multipartnered fertility among urban U.S. Parents. *Journal of Marriage and Family* 68(3):718-732.

Center for Effective Discipline. 2013. *Family and child care laws*. http://www.stophitting.com/index.php?page=statelegislation (accessed September 4, 2013).

Chaffin, M., K. Kelleher, and J. Hollenberg. 1996. Onset of physical abuse and neglect: Psychiatric, substance abuse, and social risk factors from prospective community data. *Child Abuse & Neglect* 20(3):191-203.

Champagne, F., and M. J. Meaney. 2001. Like mother, like daughter: Evidence for non-genomic transmission of parental behavior and stress responsivity. *Progress in Brain Research* 133:287-302.

Champagne, F. A., D. D. Francis, A. Mar, and M. J. Meaney. 2003. Variations in maternal care in the rat as a mediating influence for the effects of environment on development. *Physiology & Behavior* 79(3):359-371.

Chen, H. Y., T. W. Hou, and C. H. Chuang. 2010. Applying data mining to explore the risk factors of parenting stress. *Expert Systems with Applications* 37(1):598-601.

Cherlin, A. J. 2010. Demographic trends in the United States: A review of research in the 2000s. *Journal of Marriage and Family* 72(3):403-419.

Cicchetti, D., and M. Lynch. 1993. Toward an ecological/transactional model of community violence and child maltreatment: Consequences for children's development. *Psychiatry-Interpersonal and Biological Processes* 56(1):96-118.

Cicchetti, D., and S. L. Toth. 1998. Perspectives on research and practice in developmental psychopathology. In *Handbook of child psychology*, 5th ed., Vol. 4, edited by W. Damon, I. E. Sigel, and K. A. Renninger. Hoboken, NJ: John Wiley & Sons, Inc. Pp. 479-583.

Cicchetti, D., and K. Valentino. 2006. An ecological transactional perspective on child maltreatment: Failure of the average expectable environment and its influence upon child development. In *Developmental psychopathology: Risk, disorder, and adaptation*, 2nd ed., Vol. 3, edited by D. Cicchetti and D. J. Cohen. New York: John Wiley & Sons, Inc. Pp. 129-201.

Connelly, C. D., and M. A. Straus. 1992. Mother's age and risk for physical abuse. *Child Abuse & Neglect* 16(5):709-718.

Coohey, C. 1995. Neglectful mothers, their mothers, and partners: The significance of mutual aid. *Child Abuse & Neglect* 19(8):885-895.

Coohey, C. 1996. Child maltreatment: Testing the social isolation hypothesis. *Child Abuse & Neglect* 20(3):241-254.

Coohey, C. 1998. Home alone and other inadequately supervised children. *Child Welfare* 77(3):291-310.

Coohey, C. 2001. The relationship between familism and child maltreatment in Latino and Anglo families. *Child Maltreatment* 6(2):130-142.

Coohey, C., and N. Braun. 1997. Toward an integrated framework for understanding child physical abuse. *Child Abuse & Neglect* 21(11):1081-1094.

Coulton, C. J., J. E. Korbin, and M. Su. 1999. Neighborhoods and child maltreatment: A multi-level study. *Child Abuse & Neglect* 23(11):1019-1040.

Coulton, C. J., D. S. Crampton, M. Irwin, J. C. Spilsbury, and J. E. Korbin. 2007. How neighborhoods influence child maltreatment: A review of the literature and alternative pathways. *Child Abuse & Neglect* 31(11-12):1117-1142.

Crosse, S., K. Elyse, and A. Ratnofsky. 1993. *A report on the maltreatment of children with disabilities*. Washington, DC: National Center on Child Abuse and Neglect, U.S. Department of Health and Human Services.

Damashek, A. L., and M. J. Chaffin. 2012. Child abuse and neglect. In *Handbook of evidence-based practice in clinical psychology*, edited by P. Sturmey and M. Hersen. New York: John Wiley & Sons, Inc. Pp. 647-678.

Davidson, H. 1997. The legal aspects of corporal punishment in the home: When does physical discipline cross the line to become child abuse? *Children's Legal Rights Journal* 17:18-29.

DePanfilis, D. 1996. Social isolation of neglectful families: A review of social support assessment and intervention models. *Child Maltreatment* 1(1):37-52.

Dettlaff, A. J., I. Earner, and S. D. Phillips. 2009. Latino children of immigrants in the child welfare system: Prevalence, characteristics, and risk. *Children and Youth Services Review* 31(7):775-783.

Dixon, L., K. Browne, and C. Hamilton-Giachritsis. 2005. Risk factors of parents abused as children: A mediational analysis of the intergenerational continuity of child maltreatment (Part I). *Journal of Child Psychology and Psychiatry* 46(1):47-57.

Dore, M. M., and J. M. Lee. 1999. The role of parent training with abusive and neglectful parents. *Family Relations* 48(3):313-325.

Downey, G., and J. C. Coyne. 1990. Children of depressed parents: An integrative review. *Psychological Bulletin* 108(1):50-76.

Drake, B., and S. Pandey. 1996. Understanding the relationship between neighborhood poverty and specific types of child maltreatment. *Child Abuse & Neglect* 20(11):1003-1018.

Dubowitz, H. 1999. *Neglected children: Research, practice, and policy*. Thousand Oaks, CA: Sage Publications.

Dubowitz, H., J. Kim, M. M. Black, C. Weisbart, J. Semiatin, and L. S. Magder. 2011. Identifying children at high risk for a child maltreatment report. *Child Abuse & Neglect* 35(2):96-104.

Dufour, S., C. Lavergne, M. C. Larrivée, and N. Trocmé. 2008. Who are these parents involved in child neglect? A differential analysis by parent gender and family structure. *Children and Youth Services Review* 30(2):141-156.

Duncan, G. J., W. J. Yeung, J. Brooks-Gunn, and J. R. Smith. 1998. How much does childhood poverty affect the life chances of children? *American Sociological Review* 63(3):406-423.

Dunlap, E., A. Golub, B. D. Johnson, and E. Benoit. 2009. Normalization of violence: Experiences of childhood abuse by inner-city crack users. *Journal of Ethnicity in Substance Abuse* 8(1):15-34.

Eckenrode, J., E. Rowe, M. Laird, and J. Brathwaite. 1995. Mobility as a mediator of the effects of child maltreatment on academic performance. *Child Development* 66(4):1130-1142.

Edleson, J. L. 1999. The overlap between child maltreatment and woman battering. *Violence Against Women* 5(2):134-154.

Egeland, B., and A. Susman-Stillman. 1996. Dissociation as a mediator of child abuse across generations. *Child Abuse & Neglect* 20(11):1123-1132.

Egeland, B., D. Jacobvitz, and L. A. Sroufe. 1988. Breaking the cycle of abuse. *Child Development* 59(4):1080-1088.

Ertem, I. O., J. M. Leventhal, and S. Dobbs. 2000. Intergenerational continuity of child physical abuse: How good is the evidence? *Lancet* 356(9232):814-819.

Éthier, L. S., C. Lacharité, and G. Couture. 1995. Childhood adversity, parental stress, and depression of negligent mothers. *Child Abuse & Neglect* 19(5):619-632.

Fergusson, D. M., J. M. Boden, and L. J. Horwood. 2006. Examining the intergenerational transmission of violence in a New Zealand birth cohort. *Child Abuse & Neglect* 30(2):89-108.

Fox, K. 2004. Are they really neglected? A look at worker perceptions of neglect through the eyes of a national data system. *First Peoples Child and Family Review* 1(1):73-82.

Freisthler, B., D. H. Merritt, and E. A. LaScala. 2006. Understanding the ecology of child maltreatment: A review of the literature and directions for future research. *Child Maltreatment* 11(3):263-280.

Freisthler, B., E. Bruce, and B. Needell. 2007. Understanding the geospatial relationship of neighborhood characteristics and rates of maltreatment for black, Hispanic, and white children. *Social Work* 52(1):7-16.

Fryer, G. E., and T. J. Miyoshi. 1996. The role of the environment in the etiology of child maltreatment. *Aggression and Violent Behavior* 1(4):317-326.

Gale, J., R. J. Thompson, T. Moran, and W. H. Sack. 1988. Sexual abuse in young children: Its clinical presentation and characteristic patterns. *Child Abuse & Neglect* 12(2):163-170.

Garbarino, J., and G. Gilliam. 1980. *Understanding abusive families*. Lexington, MA: Lexington Books.

Garbarino, J., and K. Kostelny. 1992. Child maltreatment as a community problem. *Child Abuse & Neglect* 16(4):455-464.

Garmezy, N. 1991. Resilience in children's adaptation to negative life events and stressed environments. *Pediatric Annals* 20(9):459-460, 463-466.

Gelles, R. J. 1997. *Intimate violence in families*, 3rd ed. Newbury Park, CA: Sage Publications.

Gilbert, R., C. S. Widom, K. Browne, D. Fergusson, E. Webb, and S. Janson. 2009. Burden and consequences of child maltreatment in high-income countries. *Lancet* 373(9657):68-81.

Gillham, B., G. Tanner, B. Cheyne, I. Freeman, M. Rooney, and A. Lambie. 1998. Unemployment rates, single parent density, and indices of child poverty: Their relationship to different categories of child abuse and neglect. *Child Abuse & Neglect* 22(2):79-90.

Glenn, E. N. 2009. *Shades of difference: Why skin color matters*. Stanford, CA: Stanford University Press.

Govindshenoy, M., and N. Spencer. 2007. Abuse of the disabled child: A systematic review of population-based studies. *Child: Care, Health and Development* 33(5):552-558.

Gracia, E., and G. Musitu. 2003. Social isolation from communities and child maltreatment: A cross-cultural comparison. *Child Abuse & Neglect* 27(2):153-168.

Guterman, N. B., S. J. Lee, C. A. Taylor, and P. J. Rathouz. 2009. Parental perceptions of neighborhood processes, stress, personal control, and risk for physical child abuse and neglect. *Child Abuse & Neglect* 33(12):897-906.

Hall, J. E. 2010. Manifestations and effects of violence and social and economic disadvantage. Foreword. *Family and Community Health* 33(2):80-81.

Hardt, J., and M. Rutter. 2004. Validity of adult retrospective reports of adverse childhood experiences: Review of the evidence. *Journal of Child Psychology and Psychiatry* 45(2):260-273.

Harknett, K., and J. Knab. 2007. More kin, less support: Multipartnered fertility and perceived support among mothers. *Journal of Marriage and Family* 69(1):237-253.

Haskett, M. E., Scott, S. S., and Fann, K. D. 1995. Child abuse potential inventory and parenting behavior: Relationships with high-risk correlates. *Child Abuse & Neglect* 19(12):1483-1495.

Henry, B., T. E. Moffitt, A. Caspi, J. Langley, and P. A. Silva, 1994. On the "remembrance of things past": A longitudinal evaluation of the retrospective method. *Psychological Assessment* 6(2):92-101.

Herring, C., V. M. Keith, and H. D. Horton, Eds. 2004. *Skin deep: How race and complexion matter in the "color-blind" era.* Chicago: University of Illinois Press.

Hill, A. B. 1965. The environment and disease: Association or causation? *Proceedings of the Royal Society of Medicine* 58:295-300.

Hunter, M. 2007. The persistent problem of colorism: Skin tone, status, and inequality. *Sociology Compass* 1(1):237-254.

IOM (Institute of Medicine) and NRC (National Research Council). 2012. *Child maltreatment research, policy, and practice for the next decade: Workshop summary.* Washington, DC: The National Academies Press.

Jackson, R., F. Triber, J. Turner, H. Davis, and W. Strong. 1999. Effects of race, sex, and socioeconomic status upon cardiovascular stress responsivity and recovery youth. *International Journal of Psychophysiology* 31(2):111-119.

Johns, J. M., P. W. Joyner, M. S. McMurray, D. L. Elliott, V. E. Hofler, C. L. Middleton, K. Knupp, K. W. Greenhill, L. M. Lomas, and C. H. Walker. 2005. The effects of dopaminergic/serotonergic reuptake inhibition on maternal behavior, maternal aggression, and oxytocin in the rat. *Pharmacology Biochemistry and Behavior* 81(4):769-785.

Johns, J. M., M. S. McMurray, P. W. Joyner, T. M. Jarrett, S. K. Williams, E. T. Cox, M. A. Black, C. L. Middleton, and C. H. Walker. 2010. Effects of chronic and intermittent cocaine treatment on dominance, aggression, and oxytocin levels in post-lactational rats. *Psychopharmacology* 211(2):175-185.

Jones, E. D., and K. McCurdy. 1992. The links between types of maltreatment and demographic characteristics of children. *Child Abuse & Neglect* 16(2):201-215.

Jonson-Reid, M., B. Drake, J. Kim, S. Porterfield, and L. Han. 2004. A prospective analysis of the relationship between reported child maltreatment and special education eligibility among poor children. *Child Maltreatment* 9(4):382-394.

Jonson-Reid, M., S. Chung, I. Way, and J. Jolley. 2010. Understanding service use and victim patterns associated with re-reports of alleged maltreatment perpetrators. *Children and Youth Services Review* 32(6):790-797.

Jouriles, E. N., R. McDonald, A. M. S. Slep, R. E. Heyman, and E. Garrido. 2008. Child abuse in the context of domestic violence: Prevalence, explanations, and practice implications. *Violence and Victims* 23(2):221-235.

Kaufman, J., and E. Zigler. 1987. Do abused children become abusive parents? *American Journal of Orthopsychiatry* 57(2):186-192.

Kaufman, J., P. M. Plotsky, C. B. Nemeroff, and D. S. Charney. 2000. Effects of early adverse experiences on brain structure and function: Clinical implications. *Biological Psychiatry* 48(8):778-790.

Kelleher, K., M. Chaffin, J. Hollenberg, and E. Fischer. 1994. Alcohol and drug disorders among physically abusive and neglectful parents in a community-based sample. *American Journal of Public Health* 84(10):1586-1590.

Kelley, M. L., T. G. Power, and D. D. Wimbush. 1992. Determinants of disciplinary practices in low-income black mothers. *Child Development* 63(3):573-582.

Killeen, P. R. 2001. The four causes of behavior. *Current Directions in Psychological Science* 10(4):136-140.

Kim, J. 2009. Type-specific intergenerational transmission of neglectful and physically abusive parenting behaviors among young parents. *Children and Youth Services Review* 31(7):761-767.

Kim, K., P. K. Trickett, and F. W. Putnam. 2010. Childhood experiences of sexual abuse and later parenting practices among non-offending mothers of sexually abused and comparison girls. *Child Abuse & Neglect* 34(8):610-622.

Klerman, L. V. 1993. The relationship between adolescent parenthood and inadequate parenting. *Children and Youth Services Review* 15(4):309-320.

Knutson, J. F., and H. A. Schartz. 1997. Physical abuse and neglect of children. In *DSM-IV sourcebook,* Vol. 3, edited by T. A. Widiger, A. J. Frances, H. A. Pincus, R. Ross, M. B. First, and W. Davis. Washington, DC: American Pyschiatric Association. Pp. 713-804.

Koenig, A. L., D. Cicchetti, and F. A. Rogosch. 2000. Child compliance/noncompliance and maternal contributors to internalization in maltreating and nonmaltreating dyads. *Child Development* 71(4):1018-1032.

Korbin, J. E. 1980. The cross-cultural context of child abuse and neglect. In *The Battered Child,* 3rd ed., edited by C. H. Kempe and R. E. Helfer. Chicago: University of Chicago Press. Pp. 21-35.

Korbin, J. E., C. J. Coulton, S. Chard, C. Platt-Houston, and M. Su. 1998. Impoverishment and child maltreatment in African American and European American neighborhoods. *Development and Psychopathology* 10(2):215-233.

Korbin, J. E., C. J. Coulton, H. Lindstrom-Ufuti, and J. Spilsbury. 2000. Neighborhood views on the definition and etiology of child maltreatment. *Child Abuse & Neglect* 24(12):1509-1527.

Kotch, J. B., D. C. Browne, C. L. Ringwalt, P. W. Stewart, E. Ruina, K. Holt, B. Lowman, and J. W. Jung. 1995. Risk of child abuse or neglect in a cohort of low-income children. *Child Abuse & Neglect* 19(9):1115-1130.

Kotch, J. B., D. C. Browne, C. L. Ringwalt, V. Dufort, E. Ruina, P. W. Stewart, and J. W. Jung. 1997. Stress, social and substantiated maltreatment in the second and third years of life. *Child Abuse & Neglect* 21(11):1025-1037.

Kotch, J. B., D. Browne, V. Dufort, J. Winsor, and D. Catellier. 1999. Predicting child maltreatment in the first four years of life from characteristics assessed in the neonatal period. *Child Abuse & Neglect* 23(4):305-319.

Lee, S. J., N. B. Guterman, and Y. Lee. 2008. Risk factors for paternal physical child abuse. *Child Abuse & Neglect* 32(9):846-858.

Lee, S. J., J. Kim, C. A. Taylor, and B. E. Perron. 2011. Profiles of disciplinary behaviors among biological fathers. *Child Maltreatment* 16(1):51-62.

Lee, Y. 2009. Early motherhood and harsh parenting: The role of human, social, and cultural capital. *Child Abuse & Neglect* 33(9):625-637.

Leung, S. M. R., and J. E. Carter. 1983. Cross cultural study of child abuse among Chinese, Native Indians, and Anglo-Canadian children. *Journal of Psychiatric Treatment and Evaluation* 5:37-44.

Lynch, M., and D. Cicchetti. 1998. An ecological-transactional analysis of children and contexts: The longitudinal interplay among child maltreatment, community violence, and children's symptomatology. *Development and Psychopathology* 10(2):235-257.

Maestripieri, D. 2005. Early experience affects the intergenerational transmission of infant abuse in rhesus monkeys. *Proceedings of the National Academy of Sciences of the United States of America* 102(27):9726-9729.

Maestripieri, D., J. D. Higley, S. G. Lindell, T. K. Newman, K. M. McCormack, and M. M. Sanchez. 2006. Early maternal rejection affects the development of monoaminergic systems and adult abusive parenting in rhesus macaques (*Macaca mulatta*). *Behavioral Neuroscience* 120(5):1017-1024.

Massat, C. R. 1995. Is older better? Adolescent parenthood and maltreatment. *Child Welfare* 74(2):325-336.

Masten, A. S. 2001. Ordinary magic: Resilience processes in development. *American Psychologist* 56(3):227-238.

Masten, A. S. 2011. Resilience in children threatened by extreme adversity: Frameworks for research, practice, and translational synergy. *Development and Psychopathology* 23(2):141-154.

Masten, A. S., K. M. Best, and N. Garmezy. 1990. Resilience and development: Contributions from the study of children who overcome adversity. *Development and Psychopathology* 2(4):425-444.

Mayer, S. E., and L. M. Lopoo. 2001. Trends in the intergenerational economic mobility of sons and daughters. In *Generational income mobility in North America and Europe*, edited by M. Corak. Cambridge, UK: Cambridge University Press. Pp. 90-121.

McCormack, K., T. K. Newman, J. D. Higley, D. Maestripieri, and M. M. Sanchez. 2009. Serotonin transporter gene variation, infant abuse, and responsiveness to stress in rhesus macaque mothers and infants. *Hormones and Behavior* 55(4):538-547.

Meyer, D. R., and M. Cancian. 2011. "I'm not supporting his kids": Nonresident fathers' contributions given mothers' new fertility. *Journal of Marriage and Family* 74(1):132-151.

Miller, B. A., E. Maguin, and W. R. Downs. 1997. Alcohol, drugs, and violence in children's lives. In *Recent developments in alcoholism*, Vol. 13, edited by M. Galanter. New York: Plenum Press. Pp. 357-385.

Moss, H. B., and R. E. Tarter. 1993. Substance abuse, aggression and violence. *The American Journal on Addictions* 2(2):149-160.

Muehrer, P., and D. S. Koretz. 1992. Issues in preventive intervention research. *Current Directions in Psychology Science* 1(3):109-112.

Nolen-Hoeksema, S., A. Wolfson, D. Mumme, and K. Guskin. 1995. Helplessness in children of depressed and nondepressed mothers. *Developmental Psychology* 31(3):377-387.

NRC (National Research Council). 1993. *Understanding child abuse and neglect*. Washington, DC: National Academy Press.

Offer, D., M. Kaiz, K. I. Howard, and E. S. Bennett. 2000. The altering of reported experiences. *Journal of the American Academy of Child and Adolescent Psychiatry* 39(6):735-742.

Ondersma, S. J. 2002. Predictors of neglect within low-SES families: The importance of substance abuse. *American Journal of Orthopsychiatry* 72(3):383-391.

Parrish, J. W., M. B. Young, K. A. Perham-Hester, and B. D. Gessner. 2011. Identifying risk factors for child maltreatment in Alaska: A population-based approach. *American Journal of Preventive Medicine* 40(6):666-673.

Pears, K. C., and D. M. Capaldi. 2001. Intergenerational transmission of abuse: A two-generational prospective study of an at-risk sample. *Child Abuse & Neglect* 25(11):1439-1461.

Persico, N., A. Postlewaite, and D. Silverman. 2004. The effect of adolescent experience on labor market outcomes: The case of height. *Journal of Political Economy* 112(5):1019-1053.

Putnam-Hornstein, E., and B. Needell. 2011. Predictors of child protective service contact between birth and age five: An examination of California's 2002 birth cohort. *Children and Youth Services Review* 33(8):1337-1344.

Reid, J. B., K. Kavanagh, and D. V. Baldwin. 1987. Abusive parents' perceptions of child problem behaviors: An example of parental bias. *Journal of Abnormal Child Psychology* 15(3):457-466.

Renner, L. M., and K. S. Slack. 2006. Intimate partner violence and child maltreatment: Understanding intra- and intergenerational connections. *Child Abuse & Neglect* 30(6):599-617.

Ross, M. 1989. Relation of implicit theories to the construction of personal histories. *Psychological Review* 96:341-357.

Rumm, P., P. Cummings, M. Krauss, M. Bell, and F. Rivara. 2000. Identified spouse abuse as a risk factor for child abuse. *Child Abuse & Neglect* 24(11):1375-1381.

Sanchez, M. M., and S. D. Pollak. 2009. Socioemotional development following early abuse and neglect: Challenges and insights from translational research. In *Handbook of developmental social neuroscience*, edited by M. de Haan and M. R. Gunnar. New York: Guilford Press. Pp. 497-520.

Sanchez, M. M., K. M. McCormack, and D. Maestripieri. 2010. Ethological case study: Infant abuse in rhesus macaques. In *Formative experiences: The interaction of caregiving, culture, and developmental psychobiology*, edited by C. M. Worthman, P. M. Plotsky, D. S. Schechter, and C. Cummings. New York: Cambridge University Press. Pp. 224-237.

Schuck, A. M., and C.S. Widom. 2001. Childhood victimization and alcohol symptoms in females: Causal inferences and hypothesized mediators. *Child Abuse & Neglect* 25(8):1069-1092.

Sedlak, A. J., J. Mettenburg, M. Basena, I. Petta, K. McPherson, A. Greene, and S. Li. 2010. *Fourth National Study of Child Abuse and Neglect (NIS-4): Report to Congress executive summary.* Washington, DC: U.S. Department of Health and Human Services.

Shahar, G. G. 2001. Maternal personality and distress as predictors of child neglect. *Journal of Research in Personality* 35(4):537-545.

Shipler, D. K. 2004. *The working poor: Invisible in America.* New York: Alfred Knopf.

Shipman, K. L., B. B. R. Rossman, and J. C. West. 1999. Co-occurrence of spousal violence and child abuse: Conceptual implications. *Child Maltreatment* 4(2):93-102.

Sidebotham, P., J. Golding, and A. S. Team. 2001. Child maltreatment in the "children of the nineties." A longitudinal study of parental risk factors. *Child Abuse & Neglect* 25(9):1177-1200.

Simkins, L. 1984. Consequences of teenage pregnancy and motherhood. *Adolescence* 19(3):39-54.

Slack, K. S., J. Holl, L. Altenbernd, M. McDaniel, and A. B. Stevens. 2003. Improving the measurement of child neglect for survey research: Issues and recommendations. *Child Maltreatment* 8(2):98-111.

Slack, K. S., J. Holl, M. McDaniel, J. Yoo, and K. Bolger. 2004. Understanding the risks of child neglect: An exploration of poverty and parenting characteristics. *Child Maltreatment* 9(4):395-408.

Spiegel, D., R. Loewenstein, R. Lewis-Fernandez, V. Sar, D. Simeon, E. Vermetten, E., D. Simeon, and M. Friedman. 2011. Dissociative disorders in DSM-5. *Depression and Anxiety* 28:824-825.

Squire, L. R. 1989. On the course of forgetting in very long-term memory. *Journal of Experimental Psychology: Learning, Memory, and Cognition* 15(2):241-245.

Stith, S. M., T. Liu, L. C. Davies, E. L. Boykin, M. C. Alder, J. M. Harris, A. Sorn, M. McPherson, and J. E. Dees. 2009. Risk factors in child maltreatment: A meta-analytic review of the literature. *Aggression and Violent Behavior* 14(1):13-29.

Straus, M. A., and J. H. Stewart. 1999. Corporal punishment by American parents: National data on prevalence, chronicity, severity, and duration, in relation to child and family characteristics. *Clinical Child and Family Psychology Review* 2(2):55-70.

Straus, M. A., R. J. Gelles, and S. K. Steinmetz. 1980. *Behind closed doors: Violence in the American family.* Garden City, NY: Anchor Press.

Sullivan, P. M., and J. F. Knutson. 1998. The association between child maltreatment and disabilities in a hospital-based epidemiological study. *Child Abuse & Neglect* 22(4): 271-288.

Sullivan, P. M., and J. F. Knutson. 2000. Maltreatment and disabilities: A population-based epidemiological study. *Child Abuse & Neglect* 24(10):1257-1273.

Suomi, S. J. 1997. Early determinants of behaviour: Evidence from primate studies. *British Medical Bulletin* 53(1):170-184.

Sweeney, M. M. 2010. Remarriage and stepfamilies: Strategic sites for family scholarship in the 21st century. *Journal of Marriage and Family* 72(3):667-684.

Tach, L., R. Mincy, and K. Edin. 2010. Parenting as a "package deal": Relationships, fertility, and nonresident father involvement among unmarried parents. *Demography* 47(1): 181-204.

Thomas, R., and M. J. Zimmer-Gembeck. 2011. Accumulating evidence for parent-child interaction therapy in the prevention of child maltreatment. Child Development 82(1): 177-192.

Thompson, R. A. 1995. *Preventing child maltreatment through social support: A critical analysis.* Thousand Oaks, CA: Sage Publications.

Thompson, R. A. 2006. Exploring the link between maternal history of childhood victimization and child risk of maltreatment. *Journal of Trauma Practice* 5(2):57-72.

Thornberry, T. P., K. E. Knight, and P. J. Lovegrove. 2012. Does maltreatment beget maltreatment? A systematic review of the intergenerational literature. *Trauma, Violence, and Abuse* 13(3):135-152.

Timmer, S. G., A. J. Urquiza, N. M. Zebell, and J. M. McGrath. 2005. Parent-child interaction therapy: Application to maltreating parent-child dyads. *Child Abuse & Neglect* 29(7):825-842.

Turner, H. A., J. Vanderminden, D. Finkelhor, S. Hamby, and A. Shattuck. 2011. Disability and victimization in a national sample of children and youth. *Child Maltreatment* 16(4):275-286.

Vogeltanz, N. D., S. C. Wilsnack, T. R. Harris, R. W. Wilsnack, S. A. Wonderlich, and A. F. Kristjanson. 1999. Prevalence and risk factors for childhood sexual abuse in women: National survey findings. *Child Abuse & Neglect* 23(6):579-592.

Weissman, A. M., G. J. Jogerst, and J. D. Dawson. 2003. Community characteristics associated with child abuse in Iowa. *Child Abuse & Neglect* 27(10):1145-1159.

White, H. R., C. S. Widom, and P.-H. Chen. 2007. Congruence between adolescents' self-reports and their adult retrospective reports regarding parental discipline practices during their adolescence. *Psychological Reports* 101(3, Pt. 2):1079-1094.

Widom, C. S. 1989. Does violence beget violence? A critical examination of the literature. *Psychological Bulletin* 106(1):3-28.

Widom, C. S., T. Ireland, and P. J. Glynn. 1995. Alcohol abuse in abused and neglected children followed-up: Are they at increased risk? *Journal of Studies on Alcohol* 56(2):207-217.

Williams, L. M. 1994. Recall of childhood trauma: A prospective study of women's memories of child sexual abuse. *Journal of Consulting and Clinical Psychology* 62(6):1167-1176.

Wolfe, D. A. 1999. *Child abuse: Implications for child development and psychopathology,* 2nd ed. Thousand Oaks, CA: Sage Publications.

Woodward, L. J., and D. M. Fergusson. 2002. Parent, child, and contextual predictors of childhood physical punishment. *Infant & Child Development* 11(3):213-235.

Yampolskaya, S., and S. M. Banks. 2006. An assessment of the extent of child maltreatment using administrative databases. *Assessment* 13(3):342-355.

Zolotor, A. J., A. D. Theodore, T. Coyne-Beasley, and D. K. Runyan. 2007. Intimate partner violence and child maltreatment: Overlapping risk. *Brief Treatment and Crisis Intervention* 7(4):305-321.

Zolotor, A. J., A. D. Theodore, D. K. Runyan, J. J. Chang, and A. L. Laskey. 2011. Corporal punishment and physical abuse: Population-based trends for three-to-11-year-old children in the United States. *Child Abuse Review* 20(1):57-66.

4

Consequences of
Child Abuse and Neglect

Since the 1993 National Research Council (NRC) report on child abuse and neglect was issued, dramatic advances have been made in understanding the causes and consequences of child abuse and neglect, including advances in the neural, genomic, behavioral, psychologic, and social sciences. These advances have begun to inform the scientific literature, offering new insights into the neural and biological processes associated with child abuse and neglect and in some cases, shedding light on the mechanisms that mediate the behavioral sequelae that characterize children who have been abused and neglected. Research also has expanded understanding of the physical and behavioral health, academic, and economic consequences of child abuse and neglect. Knowledge of sensitive periods—the idea that for those aspects of brain development that are dependent on experience, there are stages in which the normal course of development is more susceptible to disruption from experiential perturbations—also has increased exponentially. In addition, research has begun to explore differences in individual susceptibility to the adverse outcomes associated with child abuse and neglect and to uncover the factors that protect some children from the deleterious consequences explored throughout this chapter. An important message is that factors relating to the individual child and to the familial and social contexts in which the child lives, as well as the severity, chronicity, and timing of abuse and neglect experiences, all conspire to impact, to varying degrees, the neural, biological, and behavioral sequelae of abuse and neglect.

This chapter begins by exploring background topics that are important to an understanding of research on the consequences of child abuse and

111

neglect, including an ecological framework and methodological attributes of studies in this field. Next is a review of the research surrounding specific outcomes across the neurobiological, cognitive, psychosocial, behavioral, and health domains, many of which can be seen in childhood, adolescence, and adulthood. The chapter then examines outcomes that are specific to adolescence and adulthood, reviews factors that contribute to individual differences in outcomes, and considers the economic burden of child abuse and neglect. The final section presents conclusions.

CASCADING CONSEQUENCES

Newborns are almost fully dependent upon parents to help them regulate physiology and behavior. Under optimal conditions, parents buffer young children from stress and serve as "co-regulators" of behavior and physiology (Hertsgaard et al., 1995; Hofer, 1994, 2006). Over time, children raised by such parents gradually assume these regulatory capacities. They typically enter school well regulated behaviorally, emotionally, and physiologically; thus, being prepared for the tasks of learning to read, write, and interact with peers.

For some children, parents cannot fill these roles as buffer and co-regulator effectively. When children have caregivers who cannot buffer them from stress or who cannot serve as co-regulators, they are vulnerable to the vicissitudes of a challenging environment. Although children can cope effectively with mild or moderate stress when supported by a caregiver, conditions that exceed their capacities to cope adaptively often result in problematic short- or long-term consequences.

Studies conducted with some nonhuman primate species and rodents have shown that the young are dependent on the parent for help in regulating behavior and physiology (Moriceau et al., 2010). Thus, young infants are dependent on parents fulfilling the functions of carrying, holding, and feeding. The period of physical immaturity and dependence lasts an extended time in humans. Even beyond the point at which young children are physically dependent, they remain psychologically dependent throughout childhood and adolescence. Thus, inadequate or abusive care can have considerable consequences in terms of children's health and social, psychological, cognitive, and brain development.

Children who have experienced abuse and neglect are therefore at increased risk for a number of problematic developmental, health, and mental health outcomes, including learning problems (e.g., problems with inattention and deficits in executive functions), problems relating to peers (e.g., peer rejection), internalizing symptoms (e.g., depression, anxiety), externalizing symptoms (e.g., oppositional defiant disorder, conduct disorder, aggression), and posttraumatic stress disorder (PTSD). As adults, these children continue to show increased risk for psychiatric disorders, substance use, serious medical illnesses, and lower economic productivity.

This chapter highlights research supporting the association between these outcomes, among others, and experiences of child abuse and neglect. The potential dramatic and pervasive consequences of child abuse and neglect underscore the need for research to illuminate the myriad pathways by which these ill effects manifest in order to guide treatment and intervention efforts. However, it is important to note at the outset that not all abused and neglected children experience problematic outcomes. As discussed in the section on individual differences later in this chapter, a body of research is devoted to uncovering the factors that distinguish children who do not experience problematic outcomes despite facing significant adversity in the form of abuse or neglect. Further, as discussed in Chapter 6, the past two decades have seen substantial growth in proven models for treatment of the consequences of child abuse and neglect, indicating that these effects are potentially reversible and that there is opportunity to intervene throughout the life course.

BACKGROUND

Several key concepts need to be considered in attempting to understand potential pathways that lead from abuse and neglect to the various consequences discussed in this chapter and the context in which those consequences manifest. First, positive and negative influences found among individual child characteristics, within the family environment, and in the child's broader social context all interact to predict outcomes related to child abuse and neglect. Second, child abuse and neglect occur in the context of a child's brain development, and their potential effects on developing brain structures can help explain the onset of certain negative outcomes. Finally, abused and neglected children often are exposed to multiple stressors in addition to experiences of abuse and neglect, and potential consequences may manifest at different points in a child's development. Therefore, the most rigorous research on this topic attempts to account for the many factors that may be confounded with abuse or neglect.

Ecological Framework

Since 1993, transactional-bioecological or ecological models have guided attempts to conceptualize the relative contributions of risk and protective factors to children's developmental outcomes, particularly in relation to child abuse and neglect (Belsky, 1993; Cicchetti and Lynch, 1993; Cicchetti and Toth, 1998). Versions of this approach consider the development of the child in the context of the broader social environment in which he or she functions, within the context of a family; in turn, children and families are embedded in a larger social system that includes communities, neighborhoods, and cultures. The assumption underlying these models is that behavior is complex, and development is multiply determined by characteristics of the individual, parents and family, and neighborhood and/or community and their interactions.

In examining the role of contextual factors in the onset of consequences due to child abuse and neglect, Cicchetti and Lynch's (1993) ecological/transactional model is particularly useful because it successfully incorporates multiple etiological frameworks (Lynch and Cicchetti, 1998). This model is based on Belsky's (1980, 1993) ecological model and Cicchetti and Rizley's (1981) transactional model. It expands on these models by highlighting the nature of interaction among risk factors and the ecology in which child maltreatment occurs. The ecological/transactional model describes four interrelated, mutually embedded categories that contribute to abuse and neglect and the potential associated consequences:

- Ontogenic development—Reflects factors within the individual that influence the achievement of competence and adaptation.
- Microsystem—Defined as the "immediate context" (i.e., the family) in which the child experiences abuse or neglect, including the bidirectional influence of parent and child characteristics and other relationships (such as marriage) that may impact parent-child interactions directly or indirectly.
- Exosystem—The exo- and macrosystemic levels reflect social or cultural forces that contribute to and maintain abuse or neglect. The exosystem encompasses the effects of broader societal systems (e.g., employment, neighborhoods) on parent and child functioning.
- Macrosystem—Mirrors temporally driven, sociocultural ideologies (e.g., cultural views of corporal punishment), or a "larger cultural fabric," that inevitably shape functioning at all other levels. It is represented by social attitudes (such as attitudes toward violence or the value of children).

The model is based on the fact that a child's multiple ecologies influence one another, affecting the child's development. Thus, the combined influence of the individual, family, community, and larger culture affect the child's developmental outcomes. Parent, child, and environmental characteristics combine to shape the probabilistic course of the development of abused and neglected children.

At higher, more distal levels of the ecology, risk factors increase the likelihood of child maltreatment. These environmental systems also influence what takes place at more proximal ecological levels, such as when risk and protective factors determine the presence or absence of maltreatment within the family environment. Overall, concurrent risk factors at the various ecological levels (e.g., cultural sanction of violence, community violence, low socioeconomic status, loss of job, divorce, parental substance abuse, maladaptation, and/or child psychopathology) act to increase or decrease the likelihood that abuse will occur.

The manner in which children handle the challenges associated with maltreatment is seen in their own ontogenic development, which shapes their ultimate adaptation or maladaptation. Although the overall pattern is that risk factors outweigh protective factors, there are infinite permutations of these risk variables across and within each level of the ecology, providing multiple pathways to the sequelae of child abuse and neglect.

Types of Evidence

Many studies of the consequences of abuse and neglect have been conducted with methodologies ranging from prospective to retrospective designs, from observational measures to self-report, and from experimental to case-controlled designs to no-control designs. The strongest conclusions could be reached with experimental designs whereby children would be randomly assigned to different abusive or neglectful experiences; however, this is obviously neither desirable nor possible.

Nonhuman studies involving primates and other species have allowed experimental assessment of different rearing conditions that may parallel human conditions of neglect and abuse (e.g., Sanchez, 2006; Suomi, 1997). One salient human study involved random assignment of children abandoned to institutions to high-quality foster care (a randomized controlled trial of foster care as an alternative to institutional care) (Nelson, 2007). In this prospective, longitudinal study, known as the Bucharest Early Intervention Project, 136 children abandoned at or around the time of birth and then placed in state-run institutions were extensively studied when they ranged in age from 6 to 31 months (mean age = 21 months), as was a sample of 72 never-institutionalized children who lived with their families in the greater Bucharest community. Following the baseline assessment, half of the institutionalized children were randomly assigned to a high-quality foster care program that the investigators created, financed, and maintained, and half were randomly assigned to remain in care as usual (institutional care). These children were followed extensively through age 12 (for discussion, see Fox et al., 2013; Nelson et al., 2007a,b; Zeanah et al., 2003). Although at first glance it may not be obvious why the study of children reared in institutions is relevant to a report on child abuse and neglect, institutional care, which affects as many as 8 million children around the world, can involve an extreme and specific form of neglect—broad-spectrum psychosocial deprivation. Therefore, neglectful institutional care settings can serve as a model system for understanding the effects of neglect on brain development. The neglect experienced by children in such settings should not serve as a proxy for the type of neglect experienced by noninstitutionalized children in the United States, who are more likely to experience neglect in such domains as food, shelter, clothing, or medical care rather than broad-spectrum psychosocial deprivation. Nevertheless, this study can provide important insight into the effects of neglect on behavioral and neurological development because of its randomized, controlled, and longitudinal nature.

The discussion in this chapter necessarily relies primarily (although not exclusively) on the strongest nonexperimental studies conducted. These studies involve longitudinal prospective designs, which assess child abuse and neglect objectively at the time of occurrence and assess outcomes longitudinally. A good example is the study of Widom and colleagues (1999), which followed a large cohort of abused and neglected children and a matched comparison sample from childhood into adulthood. Other examples include the studies of Johnson and colleagues (1999, 2000), Noll and colleagues (2007), and Jonson-Reid and colleagues (2012). Retrospective designs that ask participants to recall whether abuse and neglect were experienced are more troublesome because recall of child abuse and neglect can be affected by a variety of factors and open to a number of potential biases (Briere, 1992; Offer et al., 2000; Ross, 1989; Widom, 1988). Results of studies based on treatment samples of adults who experienced maltreatment as children may be potentially biased because not all victims of child abuse and neglect seek treatment as adults, and because people who do seek treatment may have higher rates of problems than people who do not seek treatment (Widom et al., 2007a). When participants are asked to report on conditions such as current depression and previous history of child abuse and neglect, the added problem of shared method variance arises. On the other hand, use of official records raises the problem of underreporting (Gilbert et al., 2009a).

The federal government has supported an effort, launched since the 1993 NRC report was issued—the National Survey of Child and Adolescent Well-Being (NSCAW)—to expand understanding of the consequences of child abuse and neglect. This study includes use of multiple data sources and record reviews, as well as interviews with children and youth who have experienced child abuse and neglect, their caretakers, and child welfare workers. Several of its findings are discussed in Chapter 5.

This chapter contains an extensive review of the more recent biologically based studies of child abuse and neglect because of the important advances that have been made in this area. To the extent possible, the discussion relies on findings from studies characterized by the greatest methodological rigor.

Despite recent methodological advances, researchers face many challenges in attempting to understand the short- and long-term consequences of the various types of child abuse and neglect (e.g., physical abuse, sexual abuse, neglect from caregivers) for child functioning and development. One of those challenges is teasing apart the impact of child abuse and neglect from that of other co-occurring factors. For example, children involved with child protective services because of neglect or abuse often face a number of overlapping and concurrent risk factors, including poverty, prenatal substance exposure, and parent psychopathology, among others (Dubowitz et al., 1987; Lyons et al., 2005; McCurdy, 2005). These concurrent risk factors can make it particularly difficult to draw causal inferences about the specific consequences of abuse and neglect for children's functioning, but need to be disentangled from the specific effects of abuse and neglect (Widom et al., 2007a). Controlling for other relevant variables becomes vital, since failure to take such family variables into account may result in reporting spurious relationships (Widom et al., 2007a). Some studies consider and covary other risk factors, and some do not. Considering the course of abuse and neglect may also be particularly important, as Jonson-Reid and colleagues (2012) found that the number of child abuse and neglect reports powerfully predicted adverse outcomes across a range of domains.

> *Finding:* Risk factors that co-occur with child abuse and neglect, such as poverty, prenatal substance exposure, and parent psychopathology, can confound attempts to draw causal inferences about the specific consequences of abuse and neglect for children's functioning. These factors need to be controlled for in studies seeking to identify the specific consequences of child abuse and neglect.

NEUROBIOLOGICAL OUTCOMES

An adequate caregiver is needed to support developing brain architecture and the developing ability to regulate behavior, emotions, and physiology for young children. When children experience abuse or neglect, such development can be compromised. The effects of abuse and neglect are seen especially in brain regions that are dependent on environmental input for optimal development, and on aspects of functioning especially susceptible to environmental input. Early in development, infants are completely reliant on input from their caregivers for help in regulating arousal, neuroendocrine functioning, temperature, and other basic functions. With time and with successful experiences in co-regulation, children increasingly take over these functions themselves. Abuse and neglect represent the absence of adequate input (as in the case of neglect) or the presence of threatening input (as in the case of abuse), either of which can compromise development. The following sections present a review of evidence with respect to key neurobiological systems that are altered as a result of abuse and neglect early in life: the hypothalamic-pituitary-adrenal (HPA) axis of the stress response system; the amygdala, involved in emotion processing and emotion regulation; the hippocampus, involved in learning and memory; the corpus callosum, involved in integrating functions between hemispheres; and the prefrontal cortex, involved in higher-order cognitive functions. The discussion begins, however, with a brief overview of brain development.

Overview of Neurobiological Development

The Construction of the Brain

Brain development begins just a few weeks after conception, starting with the construction of the neural tube. This is followed by the generation of different classes of brain cells—neurons and glia. Once formed, these immature neurons begin their migratory phase (generally away from the ventricular zone, which is their point of origin) to build the cerebral cortex. Much of cell migration is completed by the end of the second trimester of pregnancy, eventually leading to the construction of the six-layered cerebral cortex. After these immature cells have migrated to their target destination, they can differentiate; that is, they develop cell bodies and processes (axons and dendrites). Once processes have been formed, synapses begin to form; synapses are the connections between neurons that allow for the transmission of signals across the synaptic cleft, which is the small space that exists between two adjacent brain cells, generally between a dendrite and an axon. The synapse permits one neuron to communicate with another, and eventually, entire circuits are built, followed by neural networks (i.e., organized units). Finally, some axons in the brain develop a coating called myelin that speeds the flow of information along the length of the axon. Sensory and motor pathways begin to myelinate during the last trimester of pregnancy, whereas association areas of the brain, particularly the prefrontal cortex, continue to myelinate through the second decade of life. Neural elements (e.g., axons) that are coated with myelin are referred to as *white matter*, whereas most of the rest of the brain is referred to as *grey matter*.

Many aspects of brain development (particularly those that occur before birth) fall under genetic control (although some are affected by experience—prenatal exposure to neurotoxins such as alcohol being but one example). After birth, however, much of brain development becomes dependent on experience. For example, although the generation of synapses—which are massively overproduced early in development—is largely under genetic control, the pruning of synapses—which occurs primarily after birth—is largely under experiential control. Thus the prefrontal cortex of the 1-year-old child has many more synapses than the adult brain, but over the next one to two decades, these synapses are pruned back to adult numbers, based largely on experience (Nelson et al., 2011).

Neural Plasticity and Sensitive Periods

Many aspects of brain development depend on experiences occurring during particular time periods, often the first few years of life. These so-called *sensitive* or *critical periods* represent vital inflection points in the course of development, such that if specific experiences fail to occur within some narrow window of time (or the *wrong* experiences occur), development can go awry. This leads to the concept that plasticity "cuts both ways," meaning that if the child is exposed to *good* experiences, the brain benefits, but if the child is exposed to *bad* experiences or inadequate input, the brain may suffer (Nelson et al., 2011). Prenatally, an example of a bad experience is exposure to neurotoxins such as alcohol or drugs of abuse. An example of a good experience is access to good nutrition, including the many micronutrients that facilitate brain development (e.g., iron, zinc). Postnatally, the topic of this report represents examples of bad experience (i.e., abuse and neglect). Conversely, examples of good experiences include providing a child with consistent, sensitive caregiving; a nurturing home in general; and adequate stimulation.

The Time Course of Development

In general, most sensory systems develop early in life; thus the ability to see and to discriminate and recognize faces and speech sounds come on line in the first months and years of life, based on appropriate experiences occurring during that time window (e.g., exposure to faces, to speech). This is not surprising given how vitally important these functions are to subsequent development (e.g., language is not learned until children can discriminate the basic units of sound, such as one consonant from another). Critical to the discussion in this chapter, however, is that the functions subserved by some other regions of the brain, most notably the prefrontal cortex—executive control, planning, cognitive flexibility, emotion regulation—have a much more protracted course of development for the simple reason that both synaptogenesis

Human Brain Development

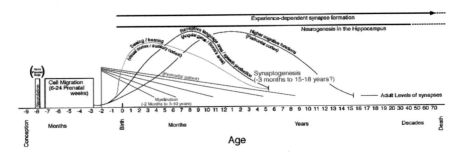

FIGURE 4-1 The time course of key aspects of brain development.
SOURCE: Thompson and Nelson, 2001 (reprinted with the permission of *American Psychologist*).

and myelination of these cortical regions do not mature until mid- to late adolescence, perhaps even a bit later. As a result, the sensitive period for prefrontal cortical functions may be far more prolonged than is the case for sensory functions, extending well into the adolescent period. One example of the differential time course of different brain regions, and perhaps their corresponding sensitive periods, is illustrated in Figure 4-1.

These concepts are important to the study of the neurobiological toll of early childhood abuse and neglect because children who experience considerable adversity early in life may be exposed to environments/experiences that the species has not come to expect (such as abusive caregivers) or worse, environments that are largely lacking in key experiences (i.e., neglect). In both cases, when the expectable environment is violated by either gross alterations in the type of care received or a complete lack of care, subsequent development can be seriously derailed.

Hypothalamic-Pituitary-Adrenocortical (HPA) Axis and Biological Regulation

There is strong evidence across species that the HPA axis is affected by experiences of early childhood abuse and neglect (e.g., Bruce et al., 2009; Gunnar and Vazquez, 2001; Levine et al., 1993; Shonkoff et al., 2012). Glucocorticoids (cortisol in humans, corticosterone in rodents) are steroid hormones produced as an end product of the HPA system. The HPA axis serves two orthogonal functions: mounting a stress response and maintaining a diurnal rhythm. A cascade of events is designed to promote survival behavior by directing energy to processes that are critical to immediate survival (e.g., metabolism of glucose) and away from processes that are less critical to immediate survival, such as immune functioning, growth, digestion, and reproduction (Gunnar and Cheatham, 2003).

Glucocorticoids also serve an important role in maintaining circadian patterns of daily activity, such as waking up, sleeping, and energy regulation (Gunnar and Cheatham, 2003). Diurnal species, including humans, have a diurnal pattern of cortisol production that enhances the likelihood of being awake at the same time in the day. In humans, diurnal cortisol levels peak about 30 minutes after waking up, decrease sharply by mid-morning, and continue to decrease gradually until bedtime (Gunnar and Donzella, 2002). The higher morning values of cortisol reflect greater metabolism of glucose early in the day, providing energy for the day's activities.

The HPA axis is highly sensitive to the effects of early experiences. Diurnal effects typically have been examined as wake-up values and bedtime values because those time points allow assessments of change from nearly the highest reliable waking time point (with 30 minutes post wake-up being the highest) to the lowest waking time point. Daytime values are affected by a number of factors, such as exercise, naps, and travel to work (Larson et al., 1991; Watamura et al., 2002). The most consistent findings involve flatter, more blunted patterns of diurnal regulation among abused or neglected children relative to low-risk children (Bernard et al., 2010; Bruce et al., 2009; Dozier et al., 2006; Fisher et al., 2007; Gunnar and Vazquez, 2001). Similar flattened diurnal rhythms have been found in institutionalized children (Bruce et al., 2000; Carlson and Earls, 1997). Flattened diurnal cortisol patterns may reflect down-regulation of HPA axis activity following earlier hyperactivation (Carpenter et al., 2009; Fries et al., 2005).

Cicchetti and colleagues (Cicchetti and Rogosch, 2001a,b) examined changes across the day among abused and neglected children attending summer camp. The time points included when children first arrived at camp (at about 9 AM) and before they left camp for the day (at about 4 PM), likely tapping diurnal change within a challenging environment. The authors report complex findings regarding cortisol in this setting. Differences were found in some studies related to subtype and/or psychopathology and/or aggression (Cicchetti and Rogosch, 2001b; Murray-Close et al., 2008).

Animal models have been used to study experimentally the effects of neglect and abuse on HPA functioning (e.g., Levine et al., 1993). Experiences of abuse or neglect, depending on age of pup/infant, duration, chronicity, and subsequent response of dam/mother differentially affect short- and long-term effects on the HPA axis (Sanchez, 2006). Under naturally occurring conditions (about 10 percent of rhesus monkeys abuse their infants), a 1-year-old rhesus monkey that was abused (primarily in the first month of life) showed higher cortisol levels under basal and stress conditions than a 1-year-old that had not been abused. These effects were not seen at older ages. (The age translation from rhesus to human is about 1 to 4, so a 1-year-old rhesus is developmentally similar to about a 4-year-old human child.) In other studies that have manipulated rearing conditions (such as isolation rearing), differences between conditions of abuse or neglect have been inconsistent. In some studies, higher cortisol values were observed in basal and/or stress conditions; in some, lower basal and/or stress conditions; and in some, no differences between the monkeys that had undergone deprivation and those that had not (Champoux et al., 1989; Clarke, 1993; Higley et al., 1992; Shannon et al., 1998).

Disrupted HPA axis regulation may have negative effects on a number of other biological systems. High levels of circulating cortisol resulting from early life stress may cause damage to developing brain regions (Teicher et al., 2003; Twardosz and Lutzker, 2010). Several brain regions, including limbic regions such as the amygdala and hippocampus and prefrontal regions, may be particularly susceptible to the effects of high levels of circulating cortisol because of the high number of glucocorticoid receptors in these areas (Brake et al., 2000; Schatzberg and Lindley, 2008; Wellman, 2001).

High levels of circulating cortisol may affect telomere length as well. Telomeres are the repeated sequences of DNA that cap the ends of chromosomes. Telomeres shorten each time cells divide, a process generally associated with aging, but also with stress (Epel et al., 2004). If telomeres become too short, the cell may become senescent (grow old) or may become malfunctional, for example, triggering inflammation or tumor development. Children who have been exposed to neglect show shortened telomeres (Asok et al., 2013; Drury et al., 2011). Drury and colleagues (2011) found shorter telomeres among children in institutional care. Similarly, Asok and colleagues (2013) found that children living in highly challenging environments showed shorter telomeres than comparison children, but that mothers could buffer children from the environment challenge. When mothers of neglected children were sensitive to challenging environments, their children's telomeres were as long as those of low-risk children, but when mothers were insensitive, children's telomeres were shorter. Clearly, then, sensitive caregiving serves as a protective factor even under difficult conditions of adversity.

There is as yet no compelling empirical evidence among humans that high levels of cortisol result from abuse or neglect and persist long enough to affect brain development adversely, leaving these arguments speculative. Nonetheless, the evidence is compelling that the HPA axis is perturbed in many cases, and perturbations are associated with a range of health and mental health problems (McEwen, 1998; Yehuda et al., 2002).

Studies (e.g., McGowan et al., 2008, 2009, 2011; Meaney and Szyf,

2005; Weaver et al., 2004) have found that the effects of abuse on the stress response are mediated by epigenetic programming of glucocorticoid receptor expression. Differential methylation of the glucocorticoid receptor gene promoter in the hippocampus was found to be associated with different rearing conditions in rodents, and was reversed by changes in caregiving conditions (McGowan et al., 2008). Paralleling these findings among rodents are nonexperimental findings among humans examined in postmortem analyses (McGowan et al., 2009; Szyf and Bick, 2013). Adult suicide victims who had experienced abuse as children differed in glucocorticoid receptor mRNA from adult suicide victims who had not experienced abuse as children and from controls. These findings are consistent with the experimental rodent findings, and suggest that methylation of receptor sites mediates the association between early care and stress responsiveness.

Amygdala

The amygdala performs a primary role in the formation and storage of memories associated with emotional events. The amygdala undergoes rapid development within the first several years of life and is particularly susceptible to early adversity (e.g., Chareyron et al., 2012). Relative to low-risk children, abused and neglected children show behavioral and emotional difficulties that are consistent with effects on the amygdala, such as internalizing problems, heightened anxiety, and emotional reactivity (Ellis et al., 2004; Kaplow and Widom, 2007; Tottenham et al., 2009; van Ijzendoorn and Juffer, 2006; Zeanah et al., 2009) and deficits in emotional processing (Dalgeish et al., 2001; Pollak et al., 2000; Vorria et al., 2006). Figure 4-2 illustrates structures in the medial temporal lobe critically involved in emotion (amygdala) and learning and memory (hippocampus).

Most studies have found no evidence that the structure of the amygdala is affected by abuse or neglect (De Bellis et al., 2001b; Tottenham and Sheridan, 2010; Woon and Hedges, 2008). However, Tottenham and colleagues (2010) and Mehta and colleagues (2009) found that amygdala volume was enlarged among children following institutionalized care, although this finding was not replicated by Sheridan and colleagues (2012) among a similar population. Importantly, both the Mehta et al. and Sheridan et al. studies did find a dramatic reduction in total brain volume, meaning that these children had physically smaller brains.

Functional magnetic resonance imaging (fMRI) studies have shown that early adversity leads to a sensitized amygdala. Relative to comparison children, previously institutionalized children showed heightened amygdala activity in response to fearful faces compared with neutral faces (Tottenham et al., 2011). Similarly, Maheu and colleagues (2010) found that children

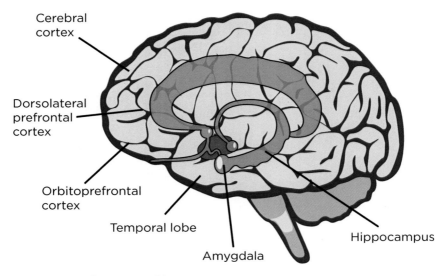

Cerebral cortex

Dorsolateral prefrontal cortex

Orbitoprefrontal cortex

Temporal lobe

Amygdala

Hippocampus

FIGURE 4-2 Illustration of brain structures.

with a history of abuse or neglect showed greater activation of the left amygdala in response to fearful and angry relative to neutral faces.

Hippocampus, Learning, and Memory

The hippocampus (see Figure 4-2) plays an important role in learning and memory (Andersen et al., 2007; Ghetti et al., 2010; Otto and Eichenbaum, 1992) and, like the amygdala, matures rapidly over the first months and years of life (Lavenex et al., 2007). The hippocampus appears to be particularly susceptible to stress early in life (Gould and Tanapat, 1999; Sapolsky et al., 1990) and plays a role in modulating the response of the HPA axis to stressors, as binding of cortisol to hippocampal receptors serves to turn off the HPA axis response (Kim and Yoon, 1998). Damage to the hippocampus due to abuse or neglect can have negative consequences for its roles in regulation of the stress response system and in memory formulation (de Quervain et al., 1998; Sheridan et al., 2012).

Most studies have found no evidence of hippocampal volume deficits among abused children compared with healthy, nonabused control children (De Bellis et al., 1999, 2001a, 2002). Among adults, however, decreased hippocampal volume has been linked with the experience of childhood physical and sexual abuse (Andersen and Teicher, 2004; Andersen et al., 2008; Schmahl et al., 2003; Woon and Hedges, 2008). Nonetheless, relatively smaller hippocampal volumes in abused adults may be specific to PTSD rather than abuse itself (Kitayama et al., 2005).

Prefrontal Cortex and Executive Functions

The prefrontal cortex (see Figure 4-2) is responsible for a variety of higher-order "executive" functions (Miller and Cohen, 2001). The development of the prefrontal cortex is protracted, extending from birth into the third decade of life (Gogtay et al., 2004; Rubia et al., 2006; Sowell et al., 2003). Prefrontal systems are especially sensitive to experiences of early adversity (Hart and Rubia, 2012; McLaughlin et al., 2010).

Evidence is mixed with regard to structural changes in the prefrontal cortex following abuse and neglect, with some studies showing smaller volumes of the right orbitofrontal cortex, right ventral-medial prefrontal cortex, and dorsolateral prefrontal cortex (Hanson et al., 2010); some showing decreased grey matter volume in the prefrontal cortex in children with interpersonal trauma and PTSD symptoms (Carrion et al., 2008); some showing the opposite effect (Carrion et al., 2009; Richert et al., 2006); and still others showing no effect after controlling for total brain volume (De Bellis et al., 2002). Despite mixed evidence regarding structural changes in the prefrontal cortex, a number of studies suggest that abuse and neglect are associated with functional changes in the prefrontal cortex and related brain regions. In particular, children with trauma experiences show patterns of neural activation during tasks requiring executive function that are similar to patterns observed in children with attention-deficit hyperactivity disorder (ADHD) (e.g., Carrion et al., 2008).

Consistent with these findings among abused and neglected children, previously institutionalized children and adolescents have been found to demonstrate disruptions in the prefrontal network that is associated with inhibitory control. For example, Mueller and colleagues (2010) found that children with a history of neglect or institutional care showed greater activation in several regions of the prefrontal cortex (e.g., left inferior frontal cortex, anterior cingulate cortex) during response inhibition trials of a go/no-go task compared with children without a history of neglect. Similar findings have been reported by McDermott and colleagues (2012) and Loman and colleagues (2009) among currently and previously institutionalized children.

Corpus Callosum

The corpus callosum facilitates communication between the two hemispheres of the brain (Giedd et al., 1996a,b; Kitterle, 1995). The white matter fibers composing the corpus callosum are myelinated throughout childhood and adulthood (Giedd et al., 1996a; Teicher et al., 2004), which allows faster, more efficient transmission (Bloom and Hynd, 2005). Myelinated regions such as the corpus callosum are susceptible to the impacts of early exposure to high levels of cortisol, which suppress the glial cell division critical for myelination.

Retrospective/cross-sectional studies have found abuse and neglect to be associated with structural changes in the corpus callosum. Teicher and colleagues (2004) compared corpus callosum volume in adults with different abuse and neglect experiences. The total corpus callosum area of the abused children was smaller than that of both healthy control children and children with psychiatric disorders and no abuse or neglect. Other findings suggest that gender may moderate these effects, with the effects being more pronounced among males than females (De Bellis and Keshavan, 2003; De Bellis et al., 1999, 2002; Teicher et al., 1997). Sheridan and colleagues (2012) performed structural MRIs on children enrolled in the Bucharest Early Intervention Project, described previously in this chapter. In a follow-up of 8- to 11-year-olds, Sheridan and colleagues (2012) found smaller total white and gray matter volume and smaller posterior corpus callosum volume among children who had been institutionalized relative to those who had never been institutionalized. By middle childhood, however, there were no significant differences in total white matter volume or posterior corpus callosum volume between the never-institutionalized (community) children and the foster care children. These early differences in corpus callosum may be associated with less efficient cognitive functioning among children who experience early adversity.

Influence of Early Profound Neglect on Brain Electrical Activity

The influence of profound neglect early in life has been examined using electroencephalography (EEG) and event-related potentials (ERPs).

Electroencephalography

EEG measurements of the brain's electrical activity can serve as a coarse metric for brain development. Most work on EEG in the context of neglect has been performed on children with a history of institutional care. The most extensive study of brain electrical activity among children with a history of institutional care was conducted with the children enrolled in the prospective, longitudinal Bucharest Early Intervention Project. At baseline (mean age 20 months), prior to random assignment to continued institutional care or foster care, institutionalized children showed higher levels of theta power (low-frequency brain activity) and lower levels of alpha and beta power (high-frequency activity) compared with children who were not institutionalized (Marshall et al., 2004). The pattern of activity observed in institutionalized children suggests a maturational delay or deficit in cortical development associated with an extreme form of neglect (Marshall et al., 2004). The profiles are similar to patterns found among children with ADHD (Barry et al., 2003; Harmony et al., 1990).

At follow-up, as a group, children assigned to foster care did not differ from the care-as-usual group (Marshall et al., 2008). However, the subset of children placed in foster care before 2 years of age showed EEG activity that more closely resembled that of the never-institutionalized group than the care-as-usual group. Overall, then, "institutionalization led to dramatic reductions in brain activity (as reflected in the EEG), whereas placement in foster care before 2 years of age led to a more normal pattern of EEG activity" (Nelson et al., 2011, p. 139). This last finding was replicated when the children were 8 years old (Vanderwert et al., 2010). Specifically, previously institutionalized children placed in foster care before about 2 years of age had patterns of brain activity that resembled those of never-institutionalized children, whereas children placed in foster care after 2 years of age had patterns of brain activity that resembled those of children randomly assigned to institutional care.

Event-Related Potentials

ERPs measure changes in the brain's electrical activity in response to an internal or external stimulus or event. The components of the ERP (i.e., positive and negative deflections) can be quantified in terms of latency, amplitude, and location/distribution on the scalp. The P300 (i.e., positive deflection occurring approximately 300 ms after a stimulus) is associated with attention to emotionally evocative visual stimuli, such as emotional faces (Eimer and Holmes, 2007; Olofsson et al., 2008). Whereas nonabused children show similar P300 activity across emotional expressions, abused children show larger P300s to angry target faces (Pollak et al., 1997, 2001), a finding consistent with behavioral evidence of enhanced attention to angry faces among abused children.

Finding: Across human and nonhuman primate studies, perturbations to the HPA system often are seen to be associated with child abuse and neglect. The findings are complex, moderated by a number of factors and seen at some ages and not others. Further, the perturbations sometimes are reflected in atypically high production of cortisol across either basal or reactive contexts and sometimes in atypically low production. Recent work in epigenetics suggests that this may well be an area of future inquiry into the mechanisms whereby abuse or neglect alters gene expression and, in turn, behavior.

Finding: Abused and neglected children show behavioral and emotional difficulties that are consistent with effects on the amygdala, such as internalizing problems, heightened anxiety and emotional reactivity, and deficits in emotional processing. Most studies have found no evidence that the structure of the amygdala is affected by abuse or neglect; however, fMRI studies have shown that early adversity leads to a sensitized amygdala.

Finding: Despite mixed evidence regarding structural changes in the prefrontal cortex, a number of studies suggest that abuse and neglect are associated with functional changes in the prefrontal cortex and associated brain regions, often affecting inhibitory control.

Finding: Examination of patterns of brain electrical activity in institutionalized children suggests that extreme forms of neglect are associated with a maturational delay or deficit in cortical development.

COGNITIVE, PSYCHOSOCIAL, AND BEHAVIORAL OUTCOMES

Cognitive Development

There is a long history of research exploring the effects of child abuse and neglect on cognitive development. Studies have examined executive functioning and attention, as well as academic achievement.

Executive Functioning and Attention

As discussed earlier, some studies have found that child abuse and neglect have effects on the prefrontal cortex, a brain structure centrally involved in executive functioning. Executive functioning refers to higher-order cognitive processes that aid in the monitoring and control of emotions and behavior (Lewis-Morrarty et al., 2012). Included among executive functions are "holding information in working memory, inhibiting impulses, planning, sustaining attention amid distraction, and flexibly shifting attention to achieve goals" (Lewis-Morrarty et al., 2012, p. 2). Executive functioning abilities develop rapidly between the ages of 3 and 6 years, but continue to develop through at least the second decade of life.

Children who experience abuse and neglect appear to be especially at risk for deficits in executive functioning, which have implications for behavioral regulation. Extreme neglect, as seen in institutional care, has been related to executive functioning in a number of studies conducted by the Bucharest Early Intervention Project team (McDermott et al., 2012). For example, McDermott and colleagues (2012) found that children who were randomly assigned to foster care showed better performance on an executive functioning task (i.e., a go/no-go task requiring inhibitory control) than children who were randomly assigned to treatment as usual. The assessments of executive functioning were conducted when children were 8 years old. Similar findings among comparably aged internationally adopted children (with histories of institutionalization) have been reported (e.g., Loman et al., 2013). These findings suggest that extreme forms of neglect may interfere with the development of executive functioning.

Problems in regulating attention represent one of the most striking deficits seen among children who have experienced severe early deprivation in institutional settings (Gunnar et al., 2007; Kreppner et al., 2001). Gunnar and colleagues (2007) found that problems with inattention or overactivity were more pronounced among children who had experienced early institutional care than among those who had been adopted internationally without early institutional care. Kreppner and colleagues (2007) found that many children who had been adopted following institutional care showed problems with inattention or overactivity, but that such problems were usually seen in combination with reactive attachment disorder, quasi-autistic behaviors, or severe cognitive impairment.

Using NSCAW data, Heneghan and colleagues (2013) examined mental health problems in teens older than age 12 who were the subject of a child welfare agency investigation. They found that 18.6 percent of abused and neglected teens scored positively for ADHD, compared with 5 percent of children and 2.5 percent of adults in the general U.S. population (APA, 2013c). Likewise, Briscoe-Smith and Hinshaw (2006) studied a sample of 228 girls with and without ADHD and with and without a history of abuse and neglect, finding that the girls with ADHD had a statistically significant heightened risk of having a documented history of abuse or neglect, as indicated by substantiated child protective services, parental, or school report. Some studies have found preliminary differences in the characteristics of ADHD displayed by children with and without a history of abuse or neglect (Webb, 2013). For example, Becker-Blease and Freyd (2008) studied a small community sample of 8- to 11-year-old children in which ADHD and abuse history were assessed by parent report. They found that children with a history of abuse displayed more severe impulsivity and inattention than nonabused children with ADHD, but the groups did not differ on measures of hyperactivity (Becker-Blease and Freyd, 2008).

A number of studies have found evidence that children who experience abuse and neglect show deficits in executive functioning and attention (Arseneault et al., 2011; De Bellis et al., 2009; Fisher et al., 2011; Lewis et al., 2007; Spann et al., 2012). Pears and colleagues (2008) found that abuse and neglect were associated with generally lower cognitive functioning among preschoolers. Lewis and colleagues (2007) found that 4-year-old children who had experienced abuse or neglect and were in foster care showed poorer inhibitory control on a Stroop-like task relative to comparison children, despite similar levels of performance on a control task. Spann and colleagues (2012) found that physical abuse and neglect were associated with diminished cognitive flexibility on the Wisconsin Card Sorting Task among adolescents.

Academic Achievement

Abuse and neglect increase children's risk for experiencing academic problems. Several studies suggest that abuse versus neglect matters, with neglect being especially predictive of academic underachievement (Briere et al., 1996; Jonson-Reid et al., 2004; Nikulina et al., 2011). Other studies failed to find differences between abuse and neglect, with both predicting achievement problems (e.g., Barnett et al., 1996; Crozier and Barth, 2005; Eckenrode et al., 1993; Jaffee and Gallop, 2007; Kurtz et al., 1993; Leiter and Johnsen, 1997). On balance, the evidence suggests that both abuse and neglect are predictive of academic problems. Perez and Widom (1994) found that child abuse and neglect had a significant impact on reading ability, IQ scores, and academic achievement. For example, 42 percent of abused and neglected children completed high school, compared with two-thirds of the matched comparison group without histories of abuse and neglect. The average IQ score for the abused and neglected children was about one standard deviation below the average for the control group; this association was significant after controlling for age, race, gender, and social class (Perez and Widom, 1994). Using NSCAW data, Jaffee and Maikovich-Fong (2011) found that chronically abused or neglected children had lower IQ scores than situationally abused or neglected children. The effect of chronic abuse or neglect on IQ scores remained significant after controlling for the effects of caregiver educational level on IQ. Leiter and Johnsen (1997) found that effects of abuse and neglect on school performance were cumulative, with more episodes of abuse and neglect being associated with poorer outcomes. Abuse and neglect predicted entry into special education after controlling for early medical conditions (Jonson-Reid et al., 2004). Jonson-Reid and colleagues (2004) found that 24 percent of the abused and neglected children entered special education, compared with 14 percent of those with no record of abuse or neglect. Further, every additional report of abuse or neglect before the age of 8 led to an increase of 7 percent in entry into special education. Thompson and colleagues (2012) found that expectations of future academic success were adversely affected by previous experiences of abuse and neglect, with these expectations having powerful self-fulfilling possibilities (Ross and Hill, 2002).

Psychosocial and Behavioral Outcomes

Given that child abuse and neglect are social experiences that undermine the ability to trust in caregivers, either because caregivers are frightening (as in cases of abuse) or because they fail to protect or provide care (as in cases of neglect), it makes sense that children who experience abuse and neglect are at risk for interpersonal problems. At the most proximal level, problems are seen in children's ability to form trusting attachments to their parents. But not surprisingly, the effects also are seen in such areas as children's processing of emotion (e.g., overly vigilant of angry faces), their attributions of others' intent (e.g., assuming that intentions are malevolent when they are ambiguous), and difficulties with peers (e.g., being the victim or perpetrator of bullying or violence). Problems also are seen in internalizing symptoms, such as anxiety and depression, and externalizing symptoms, such as conduct disorder and substance use.

Attachment

Children develop secure attachments to parents who are responsive to them when they are distressed (Ainsworth, 1978). Children typically develop insecure (avoidant or resistant) attachments when parents are unresponsive or inconsistent in responsiveness, but not frightening or bizarre (e.g., Lyons-Ruth et al., 1993; Schuengel et al., 1998). Secure, avoidant, and resistant attachments are referred to as *organized* attachment strategies because they are organized around the caregiver's availability and provide a child a template for dealing with distress. On the other hand, *disorganized* attachment represents a breakdown in or a lack of strategy for dealing with distress when in the parent's presence (Main and Solomon, 1990). Disorganized attachments are the most problematic in terms of outcomes for children. Relative to organized attachment, disorganized attachment is most predictive of long-term problems, especially externalizing symptoms (Fearon et al., 2010). Fearon and colleagues (2010) found strong evidence for a link between disorganized attachment and later externalizing symptoms through a meta-analysis of 34 studies involving 3,778 participants.

Child abuse and neglect are predictive of disorganized attachment, as well as insecure attachment more generally. A meta-analysis conducted by Cyr and colleagues (2010) included the 10 studies that have examined attachment quality with samples of children who have experienced abuse and neglect. The effect size was large for both disorganized and insecure attachment. Although abuse was more strongly related to disorganized attachment and neglect to insecure attachment, both abuse and neglect were associated with both types of attachment. These results are consistent with theory and with other empirical findings suggesting that when parents are either frightening or unavailable, children fail to develop a secure attachment to them. Nonetheless, the effects of having more than five socioeconomic risk factors were comparable to those of child abuse and neglect, indicating that multiple challenges to parental functioning had significant effects on attachment regardless of whether these effects were seen in child abuse and neglect.

In early childhood, abused or neglected children may develop attachment disorders resulting from and following pathogenic care that inhibits a young child's ability to form selective attachments (Hornor, 2008). Childhood attachment disorders are phenomena distinct from insecure, disorganized, or nonexistent attachment types; they have been redefined in the *Diagnostic and Statistical Manual of Mental Disorders*, fifth edition (DSM-V) to include two distinct disorders: reactive attachment disorder and disinhibited social engagement disorder (APA, 2013a,b). Reactive attachment disorder involves inhibited or emotionally withdrawn behavior, including rarely seeking and responding to comforting; it results from a lack of or incompletely formed selective attachments to adult caregivers (APA, 2013a). Disinhibited social engagement disorder is marked by a pattern of overly familiar behavior with strangers; it may occur even in children with established or secure attachments. Previously, each attachment disorder was considered the inhibited or disinhibited type of reactive attachment disorder, respectively.

Zeanah and colleagues (2004) studied the prevalence of attachment disorders among 94 toddlers in foster care whose abuse or neglect cases had been substantiated and who were enrolled in an intervention program; they found that the prevalence of attachment disorders reached 38-40 percent. Lyons-Ruth and colleagues (2009) examined socially indiscriminate attachment behavior in a sample of mother-child dyads that included pairs referred to a clinical service because of problematic caregiving and comparison pairs matched on socioeconomic status. They found that 18-month-olds displayed socially indiscriminate attachment behavior only if they had a history of abuse or neglect, or their mother had a history of psychiatric hospitalizations. Both disorders also have been identified in children exposed to neglectful institutional care in Romania who were later adopted into middle-class families in the United Kingdom (Smyke et al., 2002; Zeanah et al., 2002), although the disinhibited type of reactive attachment disorder (as defined in DSM-IV) has been found to be much more prevalent than the inhibited type (O'Connor et al., 2003). Furthermore, findings from the Bucharest Early Intervention Project study indicate that the inhibited type of reactive attachment disorder declined significantly once institutionalized children were placed in foster care, but the disinhibited type proved more persistent (Smyke et al., 2002; Zeanah and Gleason, 2010).

Emotion Regulation

Infants have limited capacities to regulate their own emotions and are dependent on caregivers to help them deal effectively with distress (Tronick, 1989). Indeed, infants and young children are highly attuned and responsive to their parents' emotions and use parental emotional signals to guide their behavior (Klinnert et al., 1983; Malatesta and Izard, 1984). The scaffolding important for the development of emotion regulation is challenged in abusing or neglecting families. When children feel upset or distressed, parents' availability and soothing presence can help them feel that they can cope with the strong negative affect, such that they are able to develop autonomous and effective means of regulating emotions over time. When children regulate their emotions well, they react to challenge with flexible and socially acceptable responses (Cole et al., 1994; Kim and Cicchetti, 2010). Abused and neglected children, however, may not have such scaffolding experiences. It is likely that abused and neglected children experience not only a lack of modeling and support and an absence of positive affect but also harsh, inconsistent, and insensitive parenting (Shipman and Zeman, 2001). In the case of abuse, parents often respond in threatening or unpredictable ways to children's distress (Milner, 2000). In the case of neglect, parents may be unresponsive or nonempathic. As a result of either response, children are at risk of failing to develop effective strategies for regulating emotions (Cicchetti et al., 1995; Kim and Cicchetti, 2010; Rogosch et al., 1995).

An initial, key task in regulating emotions is processing of cues. Studies have examined differences among children who have experienced abuse and neglect in how readily they identify angry, sad, and happy faces (Pollak and Sinha, 2002; Pollak and Tolley-Schell, 2003; Pollak et al., 2000; Shackman et al., 2007). Pollak and Sinha (2002) found that the threshold for detecting anger in the face was lower among abused than nonabused children; there were no differences in processing happy faces. Thus, these children appear to have a bias toward angry faces rather than a general deficit in processing faces. Pollak and Sinha (2002) point out that it is useful to identify emotions in others based on less than full information. Abused children's bias toward attributing angry or sad affect may be adaptive when living with parents whose anger may be an important threat cue (Belsky et al., 2012); nonetheless, it comes at the cost of assuming hostile intent too readily under benign conditions, leading to aggressive responses that would not have been evoked had attributions been different (Dodge et al., 1995). Neglected children, on the other hand, generally are not as good as nonneglected children at identifying facial expressions, showing a general deficit (Pollak et al., 2000).

Emotion regulation can be seen as key to a number of the constructs considered in this chapter. Problems in regulating emotion are associated with externalizing behaviors, such as aggression and behavior problems (Eisenberg et al., 2001; Kim and Cicchetti, 2010); internalizing behaviors, such as depression (Cole et al., 2008; Maughan and Cicchetti, 2002); and challenges in peer relations (Kim and Cicchetti, 2010; Rogosch et al., 1995). Emotion regulation can be seen, then, to have effects both on children's own affect and on their behavioral reactions, which then have implications for their relationships with others.

Peer Relations

Children's relationships with their peers are critical to their sense of well-being. Abused and neglected children have problematic peer relations at disproportionately high rates (Kim and Cicchetti, 2010), as do children with a history of institutional care (Almas et al., 2012). Chronicity of child abuse and neglect predict peer relations, as reported by teachers, at age 8 (Graham et al., 2010). Problematic emotion regulation (Shields and Cicchetti, 2001) and higher levels of aggression and withdrawal (Rogosch et al., 1995) found in abused and neglected children can become apparent to peers when frustrations and challenges arise in school and playground environments.

Externalizing Problems

Externalizing behavior refers to problem behaviors that are manifested externally (rather than internally, as in the case of depression and anxiety). Findings from several studies indicate that children who have experienced abuse and neglect are at greater risk for a number of externalizing behaviors, including conduct disorders, aggression, and delinquency (Lansford et al., 2002, 2009; Lynch and Cicchetti, 1998; Stouthamer-Loeber et al., 2001; Thornberry et al., 2010).

Oppositional defiant disorder and conduct disorder Studies have reported significant associations between a history of childhood abuse or neglect and various conduct problems, including those classified as oppositional defiant disorder or conduct disorder. Oppositional defiant disorder is indicated by a frequent or persistent pattern of angry or irritable mood, argumentative or defiant behavior, and vindictiveness (APA, 2013a). Its symptoms usually first appear during early childhood, and it often precedes conduct disorder, anxiety disorders, or major depressive disorder. Conduct disorder is indicated by a repetitive or persistent pattern of behavior that violates the basic rights of others or major societal norms or rules, including aggression toward people or animals, destruction of property, deceitfulness or theft, and serious violations of rules (APA, 2013a). Conduct disorder can begin in childhood or adolescence; however, childhood-onset conduct disorder is more often preceded by oppositional defiant disorder, more persistent into adulthood, and more likely to include aggressive behavior than adolescence-onset conduct disorder. Both disorders also frequently co-occur with ADHD.

In a study using a community sample, Dodge and colleagues (1995) found that children who were physically abused before age 5 were 4 times more likely than nonabused children to display externalizing conduct problems in grade 3 and 4. Likewise, Kaplan and colleagues (1998) found that adolescents (aged 12-18) with substantiated cases of physical abuse were more likely to display conduct disorder or oppositional defiant disorder at the time of the study (odds ratio = 5.98) than the matched nonabused comparison group. Fergusson and colleagues (2008) found that childhood sexual abuse was associated with higher rates of conduct disorder in young adulthood. Furthermore, they found that childhood physical abuse was not associated with conduct disorder when sexual abuse was included in the model. Additional environmental and individual factors that interact with abuse or neglect to increase the likelihood of conduct disorder or oppositional defiant disorder include exposure to parental divorce (Afifi et al., 2009), interparental violence (Boden et al., 2010), and community violence (McCabe et al., 2005), as well as gender, with males more likely to display conduct disorder (Boden et al., 2010).

Aggression Manly and colleagues (2001) found that children who had experienced severe emotional abuse only as infants or severe physical abuse only as toddlers were more aggressive and showed more externalizing symptoms as school-aged children than children without a history of abuse or neglect. The severity of abuse experienced predicted aggressiveness and externalizing symptoms in middle childhood. Although abuse experienced only in early childhood had lasting effects, abuse experienced beyond early childhood also had effects on aggression and externalizing symptoms, and the most problematic effects were seen for children subjected to chronic, severe abuse (Manly et al., 2001). Rogosch and colleagues (1995) found that physically abused children showed both aggressive behaviors and social withdrawal during peer interactions. Along these lines, abused and neglected children were disproportionately likely to be both bullies and victims of aggression, effects that were mediated by emotion dysregulation (Shields and Cicchetti, 2001). At odds with these findings, Kotch and colleagues (2008) found that children who experienced neglect in their first 2 years of life showed more aggression toward peers at ages 4, 6, and 8 relative to children without a history of abuse or neglect. Indeed, in that study, other subgroups (children who were abused or who were neglected at older ages) did not show an increased likelihood of aggression.

Hostile attributional bias refers to the tendency to assume that someone intended harm when circumstances were ambiguous but a negative outcome was experienced. For example, if a peer spilled milk on a child, the child could assume that the action was benign (unintentional) or intentional, with the latter representing a hostile attributional bias. When children assume that such an action was intentional, they are likely to act aggressively in response (Dodge et al., 1995). Physically abused children are more likely than other children to show such attributional biases (Dodge et al., 1995). Price and Glad (2003) found that these effects were seen in boys only and were associated with frequency of abuse. Such biases can lead to a self-fulfilling prophecy whereby children anticipate that someone intends them harm and react in a hostile way, which then elicits a hostile response (Dodge et al., 1995).

Internalizing Problems

Internalizing problems—problems that are manifested internally—include symptoms of depression and anxiety. Child abuse and neglect have been found to put children at increased risk of internalizing symptoms from early childhood through adolescence and adulthood (Dubowitz et al., 2002; Thornberry et al., 2001; Widom et al., 2007a).

Dubowitz and colleagues (2002) found that neglect was associated with internalizing problems for 3- and 5-year-old children. Swanston and colleagues (1997) found that sexually abused children had a significantly higher average score on depression measures than a control group just 5 years after the abuse occurred, after adjusting for individual differences in age and sex, as well as contextual factors such as socioeconomic status, family functioning, mother's mental health, and number of negative life events. Trickett and colleagues (2001) found that a sample of sexually abused girls had significantly higher rates of self-reported depression than a comparison group of nonabused females. At follow-up, approximately 7 years later, rates of depression were found to be significantly higher among the sexually abused group, excluding a subset whose experience of abuse was characterized chiefly by multiple perpetrators and a relatively short duration.

The heightened risk of depression extends beyond childhood to adolescence and adulthood. Multiple studies have found clear links between child abuse and neglect and depression in adolescence (e.g., Fergusson et al., 2008; Heneghan et al., 2013; Lansford et al., 2002). Brown and colleagues (1999) found that child abuse and neglect were associated with a nearly threefold increase in the rate of depression in adolescence, although this risk was diminished after controlling for other adverse conditions. Gilbert and colleagues (2009b) cite a body of studies reporting adjusted odds ratios ranging from 1.3 to 2.4 for depression after childhood among those subjected to abuse and neglect as children. Among adults, Brown and colleagues (1999) found that the increased risk of depression associated with child abuse and neglect remained when other factors were covaried, consistent with findings that more than one-third of abused or neglected children show symptoms of major depressive disorder by their late 20s (Gilbert et al., 2009b). Likewise, Widom and colleagues (2007a) followed a group of individuals who had experienced abuse and/or neglect in childhood and a matched comparison group into young adulthood and found that experiencing childhood physical abuse and multiple types of abuse increased the lifetime risk for a diagnosis of major depressive disorder.

A growing body of research examines whether different types and combinations of abuse or neglect in childhood result in different levels of risk for the development of depressive symptoms. The results in this domain are mixed, with strong evidence that sexual and physical abuse in childhood are associated with depression later in life (e.g., Heneghan et al., 2013), but mixed evidence that neglect increases risk for depression independent of contextual factors. Many studies have found child sexual abuse to have large and independent effects on risk for depression later in life. For example, Fergusson and colleagues (2008) found that young adults who reported a history of childhood sexual abuse had mental health disorders, including depression, at a rate 2.4 times higher than that among those not exposed to such abuse. By contrast, Widom and colleagues (2007a) found that child sexual abuse was not associated with an elevated risk of major depressive disorder relative to matched controls, although physical abuse or multiple kinds of abuse did increase the risk for lifetime major depressive disorder. Additional studies have found that physical abuse increased the risk for adult depression (e.g., Brown et al., 1999). Some studies have found that neglect did not increase the risk for depression when statistical models included contextual factors (Nikulina et al., 2011), although Widom and colleagues (2007a) found that neglect increased risk for current major depressive disorder relative to matched controls in adulthood.

As discussed in the section on individual differences later in this chapter, researchers also have examined how the timing (Dunn et al., 2013; Thornberry et al., 2001) and severity (Fergusson et al., 2008) of abuse and neglect affect the risk of developing depression. Other factors throughout the life course, such as the presence or absence of social support (Sperry and Widom, 2013) and exposure to multiple traumas (Banyard et al., 2001) or stressful life events in adulthood (Power et al., 2013), have been found to interact with childhood experiences of abuse and neglect to influence the risk of developing depression later in life.

Dissociation

Dissociation is defined as a "disruption of and/or discontinuity in the normal, subjective integration of one or more aspects of psychological functioning, including—but not limited to—memory, identity, consciousness, perception, and motor control" (Spiegel et al., 2011, p. 19). Dissociation can be measured reliably and validly in children, adolescents, and adults (Briere et al., 2001; Keck Seeley et al., 2004; Lanktree et al., 2008; van Ijzendoorn and Schuengel, 1996; Wherry et al., 2009).

Child abuse and neglect have been associated with dissociation among both preschool-aged and elementary-aged children (Hulette et al., 2008, 2011; Macfie et al., 2001), as well as among adults (van Ikzendoorn and Schuengel, 1996). The existence of a subgroup of PTSD patients with high levels of dissociation has been demonstrated in clinical (Lanius et al., 2013; Putnam, 1997), psychophysiological (Griffin et al., 1997), neuroimaging (Lanius et al., 2013), and epidemiological (Stein et al., 2013) research. As a result, DSM-V is adding a dissociative subtype to the PTSD diagnosis (Spiegel et al., 2011a) (see the discussion of PTSD on p. 139).

High scores on dissociation measures have proven to be a predictor of externalizing behavior in children (Kisiel and Lyons, 2001; Shapiro et al., 2012; Yates et al., 2008). In adults, high levels of dissociation are associated with refractoriness to standard treatments for a number of psychiatric conditions, as well as increased comorbidity (Jans et al., 2008; Kleindienst et al., 2011; Wolf et al., 2012; Zanarini et al., 2011).

A meta-analysis of 55 studies (Cyr et al., 2010) links abuse with disorganized attachment. Grienenberger and colleagues (2005) found that mothers who engaged in disrupted affective communication with their infants at 4 months (as measured using the AMBIANCE scale) were more likely to have toddlers who were classified as disorganized at 14 months. In turn, disorganized attachment at 14 months predicted high dissociation scores at age 20 years (Lyons-Ruth, 2008). Disorganized attachment assessed during the child's second year predicted elevated levels of self-reported dissociation in mid-adolescence (age 16 years) (Carlson, 1998) and early adulthood (age 19) (Ogawa et al., 1997).

Based on findings from the Minnesota Mother-Child Project, Egeland and Susman-Stillman (1996) propose that dissociation may act as a mediator of child abuse across generations. In a longitudinal study of sexually abused girls followed into parenthood, Kim and colleagues (2010) found that increased dissociation, together with a history of self-reported punitive parenting as a child, predicted whether a mother would parent her own children in a harsh and punitive manner. Thus, a tentative generational loop can be hypothesized in which harsh and abusive parenting increases the risk for higher levels of dissociation in childhood and adolescence, which in turn increases the risk for impulsive behavior and harsh parenting of offspring. Further research, especially with a longitudinal design, is warranted to determine whether this hypothesized generational pattern of transmission represents an early opportunity for prevention of abuse in the next generation.

Posttraumatic Stress Disorder

In DSM-V, PTSD is classified as a trauma- and stressor-related disorder, a change from its previous classification as an anxiety disorder. PTSD develops following "exposure to actual or threatened death, serious injury, or sexual violation," including directly experiencing the traumatic event, witnessing the event firsthand, learning that an actual or threatened violent or accidental death occurred to a family member or close friend, and experiencing repeated or extreme firsthand exposure to the details of the traumatic event (APA, 2013c). Behavioral symptoms of PTSD are divided into four categories: intrusion or reexperiencing, avoidance, negative alterations in cognition and mood, and alterations in arousal and reactivity (National Center for PTSD, 2013). Experiences of child abuse and neglect involve traumatic events that are often violent, invasive, and coercive (Kearney et al., 2010). Furthermore, secondary trauma may result from experiences of child abuse and neglect, including separation from family or homelessness, which may also trigger a PTSD response (Wechsler-Zimring et al., 2012).

A number of prospective and retrospective studies have found elevated rates of PTSD among individuals with a history of abuse and neglect (Chen et al., 2010; Kearney et al., 2010; Tolin and Foa, 2006; Weich et al., 2009; Widom, 1999). Numerous studies have found that PTSD was preceded by abuse and neglect; links with sexual abuse were especially strong (Chen et al., 2010; Gregg and Parks, 1995; Kendall-Tackett et al., 1993; Tolin and Foa, 2006; Weich et al., 2009; Widom, 1999). Kearney and colleagues (2010) report PTSD rates of 20-50 percent among youth who had been sexually abused, 50 percent among youth who had been physically abused, and 33-50 percent among youth who had experienced neglect combined with exposure to domestic violence. Kolko (2010) found that nearly 20 percent of youth in out-of-home care showed posttraumatic symptoms. Widom (1999) found increased risk for PTSD among adults who had experienced abuse and neglect as children, with 23 percent of those who had been sexually abused, 19 percent of those who had been physically abused, and 17 percent of those who had been neglected meeting criteria for PTSD at age 29, compared with 10 percent of the comparison group.

Some evidence indicates that PTSD may mediate the association between childhood abuse and neglect and later adverse outcomes. Wolfe and colleagues (2004) found that boys who had been abused or neglected in childhood and displayed a greater number of PTSD symptoms were at higher risk of perpetrating emotional abuse in a dating relationship compared with abused or neglected boys who displayed fewer trauma symptoms. Weierich and Nock (2008) found that the specific PTSD symptoms of reexperiencing, avoidance, and numbing mediated the relationship between childhood experiences of abuse and neglect and nonsuicidal self-injury. In a study of adult women survivors of childhood sexual abuse, Ginzburg and colleagues (2006) found that severe childhood maltreatment, including sexual abuse as well as other types of abuse or neglect, was significantly associated with experiencing high levels of dissociation in conjunction with PTSD, while less severe childhood maltreatment was not significantly associated with the dissociative subtype. Avery and colleagues (2000) examined PTSD and key areas of functioning based on interviews with sexually abused children and their nonoffending parents. Compared with sexually abused girls with low scores on the Child Posttraumatic Stress Reaction Index, sexually abused girls with higher scores expressed more worries; reported increased problems with sleep, appetite, headaches, and stomachaches; reported increased depression and suicidal ideation; displayed more problems in school functioning; and had higher levels of family disruption.

Personality Disorders

Evidence links child abuse and neglect with personality disorders. Johnson and colleagues (1999) found that adults with a history of abuse and neglect (as indicated by records and/or self-report) had a fourfold increase in personality disorders relative to those without a history of abuse or neglect. Physical abuse was associated with elevated antisocial and depressive personality disorder symptoms; sexual abuse was associated with elevated borderline personality disorder symptoms; and neglect was associated with elevated symptoms of antisocial, avoidant, borderline, narcissistic, and passive-aggressive personality disorders, as well as with attachment difficulties and other interpersonal and psychological problems. Widom (1998) reports an increase in risk for antisocial personality disorder for both males and females with a history of abuse and neglect. In a subsequent study, Widom and colleagues (2009) report an increase in risk for borderline personality disorder in males only, suggesting that there may be sex differences in the consequences of abuse and neglect. Natsuaki and colleagues (2009) found that personality problems, although not diagnosed personality disorders, worsened as adolescence progressed.

Finding: Abuse and neglect have profound effects on selected aspects of children's cognitive development. Although many attempts have been made to disentangle the effects of abuse and neglect, the balance of findings suggests that severe neglect may interfere with the development of executive functioning, and both neglect and abuse increase the risk for attention regulation problems and ADHD, lower IQ, and poorer school performance.

Finding: As a result of abusive or neglectful responses from caregivers, children have a difficult time developing organized and secure attachments. As a result, abused and neglected children are at higher risk for the development of attachment disorders, particularly disinhibited social engagement disorder.

Finding: Abused and neglected children often fail to develop effective strategies for emotion regulation, partly as a result of differences in processing of emotional cues. Difficulties with emotion regulation can lead to further problems, including externalizing and internalizing problems and challenges in peer relations.

Finding: Children who experience abuse or neglect have been found to be at higher risk for the development of externalizing behavior problems, including oppositional defiant disorder, conduct disorder, and aggressive behaviors. Abused and neglected children also have been found to be at increased risk for internalizing problems, particularly depression, in childhood, adolescence, and adulthood.

Finding: Among preschool- and elementary school–aged children, as well as adults, a history of childhood abuse and neglect has been associated with dissociation, which increases the risk for externalizing behavior in childhood and resistance to treatment for psychiatric conditions later in life. It has been suggested that dissociation may act as a mediator of harsh or abusive parenting across generations, although this hypothesis requires further research.

Finding: A number of studies have found elevated rates of PTSD among individuals with a history of abuse and neglect. PTSD has been associated with physical, cognitive, psychological, social, and behavioral problems among youth who were abused or neglected in childhood.

HEALTH OUTCOMES

Child abuse and neglect have effects on a number of health outcomes, from growth to illness to obesity. Connections have been found between problematic neurobiological outcomes of child abuse and neglect and health. One plausible mechanism for these effects relates to the purported frequent or chronic activation of the HPA axis. As discussed previously, the HPA axis is designed for responding in crises.

Growth and Motor Development

In their most extreme forms, abuse and neglect are associated with stunted growth. Children living in institutional environments (Johnson et al., 2010) or adopted from highly neglecting institutional environments (Johnson and Gunnar, 2011) sometimes show very delayed growth in height and head circumference. Olivan (2003) found that children placed in foster care between ages 24 and 48 months were significantly below normal for height, weight, and head circumference. Similarly, Chernoff and colleagues (1994) found that most children entering foster care had an abnormal physical screen involving at least one body system, and on average weighed less and were shorter than comparison children.

Gross motor development often is delayed among children with a history of institutional care who have then been adopted internationally (Dobrova-Krol et al., 2008; Roeber et al., 2012). Roeber and colleagues (2012) found that children adopted from institutional settings showed motor system delays, with greater balance delays being predicted by length of time institutionalized and bilateral coordination delays being predicted by severity of deprivation. Rapid gains are seen after placement in adoptive homes, however (Pomerleau et al., 2005). Although somewhat canalized (less responsive to genetic or environmental variations), the development of these gross motor abilities is dependent upon opportunities to engage in motor activities. Note that these findings regarding motor delays may be limited in their application to extreme cases of neglect in which young children are left alone in their cribs or otherwise neglected for extended periods of time.

Illness

Child abuse and neglect have been linked to various forms of physical illness as well as various indicators of physical health problems. Adolescents with a history of childhood abuse or neglect report a lower rating of their own health compared with low-risk peers (Bonomi et al., 2008; Hussey et al., 2006). Likewise, more gastrointestinal symptoms were reported by adults who reported having been abused or neglected as children (Walker et al., 1999). To examine whether this association resulted from shared method variance, van Tilburg and colleagues (2010) used data collected from multiple informants among a sample of 845 children enrolled in the longitudinal, prospective Longitudinal Studies of Child Abuse and Neglect.

Across informants, youth who had experienced abuse or neglect had an increased likelihood of gastrointestinal symptoms, which often followed or coincided with sexual abuse.

In a longitudinal prospective study, childhood abuse and neglect predicted health indices among middle-aged adults (Widom et al., 2012). Both physical abuse and neglect predicted hemoglobin A1C (a biomarker for diabetes) and albumin (a biomarker for liver and kidney function); physical abuse uniquely predicted malnutrition and blood urea nitrogen (a marker for kidney function); neglect uniquely predicted poor peak airflow; and sexual abuse uniquely predicted hepatitis C (Widom et al., 2012).

Findings from the Adverse Childhood Experiences study indicate a heightened risk for liver disease, lung cancer, and ischemic heart disease among adults who report multiple adverse experiences in childhood (Brown et al., 2010; Dong et al., 2003, 2004). The adverse experiences measured in the study include emotional abuse, physical abuse, sexual abuse, emotional neglect, and physical neglect, as well as indicators of household dysfunction, such as domestic violence, parental divorce or separation, household member mental illness, household member substance abuse, and household member incarceration. Dong and colleagues (2003) found that the adjusted odds ratio for ever having liver disease ranged from 1.4 to 1.6 for different types of abuse and neglect; among individuals with more than 6 adverse childhood experiences, the adjusted odds ratio was 2.6. Notably, the risk of liver disease was substantially mediated by risk behaviors for liver disease, such as alcohol and drug use and various sexual behaviors. Brown and colleagues (2010) found an association between adverse childhood experiences and an increased risk of lung cancer, which was partially mediated by smoking behavior. In particular, exposure to a large number of adverse childhood experiences was strongly associated with premature death from lung cancer; among individuals who died from lung cancer, those with 6 or more adverse childhood experiences died an average of 13 years earlier than those with no adverse childhood experiences. Likewise, Dong and colleagues (2004) found that adverse childhood experiences increased the likelihood of ischemic heart disease. The association was substantially mediated by both traditional (diabetes, hypertension, physical inactivity, smoking, and obesity) and psychological (anger and depressed affect) risk factors, but the psychological risk factors of anger (adjusted odds ratio of 2.1) and depression (adjusted odds ratio of 2.5) had stronger associations with heart disease than the traditional risk factors.

Obesity

In various studies, different forms of child abuse and neglect have been linked with increased body mass index and higher rates of obesity in childhood, adolescence, and adulthood. Some studies link neglect but not abuse to obesity (e.g., Johnson et al., 2002; Lissau and Sorensen, 1994), and some link physical abuse but not neglect (Bentley and Widom, 2009). These differences may be the result of differences in the time points at which obesity is assessed, in sample characteristics, or in the adequacy of controls, or other factors. Knutson and colleagues (2010) found that specific types of neglect (supervisory versus care) predicted obesity at different ages. Care neglect, defined as inattention to such things as provision of adequate food and clothing, predicted body mass index at younger ages, whereas supervisory neglect, defined as parental lack of availability, predicted body mass index at older ages.

> *Finding:* Experiences of child abuse and neglect have effects on many health outcomes, including risks for long-term chronic and debilitating diseases and, in extreme cases, stunted growth.

ADOLESCENT AND ADULT OUTCOMES

While a number of the consequences of child abuse and neglect discussed previously in this chapter can be present across childhood, adolescence, and adulthood, this section focuses on behavioral outcomes that manifest specifically in either adolescence or adulthood.

Delinquency and Violence

Maxfield and Widom (1996) found that abuse and neglect experienced in childhood predicted violence and arrests in early adulthood. Adults with a history of abuse and neglect were more likely than adults without such a history to have committed nontraffic offenses (49 percent versus 38 percent) and violent crimes (18 percent versus 14 percent). Victims of childhood physical abuse and neglect were more likely to be arrested for violence (odds ratios 1.9 and 1.6, respectively) after controlling for age, race, and sex. These authors also found that abused and neglected girls were at increased risk for being arrested for violence relative to girls who had not been abused and neglected, with an odds ratio of 1.9. Smith and colleagues (2005) also found that abuse and neglect increase the risk of violent offending in late adolescence and early adulthood. Jonson-Reid and colleagues (2012) found a powerful effect for the number of child abuse reports predicting violent delinquency, with the association being linear for up to three reports. Two of these prospective longitudinal studies also found that sexual abuse increased the risk for general offending, but not violent offending (Smith et al., 2005). Physical abuse appears to be strongly related to violence in girls, as demonstrated in a meta-analysis (Hubbard and Pratt, 2002).

There is evidence that childhood abuse increases the risk for crime and delinquency. A number of large prospective investigations in different parts of the United States have documented a relationship between child-hood abuse and neglect and juvenile and/or young adult crime (English et al., 2002; Lansford et al., 2007; Maxfield and Widom, 1996; Smith and Thornberry, 1995; Stouthamer-Loeber et al., 2001; Widom, 1989; Widom and Maxfield, 2001; Zingraff et al., 1993). Despite differences in geographic region, time period, youths' age and sex, definition of child maltreatment, and assessment technique, these prospective investigations provide evidence that childhood maltreatment increases later risk for de-linquency and violence. Replication of this relationship across a number of well-designed studies supports the generalizability of and increases confi-dence in the results.

Alcohol and Substance Use

As adolescents and adults, those with a history of abuse and neglect have higher rates of alcohol abuse and alcoholism than those without a history of abuse and neglect (Gilbert et al., 2009b; Jonson-Reid et al., 2012). The effects tend to be stronger for women, being seen even when other factors are covaried (Simpson and Miller, 2002; Widom et al., 1995). For example, Widom and colleagues (1995) found no association between a history of abuse and neglect and alcohol use by young men, but found an association for women even after controlling for parental substance use and other correlated variables. A similar pattern of results emerged in a follow-up with these participants about 10 years later, when they were approximately 40 years old. Women with a documented history of child abuse and/or neglect were more likely to drink excessively in middle adult-hood than those without such a history (Widom et al., 2007b); again, this difference was not seen in men. Girls with a history of physical abuse tend to start using substances (including alcohol, marijuana, tobacco, etc.) at younger ages than youth without such a history (Lansford et al., 2010). Work by Lansford and colleagues (2010) suggests that this early initiation serves as the mechanism for later substance use in adulthood.

Evidence linking abuse and neglect to substance abuse in adulthood is mixed (Gilbert et al., 2009b; Widom et al., 1999), with retrospective and prospective findings differing. For example, Widom and colleagues (1999) describe findings based on defining child abuse and neglect prospectively and retrospectively using self-reports (i.e., following their sample forward and asking adults whether they had been abused or neglected as children). The findings based on these two types of data differed dramatically. The prospective data showed no increase in risk of substance abuse at age 29, whereas the retrospective data showed significant differences. Interestingly, a later follow-up with this sample (Widom et al., 2006) found that in middle adulthood, abused and neglected individuals compared with controls were about 1.5 times more likely to report using any illicit drug (in particular, marijuana) during the past year, and reported use of a greater number of illicit drugs and more substance use–related problems. Findings such as these provide support for the importance of longitudinal studies because without the subsequent follow-up, there would have appeared to be no increase in risk for adults who had experienced childhood abuse or neglect; these findings also illustrate the importance of contextual factors in understanding consequences.

Suicide Attempts

Experiences of abuse and neglect in childhood have a large effect on suicide attempts in adolescence and adulthood (Brown et al., 1999; Fergusson et al., 2008; Gilbert et al., 2009b; Widom, 1998). Among adults in their late 20s, Widom (1998) found that 19 percent of those with a history of abuse or neglect had made at least one suicide attempt, as compared with 8 percent of a matched community sample. Fergusson and colleagues (2008) found high rates of suicide among a New Zealand sample as well. These effects are seen for physical and sexual abuse even after accounting for other associated risk factors (Fergusson et al., 2008). Trickett and colleagues (2011) found, through a prospective design, more incidents of self-harm and suicidal behaviors among women who had been sexually abused than among a control group of women who had not been sexually abused.

Sexual Behavior

Studies have investigated the association between child abuse and neglect and several aspects of sexual behavior, including early sexual initiation and sexual risk behavior, teen pregnancy, and prostitution and the risk for commercial sexual exploitation of children and adults.

Early Sexual Initiation and Sexual Risk Behavior

Children who experience abuse and neglect may initiate sexual activity at earlier ages than other children (Lodico and DiClemente, 1994; Noll et al., 2003; Springs and Friedrich, 1992; Wilson and Widom, 2008). In addition, there is limited evidence of an association between child abuse and neglect and increased risky sexual behaviors (Jones et al., 2010; Senn et al., 2008). This association has been studied most frequently for sexual abuse; however, Jones and colleagues (2010) found that physical and emotional abuse, but not neglect, contributed to risky behaviors over and above the effects of sexual abuse. Trickett and colleagues (2011) undertook one of the most extensive longitudinal studies of developmental outcomes for female victims of sexual abuse. The majority had experienced severe sexual abuse, defined by the type of abuse (with vaginal and anal penetrative abuse seen as most severe), the length of time over which the abuse occurred, and the relationship of the abuser to the victim. In addition to earlier initiation of sexual activity among women who had been sexually abused in childhood, the authors found less use of birth control (Noll et al., 2003). For both abused and nonabused women, having a large number of male peers in childhood networks was associated with a lack of birth control use in adolescence (Trickett et al., 2011). For abused females, however, having high-quality relationships with male peers and nonpeers in childhood was associated with greater birth control use in adolescence; in the comparison group, this association was not found.

Teen Pregnancy

Evidence linking childhood sexual abuse and increased risk for teen pregnancy has been mixed. Trickett and colleagues (2011) found that severely sexually abused females reported significantly higher rates of teen pregnancy and teen motherhood than nonabused females (abused = 39 percent, nonabused = 15 percent). In a meta-analysis of previously published studies of sequelae of child sexual abuse, Noll and colleagues (2009) found an increased risk for early pregnancy among girls who had been sexually abused. In contrast, using a prospective cohort design that followed children with documented cases of abuse and neglect into young adulthood, Widom and Kuhns (1996) found no evidence that childhood sexual abuse was a significant risk factor for multiple early sexual partners or teenage pregnancy.

Prostitution and Risk for Commercial Sexual Exploitation of Children and Adults

In a prospective study, Widom and Kuhns (1996) found that sexual abuse and neglect, but not physical abuse, were associated with later prostitution. In a subsequent study, Wilson and Widom (2010) examined the role of problem behaviors as a pathway to adult prostitution and found that adult victims who had experienced child abuse and neglect were more likely than nonvictims to report having been involved in prostitution as adults or prostituted as juveniles (Wilson and Widom, 2008). Stoltz and colleagues (2007) found a significant relationship between child abuse and neglect (sexual, physical, and emotional) and later involvement in prostitution among a sample of 361 drug-using, street-involved youth in Canada.

While an important topic, evidence that child abuse and neglect increase the risk for commercial sexual exploitation of children is very limited and comes primarily from retrospective studies of sexually exploited youth. Some older studies have reported that experiences of childhood sexual abuse influenced the decision of young women to become involved in commercial sex work (Bagley and Young, 1987; Silbert and Pines, 1983). A comprehensive look at those issues will be presented in a forthcoming Institute of Medicine report from the Committee on Commercial Sexual Exploitation and Sex Trafficking of Minors in the United States.

Finding: Experiences of abuse and neglect in childhood have a large effect on delinquency, violence, and suicide attempts in adolescence and adulthood.

Finding: Adolescents and adults with a history of child abuse and neglect have higher rates of alcohol abuse and alcoholism than those without a history of abuse and neglect, although this relationship has been found most frequently in women.

Finding: Children who experience abuse and neglect may initiate sexual activity at earlier ages than comparison groups. Childhood sexual abuse also has been found to be associated with heightened risks for a range of adverse outcomes related to sexual risk-taking behaviors.

Finding: Studies seeking an association between child abuse and neglect and teen pregnancy or adult prostitution have reported mixed results.

INDIVIDUAL DIFFERENCES IN OUTCOMES

This chapter has presented extensive evidence that children who are abused or neglected, as a group, are at increased risk for a variety of problematic outcomes. However, not all children who experience abuse or neglect experience these negative consequences. Not surprisingly (given what is known about typical development), children vary in the outcomes they experience even when exposed to the same type of abuse or neglect, with outcomes ranging from the most problematic to functioning well across domains. As discussed earlier in this chapter, an ecological-transactional model is helpful for understanding outcomes related to abuse and neglect as influenced by the interplay of risk and protective factors that occur at multiple levels of a child's ecology. Through examination of compensatory resources in children and their environment, an ecological-transactional

framework can aid in understanding children who exhibit resilient outcomes despite having been abused or neglected (Cicchetti and Toth, 2009;
Luthar et al., 2000). Factors that influence resilience among abused and
neglected children have been identified at the level of the individual child,
the family, and the child's broader social context. However, neither a child's
individual strengths nor the surrounding environment alone can predict
resilient outcomes. As noted by Jaffee and colleagues (2007, p. 233), "the
fit between the child and the environment is the best predictor of children's
psychological well-being." The following sections describe research examining explanatory factors for differences in outcomes related to child abuse
and neglect.

Characteristics of Abuse or Neglect Experiences

Characteristics of a child's exposure to abuse or neglect have been
shown to influence the risk for problematic outcomes. Such characteristics
include the point within the course of a child's development at which an
experience of abuse or neglect occurs; the chronicity of abuse or neglect
experiences, taking into account their duration and frequency; the severity of the experiences; and the type of abuse or neglect (Bulik et al., 2001;
Collishaw et al., 2007; Keiley et al., 2001; Manly et al., 2001).

Among a sample of adult female twins, Bulik and colleagues (2001)
found an association between characteristics of the abuse experience (e.g.,
a high level of severity of child sexual abuse, such as attempted or completed intercourse and the use of force or threats) and certain psychiatric
disorders. In examining the effect of timing on outcomes related to child
physical abuse, Keiley and colleagues (2001) found that children who
experienced such abuse while under the age of 5 were at higher risk for
negative outcomes than those who experienced the same type of abuse at
age 5 or older. Jonson-Reid and colleagues (2012) found that nearly all
children who experienced chronic, persisting abusing or neglect showed
adverse outcomes in adulthood: 91.9 percent of children showed at least
one negative outcome if they had 12 or more reports of abuse or neglect
(Jonson-Reid et al., 2012).

Resilience

The concept of resilience serves as a useful lens for evaluating the differing outcomes of children exposed to abuse and neglect. By examining factors that contribute to whether children experience maladaptive outcomes
in response to abuse or neglect, researchers can gain a better understanding
of how better to prevent and treat these consequences. While resilience has
been defined in various ways, it can be understood as "a good outcome in

spite of high risk, sustained competence under stress, and recovery from trauma" (McGloin and Widom, 2001, p. 1022).

The study of resilience in the context of child abuse and neglect must take into account several factors. First, as shown throughout this chapter, consequences of child abuse and neglect can manifest in multiple domains of functioning. Therefore, a child's subsequent adaptation or maladaptation following abuse or neglect must be assessed in terms of multiple outcomes rather than a single indicator, such as depression (Afifi and Macmillan, 2011; McGloin and Widom, 2001). Second, resilience is not a static construct, meaning that a child can exhibit resilient outcomes at a certain point in the course of development but may still experience problematic outcomes at a later time. It follows that analysis of resilience in abused and neglected children should include a temporal component (McGloin and Widom, 2001). Third, many factors believed to promote resilience in response to child abuse and neglect can also serve to promote positive adaptation more generally in response to other childhood stressors, making it imperative for studies to include a comparison group that has not been abused or neglected (Collishaw et al., 2007). Finally, resilience might usefully be considered from the perspective of allostatic load (Danese and McEwen, 2012). That is, some children who experience abuse or neglect do not show problematic outcomes, but as abuse, neglect, and other adverse childhood experiences accumulate, they challenge children's ability to cope with the negotiation of life tasks.

Results from a study of adults who were the subjects of substantiated cases of child abuse or neglect as children indicate that 22 percent of abused and neglected individuals met the criteria for resilience, which required successful functioning in 6 of 8 domains (McGloin and Widom, 2001). A study by Collishaw and colleagues (2007) examined resilience to adult psychopathology within a representative community sample, finding that 44 percent of adults who reported abuse during childhood reported no psychiatric problems in adulthood and demonstrated positive adaptation in other domains.

Protective factors supporting resilience have been examined at the levels of the individual, family, and social environment, with resilience being measured in childhood, adolescence, and early adulthood. In a review of protective factors for resilience following child abuse and neglect, Afifi and Macmillan (2011) identify three protective factors that are best supported by findings from longitudinal and cross-sectional studies: a stable family environment, supportive familial relationships, and personality traits that support social skills.

Individual-level protective factors identified among those displaying resilience following child abuse and neglect include personality traits (e.g., high ego control, high self-esteem, internal locus of control, external attributions of blame, and attribution of success to own efforts); gender (females more resilient than males); and relationship capabilities (Afifi and Macmillan, 2011; Collishaw et al., 2007; Jaffee and Gallop, 2007; Jaffee et al., 2007). There is some evidence that intelligence or cognitive ability functions as a protective factor (Masten and Tellegen, 2012), but it has not always been found to be significant in supporting resilience (Afifi and Macmillan, 2011; Collishaw et al., 2007). Jaffee and colleagues (2007) found that children with protective individual-level characteristics were likely to be resilient in low-stress environments (59 percent), but children with the same protective individual-level characteristics were less likely to be resilient in highly challenging environments.

Family-level protective factors include a caring and safe home environment; positive changes in family structure (e.g., intervention, cessation of visiting rights, or removal to foster care); and supportive familial relationships at the time of abuse (Afifi and Macmillan, 2011; Collishaw et al., 2007; Jaffee et al., 2007). In a sample of sexually abused girls in foster care, family support was not found to be a protective factor, but peer influences, school plan certainty, and positive future orientation were (Edmond et al., 2006). Other social-level protective factors include supportive relationships with non-family members, such as teachers or camp counselors, and supportive relationships with peers in adolescence (Flores et al., 2005; Jaffee et al., 2007).

Gene x Environment Interactions

Historically, those working in the field of child abuse and neglect were unable to examine whether such adverse experiences interacted with biological risk or protective factors (e.g., so-called risk or protective genes)—specifically, whether experience interacted with underlying genetics. This situation has changed over the past 20 years as advances in molecular genetics have enabled a search for gene x environment (GxE) interactions. A number of such interactions have been studied in the last several decades in relation to early adversity generally and child abuse and neglect in particular. Critics of these approaches charge, among other things, that examining single gene and single environment combinations in interactions capitalizes on chance. In addition, some experts in genetics argue that the action of any single gene is likely to be very small, and to detect its effects will likely require very large sample sizes. Nonetheless, some GxE findings have emerged as robust and apparently replicable.

The 5-HTT gene is perhaps at the top of this list. This gene regulates reuptake of serotonin (a neurotransmitter that has various functions, including regulation of mood and sleep and some cognitive functions, such as memory and learning) at the synaptic cleft. The gene has long and short allelic variants that confer differential reuptake efficiency. Rodent, nonhuman primate, and human studies (e.g., Caspi et al., 2003) have shown that two alleles confer advantage among animals raised in stressful environments. Caspi and colleagues (2003) found that adults who had experienced stressful life events as children were more likely to have a major depressive disorder if they had one or two short alleles. Those who had two long alleles were no more likely to develop depression than individuals who had not experienced stressful life events.

A second genetic polymorphism that has received much attention is a functional polymorphism in the promoter region of the monoamine oxidase A (MAOA) gene. MAOA encodes the MAOA enzyme and selectively degrades serotonin, norepinephrine, and dopamine. Abused and neglected boys with the genotype conferring low levels of MAOA expression were found to be more likely to develop a range of externalizing behaviors, including conduct disorder, antisocial personality disorder, and violent criminality (Caspi et al., 2002). However, subsequent studies have failed to replicate these findings or have demonstrated only partial replications (Huizinga et al., 2006; Widom and Brzustowicz, 2006). For a recent review of the GxE literature concerned with child depression and abuse, see Dunn and colleagues (2011).

> *Finding:* Not all children who experience abuse or neglect show problematic outcomes. Factors that influence resilience among abused and neglected children have been identified at the level of the individual child, the family, and the child's broader social context. These factors, along with risks and stressors at each level, interact with one another to predict resilient outcomes.

> *Finding:* There is a positive association between the number of risk factors for abuse and neglect to which a child is exposed and the likelihood of experiencing adverse outcomes.

> *Finding:* The timing, chronicity, and severity of child abuse and neglect, as well as the context in which they occur, have been shown to impact the associated outcomes.

ECONOMIC BURDEN

Although the total costs of child abuse and neglect are difficult to gauge because much abuse is unreported (Waters et al., 2004), a number of studies over the last few decades have attempted to document the economic burden of child abuse and neglect on society (Corso and Fertig, 2010; Fang et al., 2012; Wang and Holton, 2007; Waters et al., 2004). Economic burden or economic impact analyses typically quantify burden by aggregating the direct medical expenditures resulting from a condition, the direct nonmedical expenditures associated with a condition, and the subsequent indirect losses in productivity potential for society. These analyses often are called *cost of illness/injury analyses.*

Examples of direct medical expenditures include inpatient and outpatient hospital care, mental health care, medical transport required in the event of an emergency, medications and medical devices, and the medical treatment of chronic conditions resulting from the abuse. Multiple studies since the 1993 NRC report was issued have assessed the direct medical costs associated with child abuse and neglect (Brown et al., 2011), particularly the inpatient costs associated with severe abuse (Courtney, 1999; Evasovich et al., 1998; Irazuzta et al., 1997; Libby et al., 2003; New and Berliner, 2000; Rovi et al., 2004).

Direct nonmedical expenditures include use of the child welfare system, law enforcement, and the criminal justice system. Studies have included nonmedical costs in their assessment of the economic burden of child abuse and neglect (Staudt, 2003; Zagar et al., 2009).

Productivity losses include the child's missing school or performing at subpar levels in school because of the abuse, parents missing work or performing at subpar levels at work because of the abuse situation or having to deal with child welfare and criminal justice services, and permanent losses in lifetime productivity potential because of premature death. Productivity losses and economic well-being have been incorporated into a number of analyses of the economic burden of child abuse and neglect (Brown et al., 2011; Corso and Fertig, 2010; Corso et al., 2011; Currie and Widom, 2010; Fang et al., 2012).

Gelles and Perlman (2012) estimate that cases of abuse or neglect impose a cumulative cost to society of $80.2 billion each year—$33.3 billion in direct costs and $46.9 billion in indirect costs. An analysis by the Centers for Disease Control and Prevention found that the average lifetime cost of a case of nonfatal child abuse and neglect is $210,012 in 2010 dollars, most of this total ($144,360) due to lost productivity but also encompassing the costs of child and adult health care, child welfare, criminal justice, and special education (Fang et al., 2012). The average lifetime cost of a case of fatal child abuse and neglect is $1.27 million, due mainly to loss of productivity.

Currie and Widom (2010) found that adults who had experienced abuse and neglect in childhood had lower levels of education, employment, and earnings and fewer assets than adults without a history of abuse and neglect. A higher percentage of adults who had been abused or neglected as children worked in menial, semiskilled positions at age 29 compared with adults who had not been abused or neglected—62 versus 45 percent, respectively. More of the abused and neglected group has been unemployed at some point during the previous 5 years (41 versus 58 percent, respectively). And fewer of those from the abused or neglected group were currently employed or had a bank account, owned a car, or owned their home. Larger effects were seen for women than for men.

Analyses of the economic burden of child abuse and neglect could be strengthened by greater transparency in the study methods, including a full accounting of all cost categories that may be impacted by abuse and neglect and transparency in the unit cost estimates for each cost category, as well as a methodologically sound choice of study design for estimating economic burden (Corso and Fertig, 2010; Corso and Lutzker, 2006; Fang et al., 2012). Several approaches could be taken to estimate economic burden, each of which has advantages and disadvantages that could potentially result in overestimating or underestimating the true economic cost of child abuse and neglect. Options include using cross-sectional data to compare the medical costs for an abused/neglected population compared with a nonabused/nonneglected population, including only those health care costs that can be explicitly linked to diagnosis-specific health care utilization (and costs) through the use of diagnosis and external cause codes used in inpatient settings, and supplementing either of these two approaches by including the costs of the fraction of other health conditions attributed to child abuse and neglect.

> *Finding:* Although the total costs of child abuse and neglect are difficult to gauge, a number of studies have attempted to document the economic burden of child abuse and neglect on society, including such measures as direct medical and nonmedical expenditures and productivity losses. One study estimates that cases of abuse or neglect impose a cumulative cost to society of $80.2 billion annually (Gelles and Perlman, 2012).

> *Finding:* Some studies have shown that adults who experienced abuse and neglect in childhood have lower levels of education, employment, and earnings and fewer assets than adults without a history of abuse and neglect.

CONCLUSIONS

Child abuse and neglect appear to influence the course of development by altering many elements of biological, cognitive, psychosocial, and behavioral development; in other words, child abuse and neglect "get under the skin" (Hertzman and Boyce, 2010) to have a profound and often lasting impact on development. Brain development is affected, as is the ability to make decisions as carefully as one's peers, or executive functioning; the ability to regulate physiology, behavior, and emotions is impaired; and the trajectory toward more problematic outcomes is impacted. Effects are seen across domains, with the interplay across brain and behavioral systems being particularly striking.

Risk and protective factors across multiple levels of a child's ecology interact to influence outcomes related to child abuse and neglect. Factors that influence resilience across these domains are important to an understanding of how to protect children from the adverse outcomes discussed in this chapter. Evidence suggests that the timing, chronicity, and severity of the abuse or neglect matter in terms of outcomes. The more times children experience abuse or neglect, the worse are the outcomes (Jonson-Reid et al., 2012). As Jonson-Reid and colleagues (2012) point out, it is not enough to know whether an event happened; one must also know how ongoing the problem is. The committee sees as hopeful the evidence that changing environments can change brain development, health, and behavioral outcomes. There is a window of opportunity, with developmental tasks becoming increasingly more challenging to negotiate with continued abuse and neglect over time.

Future research in this area needs to focus on disentangling the effects of child abuse and neglect from those of other conditions. There is a need to explore beneath the surface to understand the behavioral, neurobiological, social, and environmental mechanisms that mediate the association between exposure to abuse and neglect and their behavioral and neurobiological sequelae.

REFERENCES

Afifi, T. O., and H. L. Macmillan. 2011. Resilience following child maltreatment: A review of protective factors. *Canadian Journal of Psychiatry* 56(5):266-272.

Afifi, T. O., J. Boman, W. Fleisher, and J. Sareen. 2009. The relationship between child abuse, parental divorce, and lifetime mental disorders and suicidality in a nationally representative adult sample. *Child Abuse & Neglect* 33(3):139-147.

Ainsworth, M. D. S. 1978. *Patterns of attachment: A psychological study of the strange situation.* Hillsdale, NJ: Lawrence Erlbaum Associates.

Almas, A. N., K. A. Degnan, A. Radulescu, C. A. Nelson, 3rd, C. H. Zeanah, and N. A. Fox. 2012. Effects of early intervention and the moderating effects of brain activity on institutionalized children's social skills at age 8. *Proceedings of the National Academy of Sciences of the United States of America* 109(Suppl. 2):17228-17231.

Andersen, P., R. Morris, D. Amaral, T. Bliss, and J. O'Keefe. 2007. *The hippocampus book.* New York: Oxford University Press.

Andersen, S. L., and M. H. Teicher. 2004. Delayed effects of early stress on hippocampal development. *Neuropsychopharmacology: Official Publication of the American College of Neuropsychopharmacology* 29(11):1988-1993.

Andersen, S. L., A. Tomada, E. S. Vincow, E. Valente, A. Polcari, and M. H. Teicher. 2008. Preliminary evidence for sensitive periods in the effect of childhood sexual abuse on regional brain development. *Journal of Neuropsychiatry and Clinical Neurosciences* 20(3):292-301.

APA (American Psychiatric Association). 2013a. *Diagnostic and statistical manual of mental disorders: DSM-5.* Washington, DC: APA.

APA. 2013b. *Highlights of changes from DSM-IV-TR to DSM-V.* Washington, DC: APA.

APA. 2013c. *Posttraumatic stress disorder—DSM-V.* Washington, DC: APA.

Arseneault, L., M. Cannon, H. L. Fisher, G. Polanczyk, T. E. Moffitt, and A. Caspi. 2011. Childhood trauma and children's emerging psychotic symptoms: A genetically sensitive longitudinal cohort study. *American Journal of Psychiatry* 168(1):65-72.

Asok, A., K. Bernard, T. L. Roth, J. B. Rosen, and M. Dozier. 2013. Parental responsiveness moderates the association between early-life stress and reduced telomere length. *Development and Psychopathology* 25(3):577-585.

Avery, L., C. R. Massat, and M. Lundy. 2000. Posttraumatic stress and mental health functioning of sexually abused children. *Child and Adolescent Social Work Journal* 17(1):19-34.

Bagley, C., and L. Young. 1987. Juvenile prostitution and child sexual abuse: A controlled study. *Canadian Journal of Community Mental Health* 6(1):5-26.

Banyard, V. L., L. M. Williams, and J. A. Siegel. 2001. The long-term mental health consequences of child sexual abuse: An exploratory study of the impact of multiple traumas in a sample of women. *Journal of Traumatic Stress* 14(4):697-715.

Barnett, D., J. I. Vondra, and S. M. Shonk. 1996. Self-perceptions, motivation, and school functioning of low-income maltreated and comparison children. *Child Abuse & Neglect* 20(5):397-410.

Barry, R. J., S. J. Johnstone, and A. R. Clarke. 2003. A review of electrophysiology in attention-deficit/hyperactivity disorder: II. Event-related potentials. *Journal of Clinical Neurophysiology* 114(2):184-198.

Becker-Blease, K. A., and J. J. Freyd. 2008. A preliminary study of ADHD symptoms and correlates: Do abused children differ from nonabused children? *Journal of Aggression, Maltreatment and Trauma* 17(1):133-140.

Belsky, J. 1980. Child maltreatment: An ecological integration. *American Psychologist* 35(4): 320-335.

Belsky, J. 1993. Etiology of child maltreatment: A developmental-ecological analysis. *Psychological Bulletin* 114(3):413-434.

Belsky, J., G. L. Schlomer, and B. J. Ellis. 2012. Beyond cumulative risk: Distinguishing harshness and unpredictability as determinants of parenting and early life history strategy. *Developmental Psychology* 48(3):662-673.

Bentley, T., and C. S. Widom. 2009. A 30-year follow-up of the effects of child abuse and neglect on obesity in adulthood. *Obesity (Silver Spring)* 17(10):1900-1905.

Bernard, K., Z. Butzin-Dozier, J. Rittenhouse, and M. Dozier. 2010. Cortisol production patterns in young children living with birth parents vs children placed in foster care following involvement of child protective services. *Archives of Pediatrics and Adolescent Medicine* 164(5):438-443.

Bloom, J. S., and G. W. Hynd. 2005. The role of the corpus callosum in interhemispheric transfer of information: Excitation or inhibition? *Neuropsychology Review* 15(2):59-71.

Boden, J. M., D. M. Fergusson, and L. J. Horwood. 2010. Risk factors for conduct disorder and oppositional/defiant disorder: Evidence from a New Zealand birth cohort. *Journal of the American Academy of Child and Adolescent Psychiatry* 49(11):1125-1133.

Bonomi, A. E., M. L. Anderson, F. P. Rivara, E. A. Cannon, P. A. Fishman, D. Carrell, R. J. Reid, and R. S. Thompson. 2008. Health care utilization and costs associated with childhood abuse. *Journal of Genernal Internal Medicine* 23(3):294-299.

Brake, W. G., R. M. Sullivan, and A. Gratton. 2000. Perinatal distress leads to lateralized medial prefrontal cortical dopamine hypofunction in adult rats. *Journal of Neuroscience* 20(14):5538-5543.

Briere, J. N. 1992. *Child abuse trauma: Theory and treatment of the lasting effects.* Newbury Park, CA: Sage Publications.

Briere, J., M. F. Erickson, and B. Egeland. 1996. *The APSAC handbook on child maltreatment.* Thousand Oaks, CA: Sage Publications.

Briere, J., K. Johnson, A. Bissada, L. Damon, J. Crouch, E. Gil, R. Hanson, and V. Ernst. 2001. The Trauma Symptom Checklist for Young Children (TSCYC): Reliability and association with abuse exposure in a multi-site study. *Child Abuse & Neglect* 25(8):1001-1014.

Briscoe-Smith, A. M., and S. P. Hinshaw. 2006. Linkages between child abuse and attention-deficit/hyperactivity disorder in girls: Behavioral and social correlates. *Child Abuse & Neglect* 30(11):1239-1255.

Brown, D. S., X. Fang, and C. S. Florence. 2011. Medical costs attributable to child maltreatment: A systematic review of short- and long-term effects. *American Journal of Preventive Medicine* 41(6):627-635.

Brown, D. W., R. F. Anda, V. J. Felitti, V. J. Edwards, A. M. Malarcher, J. B. Croft, and W. H. Giles. 2010. Adverse childhood experiences are associated with the risk of lung cancer: A prospective cohort study. *BMC Public Health* 10:20.

Brown, J., P. Cohen, J. G. Johnson, and E. M. Smailes. 1999. Childhood abuse and neglect: Specificity of effects on adolescent and young adult depression and suicidality. *Journal of the American Academy of Child and Adolescent Psychiatry* 38(12):1490-1496.

Bruce, J., M. Kroupina, S. Parker, and M. R. Gunnar. 2000. *The relationships between cortisol patterns, growth retardation, and developmental delay in post-institutionalized children.* Paper presented at International Conference on Infant Studies, Brighton, England.

Bruce, J., P. A. Fisher, K. C. Pears, and S. Levine. 2009. Morning cortisol levels in preschool-aged foster children: Differential effects of maltreatment type. *Developmental Psychobiology* 51(1):14-23.

Bulik, C. M., C. A. Prescott, and K. S. Kendler. 2001. Features of childhood sexual abuse and the development of psychiatric and substance use disorders. *British Journal of Psychiatry* 179(5):444-449.

Carlson, E. A. 1998. A prospective longitudinal study of attachment disorganization/disorientation. *Child Development* 69(4):1107-1128.

Carlson, M., and F. Earls. 1997. Psychological and neuroendocrinological sequelae of early social deprivation in institutionalized children in Romania. *Annals of the New York Academy of Sciences* 807:419-428.

Carpenter, L. L., A. R. Tyrka, N. S. Ross, L. Khoury, G. M. Anderson, and L. H. Price. 2009. Effect of childhood emotional abuse and age on cortisol responsivity in adulthood. *Biological Psychiatry* 66(1):69-75.

Carrion, V. G., A. Garrett, V. Menon, C. F. Weems, and A. L. Reiss. 2008. Posttraumatic stress symptoms and brain function during a response-inhibition task: An fMRI study in youth. *Depression and Anxiety* 25(6):514-526.

Carrion, V. G., C. F. Weems, C. Watson, S. Eliez, V. Menon, and A. L. Reiss. 2009. Converging evidence for abnormalities of the prefrontal cortex and evaluation of midsagittal structures in pediatric posttraumatic stress disorder: An MRI study. *Psychiatry Research* 172(3):226-234.

Caspi, A., J. McClay, T. E. Moffitt, J. Mill, J. Martin, I. W. Craig, A. Taylor, and R. Poulton. 2002. Role of genotype in the cycle of violence in maltreated children. *Science* 297(5582): 851-854.

Caspi, A., K. Sugden, T. E. Moffitt, A. Taylor, I. W. Craig, H. Harrington, J. McClay, J. Mill, J. Martin, A. Braithwaite, and R. Poulton. 2003. Influence of life stress on depression: Moderation by a polymorphism in the 5-HTT gene. *Science* 301(5631):386-389.

Champoux, M., C. L. Coe, S. M. Schanberg, C. M. Kuhn, and S. J. Suomi. 1989. Hormonal effects of early rearing conditions in the infant rhesus monkey. *American Journal of Primatology* 19(2):111-117.

Chareyron, L. J., P. B. Lavenex, D. G. Amaral, and P. Lavenex. 2012. Postnatal development of the amygdala: A stereological study in macaque monkeys. *Journal of Comparative Neurology* 520(9):1965-1984.

Chen, L. P., M. H. Murad, M. L. Paras, K. M. Colbenson, A. L. Sattler, E. N. Goranson, M. B. Elamin, R. J. Seime, G. Shinozaki, L. J. Prokop, and A. Zirakzadeh. 2010. Sexual abuse and lifetime diagnosis of psychiatric disorders: Systematic review and meta-analysis. *Mayo Clinic Proceedings* 85(7):618-629.

Chernoff, R., T. Combs-Orme, C. Risley-Curtiss, and A. Heisler. 1994. Assessing the health status of children entering foster care. *Pediatrics* 93(4):594-601.

Cicchetti, D., and M. Lynch. 1993. Toward an ecological/transactional model of community violence and child maltreatment: Consequences for children's development. *Psychiatry-Interpersonal and Biological Processes* 56(1):96-118.

Cicchetti, D., and R. Rizley. 1981. Developmental perspectives on the etiology, intergenerational transmission, and sequelae of child maltreatment. *New Directions for Child and Adolescent Development* 1981(11):31-55.

Cicchetti, D., and F. A. Rogosch. 2001a. Diverse patterns of neuroendocrine activity in maltreated children. *Developmental Psychopathology* 13(3):677-693.

Cicchetti, D., and F. A. Rogosch. 2001b. The impact of child maltreatment and psychopathology on neuroendocrine functioning. *Developmental Psychopathology* 13(4):783-804.

Cicchetti, D., and S. L. Toth. 1998. Perspectives on research and practice in developmental psychopathology. In *Handbook of child psychology*, 5th ed., Vol. 4, edited by W. Damon, I. E. Sigel, and K. A. Renninger. Hoboken, NJ: John Wiley & Sons, Inc. Pp. 479-583.

Cicchetti, D., and S. L. Toth. 2009. The past achievements and future promises of developmental psychopathology: The coming of age of a discipline. *Journal of Child Psychology and Psychiatry* 50(1-2):16-25.

Cicchetti, D., B. P. Ackerman, and C. E. Izard. 1995. Emotions and emotion regulation in developmental psychopathology. *Development and Psychopathology* 7(1):1-10.

Clarke, A. S. 1993. Social rearing effects on HPA axis activity over early development and in response to stress in rhesus monkeys. *Developmental Psychobiology* 26(8):433-446.

Cole, P. M., M. K. Michel, and L. O. D. Teti. 1994. The development of emotion regulation and dysregulation: A clinical perspective. *Monographs of the Society for Research in Child Development* 59(2-3):73-102.

Cole, P. M., J. Luby, and M. W. Sullivan. 2008. Emotions and the development of childhood depression: Bridging the gap. *Child Development Perspectives* 2(3):141-148.

Collishaw, S., A. Pickles, J. Messer, M. Rutter, C. Shearer, and B. Maughan. 2007. Resilience to adult psychopathology following childhood maltreatment: Evidence from a community sample. *Child Abuse & Neglect* 31(3):211-229.

Corso, P. S., and A. R. Fertig. 2010. The economic impact of child maltreatment in the United States: Are the estimates credible? *Child Abuse & Neglect* 34(5):296-304.

Corso, P. S., and J. R. Lutzker. 2006. The need for economic analysis in research on child maltreatment. *Child Abuse & Neglect* 30(7):727-738.

Corso, P. S., X. Fang, and J. A. Mercy. 2011. Benefits of preventing a death associated with child maltreatment: Evidence from willingness-to-pay survey data. *American Journal of Public Health* 101(3):487-490.

Courtney, M. E. 1999. National call to action: Working toward the elimination of child maltreatment. The economics. *Child Abuse & Neglect* 23(10):975-986.

Crozier, J. C., and R. P. Barth. 2005. Cognitive and academic functioning in maltreated children. *Children & Schools* 27(4):197-206.

Currie, J., and C. S. Widom. 2010. Long-term consequences of child abuse and neglect on adult economic well-being. *Child Maltreatment* 15(2):111-120.

Cyr, C., E. M. Euser, M. J. Bakermans-Kranenburg, and M. H. van Ijzendoorn. 2010. Attachment security and disorganization in maltreating and high-risk families: A series of meta-analyses. *Development and Psychopathology* 22(1):87-108.

Dalgeish, T., A. R. Moradi, M. R. Taghavi, H. T. Neshat-Doost, and W. Yule. 2001. An experimental investigation of hypervigilance for threat in children and adolescents with post-traumatic stress disorder. *Psychological Medicine* 31(3):541-547.

Danese, A., and B. S. McEwen. 2012. Adverse childhood experiences, allostasis, allostatic load, and age-related disease. *Physiology & Behavior* 106(1):29-39.

De Bellis, M. D., and M. S. Keshavan. 2003. Sex differences in brain maturation in maltreatment-related pediatric posttraumatic stress disorder. *Neuroscience and Biobehavioral Reviews* 27(1-2):103-117.

De Bellis, M. D., M. S. Keshavan, D. B. Clark, B. J. Casey, J. N. Giedd, A. M. Boring, K. Frustaci, and N. D. Ryan. 1999. Developmental traumatology. Part II: Brain development. *Biological Psychiatry* 45(10):1271-1284.

De Bellis, M. D., J. Hall, A. M. Boring, K. Frustaci, and G. Moritz. 2001a. A pilot longitudinal study of hippocampal volumes in pediatric maltreatment-related posttraumatic stress disorder. *Biological Psychiatry* 50(4):305-309.

De Bellis, M. D., M. S. Keshavan, S. R. Beers, J. Hall, K. Frustaci, A. Masalehdan, J. Noll, and A. M. Boring. 2001b. Sex differences in brain maturation during childhood and adolescence. *Cerebral Cortex* 11(6):552-557.

De Bellis, M. D., M. S. Keshavan, H. Shifflett, S. Iyengar, S. R. Beers, J. Hall, and G. Moritz. 2002. Brain structures in pediatric maltreatment-related posttraumatic stress disorder: A sociodemographically matched study. *Biological Psychiatry* 52(11):1066-1078.

De Bellis, M. D., S. R. Hooper, E. G. Spratt, and D. P. Woolley. 2009. Neuropsychological findings in childhood neglect and their relationships to pediatric PTSD. *Journal of the International Neuropsychological Society* 15(6):868-878.

de Quervain, D. J., B. Roozendaal, and J. L. McGaugh. 1998. Stress and glucocorticoids impair retrieval of long-term spatial memory. *Nature* 394(6695):787-790.

Dobrova-Krol, N. A., M. H. van Ijzendoorn, M. J. Bakermans-Kranenburg, C. Cyr, and F. Juffer. 2008. Physical growth delays and stress dysregulation in stunted and non-stunted Ukrainian institution-reared children. *Infant Behavior and Development* 31(3):539-553.

Dodge, K. A., G. S. Pettit, J. E. Bates, and E. Valente. 1995. Social information-processing patterns partially mediate the effect of early physical abuse on later conduct problems. *Journal of Abnormal Psychology* 104(4):632-643.

Dong, M., S. R. Dube, V. J. Felitti, W. H. Giles, and R. F. Anda. 2003. Adverse childhood experiences and self-reported liver disease: New insights into the causal pathway. *Archives of Internal Medicine* 163(16):1949-1956.

Dong, M., W. H. Giles, V. J. Felitti, S. R. Dube, J. E. Williams, D. P. Chapman, and R. F. Anda. 2004. Insights into causal pathways for ischemic heart disease: Adverse childhood experiences study. *Circulation* 110(13):1761-1766.

Dozier, M., M. Manni, M. K. Gordon, E. Peloso, M. R. Gunnar, K. C. Stovall-McClough, D. Eldreth, and S. Levine. 2006. Foster children's diurnal production of cortisol: An exploratory study. *Child Maltreatment* 11(2):189-197.

Drury, S. S., K. Theall, M. M. Gleason, A. T. Smyke, I. De Vivo, J. Y. Y. Wong, N. A. Fox, C. H. Zeanah, and C. A. Nelson. 2011. Telomere length and early severe social deprivation: Linking early adversity and cellular aging. *Molecular Psychiatry* 17:719-727.

Dubowitz, H., R. L. Hampton, W. G. Bithoney, and E. H. Newberger. 1987. Inflicted and noninflicted injuries: Differences in child and familial characteristics. *American Journal of Orthopsychiatry* 57(4):525-535.

Dubowitz, H., M. A. Papas, M. M. Black, and R. H. Starr, Jr. 2002. Child neglect: Outcomes in high-risk urban preschoolers. *Pediatrics* 109(6):1100-1107.

Dunn, E. C., M. Uddin, S. V. Subramanian, J. W. Smoller, S. Galea, and K. C. Koenen. 2011. Research review: Gene-environment interaction research in youth depression—a systematic review with recommendations for future research. *Journal of Child Psychology and Psychiatry* 52(12):1223-1238.

Dunn, E. C., K. A. McLaughlin, N. Slopen, J. Rosand, and J. W. Smoller. 2013. Developmental timing of child maltreatment and symptoms of depression and suicidal ideation in young adulthood: Results from the national longitudinal study of adolescent health. *Depression and Anxiety* 30(10):955-964.

Eckenrode, J., M. Laird, and J. Doris. 1993. School performance and disciplinary problems among abused and neglected children. *Developmental Psychology* 29(1):53-62.

Edmond, T., W. Auslander, D. Elze, and S. Bowland. 2006. Signs of resilience in sexually abused adolescent girls in the foster care system. *Journal of Child Sexual Abuse* 15(1):1-28.

Egeland, B., and A. Susman-Stillman. 1996. Dissociation as a mediator of child abuse across generations. *Child Abuse & Neglect* 20(11):1123-1132.

Eimer, M., and A. Holmes. 2007. Event-related brain potential correlates of emotional face processing. *Neuropsychologia* 45(1):15-31.

Eisenberg, N., E. T. Gershoff, R. A. Fabes, S. A. Shepard, A. J. Cumberland, S. H. Losoya, I. K. Guthrie, and B. C. Murphy. 2001. Mother's emotional expressivity and children's behavior problems and social competence: Mediation through children's regulation. *Developmental Psychology* 37(4):475.

Ellis, B. H., P. A. Fisher, and S. Zaharie. 2004. Predictors of disruptive behavior, developmental delays, anxiety, and affective symptomatology among institutionally reared romanian children. *Journal of American Academy of Child and Adolescent Psychiatry* 43(10):1283-1292.

English, D. J., C. S. Widom, and C. Brandford. 2002. *Childhood victimization and delinquency, adult criminality, and violent criminal behavior: A replication and extension, final report (document no. 192291)*. https://www.ncjrs.gov/pdffiles1/nij/grants/192291.pdf (accessed September 16, 2013).

Epel, E. S., E. H. Blackburn, J. Lin, F. S. Dhabhar, N. E. Adler, J. D. Morrow, and R. M. Cawthon. 2004. Accelerated telomere shortening in response to life stress. *Proceedings of the National Academy of Sciences of the United States of America* 101(49):17312-17315.

Evasovich, M., R. Klein, F. Muakkassa, and R. Weekley. 1998. The economic effect of child abuse in the burn unit. *Burns* 24(7):642-645.

Fang, X., D. S. Brown, C. S. Florence, and J. A. Mercya. 2012. The economic burden of child maltreatment in the United States and implications for prevention. *Child Abuse & Neglect* 36:156-165.

Fearon, R. P., M. J. Bakermans-Kranenburg, M. H. van Ijzendoorn, A.-M. Lapsley, and G. I. Roisman. 2010. The significance of insecure attachment and disorganization in the development of children's externalizing behavior: A meta-analytic study. *Child Development* 81(2):435-456.

Fergusson, D. M., J. M. Boden, and L. J. Horwood. 2008. Exposure to childhood sexual and physical abuse and adjustment in early adulthood. *Child Abuse & Neglect* 32(6):607-619.

Fisher, P. A., M. Stoolmiller, M. R. Gunnar, and B. O. Burraston. 2007. Effects of a therapeutic intervention for foster preschoolers on diurnal cortisol activity. *Psychoneuroendocrinology* 32(8-10):892-905.

Fisher, P. A., B. M. Lester, D. S. DeGarmo, L. L. Lagasse, H. Lin, S. Shankaran, H. S. Bada, C. R. Bauer, J. Hammond, T. Whitaker, and R. Higgins. 2011. The combined effects of prenatal drug exposure and early adversity on neurobehavioral disinhibition in childhood and adolescence. *Development and Psychopathology* 23(3):777-788.

Flores, E., D. Cicchetti, and F. A. Rogosch. 2005. Predictors of resilience in maltreated and nonmaltreated Latino children. *Developmental Psychology* 41(2):338-351.

Fox, N. A., C. A. Nelson, III, and C. H. Zeanah, Jr. 2013. The effects of early severe psychosocial deprivation on children's cognitive and social development: Lessons from the Bucharest Early Intervention Project. In *Families and child health*, edited by N. S. Landale, S. M. McHale, and A. Booth. New York: Springer. Pp. 33-41.

Fries, E., J. Hesse, J. Hellhammer, and D. H. Hellhammer. 2005. A new view on hypocortisolism. *Psychoneuroendocrinology* 30(10):1010-1016.

Gelles, R. J., and S. Perlman. 2012. *Estimated annual cost of child abuse and neglect*. Chicago: Prevent Child Abuse America.

Ghetti, S., D. M. DeMaster, A. P. Yonelinas, and S. A. Bunge. 2010. Developmental differences in medial temporal lobe function during memory encoding. *Journal of Neuroscience* 30(28):9548-9556.

Giedd, J. N., J. M. Rumsey, F. X. Castellanos, J. C. Rajapakse, D. Kaysen, A. Catherine Vaituzis, Y. C. Vauss, S. D. Hamburger, and J. L. Rapoport. 1996a. A quantitative MRI study of the corpus callosum in children and adolescents. *Developmental Brain Research* 91(2):274-280.

Giedd, J. N., J. W. Snell, N. Lange, J. C. Rajapakse, B. J. Casey, P. L. Kozuch, A. C. Vaituzis, Y. C. Vauss, S. D. Hamburger, D. Kaysen, and J. L. Rapoport. 1996b. Quantitative magnetic resonance imaging of human brain development: Ages 4-18. *Cerebral Cortex* 6(4):551-559.

Gilbert, R., A. Kemp, J. Thoburn, P. Sidebotham, L. Radford, D. Glaser, and H. L. Macmillan. 2009a. Recognising and responding to child maltreatment. *Lancet* 373(9658):167-180.

Gilbert, R., C. S. Widom, K. Browne, D. Fergusson, E. Webb, and S. Janson. 2009b. Burden and consequences of child maltreatment in high-income countries. *Lancet* 373(9657):68-81.

Ginzburg, K., C. Koopman, L. Butler, O. Palesh, H. Kraemer, C. Classen, and D. Spiegel. 2006. Evidence for a dissociative subtype of post-traumatic stress disorder among help-seeking childhood sexual abuse survivors. *Journal of Trauma and Dissociation* 7(2):7-27.

Gogtay, N., J. N. Giedd, L. Lusk, K. M. Hayashi, D. Greenstein, A. C. Vaituzis, T. F. Nugent, III, D. H. Herman, L. S. Clasen, A. W. Toga, J. L. Rapoport, and P. M. Thompson. 2004. Dynamic mapping of human cortical development during childhood through early adulthood. *Proceedings of the National Academy of Sciences of the United States of America* 101(21):8174-8179.

Gould, E., and P. Tanapat. 1999. Stress and hippocampal neurogenesis. *Biological Psychiatry* 46(11):1472-1479.

Graham, J., D. English, A. Litrownik, R. Thompson, E. Briggs, and S. Bangdiwala. 2010. Maltreatment chronicity defined with reference to development: Extension of the social adaptation outcomes findings to peer relations. *Journal of Family Violence* 25(3):311-324.

Gregg, G. R., and E. D. Parks. 1995. Selected Minnesota Multiphasic Personality Inventory-2 scales for identifying women with a history of sexual abuse. *Journal of Nervous and Mental Disease* 183(1):53-56.

Grienenberger, J. F., K. Kelly, and A. Slade. 2005. Maternal reflective functioning, mother-infant affective communication, and infant attachment: Exploring the link between mental states and observed caregiving behavior in the intergenerational transmission of attachment. *Attachment and Human Development* 7(3):299-311.

Griffin, M. G., P. A. Resick, and M. B. Mechanic. 1997. Objective assessment of peritraumatic dissociation: Psychophysiological indicators. *American Journal of Psychiatry* 154(8):1081-1088.

Gunnar, M. R., and C. L. Cheatham. 2003. Brain and behavior interface: Stress and the developing brain. *Infant Mental Health Journal* 24(3):195-211.

Gunnar, M. R., and B. Donzella. 2002. Social regulation of the cortisol levels in early human development. *Psychoneuroendocrinology* 27(1-2):199-220.

Gunnar, M. R., and D. M. Vazquez. 2001. Low cortisol and a flattening of expected daytime rhythm: Potential indices of risk in human development. *Developmental Psychopathology* 13(3):515-538.

Gunnar, M. R., M. H. van Dulmen, T. Achenbach, E. Ames, E. Ames, M. Berry, R. Barth, G. Bohlin, L. Janols, and M. Bohman. 2007. Behavior problems in postinstitutionalized internationally adopted children. *Development and Psychopathology* 19(1):129-148.

Hanson, J. L., M. K. Chung, B. B. Avants, E. A. Shirtcliff, J. C. Gee, R. J. Davidson, and S. D. Pollak. 2010. Early stress is associated with alterations in the orbitofrontal cortex: A tensor-based morphometry investigation of brain structure and behavioral risk. *Journal of Neuroscience* 30(22):7466-7472.

Harmony, T., E. Marosi, A. E. Diaz de Leon, J. Becker, and T. Fernandez. 1990. Effect of sex, psychosocial disadvantages and biological risk factors on EEG maturation. *Electroencephalography and Clinical Neurophysiology* 75(6):482-491.

Hart, H., and K. Rubia. 2012. Neuroimaging of child abuse: A critical review. *Frontiers in Human Neuroscience* 6:52.

Heneghan, A., R. E. K. Stein, M. S. Hurlburt, J. Zhang, J. Rolls-Reutz, E. Fisher, J. Landsverk, and S. M. Horwitz. 2013. Mental health problems in teens investigated by U.S. child welfare agencies. *Journal of Adolescent Health* 52(5):634-640.

Hertsgaard, L., M. Gunnar, M. F. Erickson, and M. Nachmias. 1995. Adrenocortical responses to the strange situation in infants with disorganized/disoriented attachment relationships. *Child Development* 66(4):1100-1106.

Hertzman, C., and T. Boyce. 2010. How experience gets under the skin to create gradients in developmental health. *Annual Review of Public Health* 31:329-347.

Higley, J. D., S. J. Suomi, and M. Linnoila. 1992. A longitudinal study of CSF monoamine metabolite and plasma cortisol concentrations in young rhesus monkeys: Effects of early experience, age, sex and stress on continuity of interindividual differences. *Biological Psychiatry* 32:127-145.

Hofer, M. A. 1994. Hidden regulators in attachment, separation, and loss. *Monographs of the Society for Research in Child Development* 59(2/3):192-207.

Hofer, M. A. 2006. Psychobiological roots of early attachment. *Current Directions in Psychological Science* 15(2):84-88.

Hornor, G. 2008. Reactive attachment disorder. *Journal of Pediatric Health Care* 22(4):234-239.

Hubbard, D. J., and T. C. Pratt. 2002. A meta-analysis of the predictors of delinquency among girls. *Journal of Offender Rehabilitation* 34(3):1-13.

Huizinga, D., B. C. Haberstick, A. Smolen, S. Menard, S. E. Young, R. P. Corley, M. C. Stallings, J. Grotpeter, and J. K. Hewitt. 2006. Childhood maltreatment, subsequent antisocial behavior, and the role of monoamine oxidase a genotype. *Biological Psychiatry* 60(7):677-683.

Hulette, A. C., J. J. Freyd, K. C. Pears, H. K. Kim, P. A. Fisher, and K. A. Becker-Blease. 2008. Dissociation and posttraumatic symptoms in maltreated preschool children. *Journal of Child & Adolescent Trauma* 1(2):93-108.

Hulette, A. C., J. J. Freyd, and P. A. Fisher. 2011. Dissociation in middle childhood among foster children with early maltreatment experiences. *Child Abuse & Neglect* 35(2):123-126.

Hussey, J. M., J. J. Chang, and J. B. Kotch. 2006. Child maltreatment in the United States: Prevalence, risk factors, and adolescent health consequences. *Pediatrics* 118(3):933-942.

Irazuzta, J., J. E. McJunkin, K. Danadian, F. Arnold, and J. Zhang. 1997. Outcome and cost of child abuse. *Child Abuse & Neglect* 21(8):751-757.

Jaffee, S. R., and R. Gallop. 2007. Social, emotional, and academic competence among children who have had contact with child protective services: Prevalence and stability estimates. *Journal of the American Academy of Child and Adolescent Psychiatry* 46(6):757-765.

Jaffee, S. R., and A. K. Maikovich-Fong. 2011. Effects of chronic maltreatment and maltreatment timing on children's behavior and cognitive abilities. *Journal of Child Psychology and Psychiatry and Allied Disciplines* 52(2):184-194.

Jaffee, S. R., A. Caspi, T. E. Moffitt, M. Polo-Tomás, and A. Taylor. 2007. Individual, family, and neighborhood factors distinguish resilient from non-resilient maltreated children: A cumulative stressors model. *Child Abuse & Neglect* 31(3):231-253.

Jans, T., S. Schneck-Seif, T. Weigand, W. Schneider, H. Ellgring, C. Wewetzer, and A. Warnke. 2008. Long-term outcome and prognosis of dissociative disorder with onset in childhood or adolescence. *Child and Adolescent Psychiatry and Mental Health* 2(1):19.

Johnson, D. E., and M. R. Gunnar. 2011. IV. Growth failure in institutionalized children. *Monographs of the Society for Research in Child Development* 76(4):92-126.

Johnson, D. E., D. Guthrie, A. T. Smyke, S. F. Koga, N. A. Fox, C. H. Zeanah, and C. A. Nelson, III. 2010. Growth and associations between auxology, caregiving environment, and cognition in socially deprived Romanian children randomized to foster vs ongoing institutional care. *Archives of Pediatrics and Adolescent Medicine* 164(6):507-516.

Johnson, J. G., P. Cohen, J. Brown, E. M. Smailes, and D. P. Bernstein. 1999. Childhood maltreatment increases risk for personality disorders during early adulthood. *Archives of General Psychiatry* 56(7):600-608.

Johnson, J. G., E. M. Smailes, P. Cohen, J. Brown, and D. P. Bernstein. 2000. Associations between four types of childhood neglect and personality disorder symptoms during adolescence and early adulthood: Findings of a community-based longitudinal study. *Journal of Personality Disorders* 14(2):171-187.

Johnson, J. G., P. Cohen, S. Kasen, and J. S. Brook. 2002. Childhood adversities associated with risk for eating disorders or weight problems during adolescence or early adulthood. *American Journal Psychiatry* 159(3):394-400.

Jones, D. J., D. K. Runyan, T. Lewis, A. J. Litrownik, M. M. Black, T. Wiley, D. E. English, L. J. Proctor, B. L. Jones, and D. S. Nagin. 2010. Trajectories of childhood sexual abuse and early adolescent HIV/AIDS risk behaviors: The role of other maltreatment, witnessed violence, and child gender. *Journal of Clinical Child and Adolescent Psychology* 39(5):667-680.

Jonson-Reid, M., B. Drake, J. Kim, S. Porterfield, and L. Han. 2004. A prospective analysis of the relationship between reported child maltreatment and special education eligibility among poor children. *Child Maltreatment* 9(4):382-394.

Jonson-Reid, M., P. L. Kohl, and B. Drake. 2012. Child and adult outcomes of chronic child maltreatment. *Pediatrics* 129(5):839-845.

Kaplan, S. J., D. Pelcovitz, S. Salzinger, M. Weiner, F. S. Mandel, M. L. Lesser, and V. E. Labruna. 1998. Adolescent physical abuse: Risk for adolescent psychiatric disorders. *American Journal of Psychiatry* 155(7):954-959.

Kaplow, J. B., and C. S. Widom. 2007. Age of onset of child maltreatment predicts long-term mental health outcomes. *Journal of Abnormal Psychology* 116(1):176-187.

Kearney, C. A., A. Wechsler, H. Kaur, and A. Lemos-Miller. 2010. Posttraumatic stress disorder in maltreated youth: A review of contemporary research and thought. *Clinical Child and Family Psychology Review* 13(1):46-76.

Keck Seeley, S. M., S. L. Perosa, and L. M. Perosa. 2004. A validation study of the adolescent dissociative experiences scale. *Child Abuse & Neglect* 28(7):755-769.

Keiley, M. K., T. R. Howe, K. A. Dodge, J. E. Bates, and G. S. Petti. 2001. The timing of child physical maltreatment: A cross-domain growth analysis of impact on adolescent externalizing and internalizing problems. *Development and Psychopathology* 13(4):891-912.

Kendall-Tackett, K. A., L. M. Williams, and D. Finkelhor. 1993. Impact of sexual abuse on children: A review and synthesis of recent empirical studies. *Psychological Bulletin* 113(1):164-180.

Kim, J., and D. Cicchetti. 2010. Longitudinal pathways linking child maltreatment, emotion regulation, peer relations, and psychopathology. *Journal of Child Psychology and Psychiatry* 51(6):706-716.

Kim, J. J., and K. S. Yoon. 1998. Stress: Metaplastic effects in the hippocampus. *Trends in Neurosciences* 21(12):505-509.

Kim, K., P. K. Trickett, and F. W. Putnam. 2010. Childhood experiences of sexual abuse and later parenting practices among non-offending mothers of sexually abused and comparison girls. *Child Abuse & Neglect* 34(8):610-622.

Kisiel, C. L., and J. S. Lyons. 2001. Dissociation as a mediator of psychopathology among sexually abused children and adolescents. *American Journal of Psychiatry* 158(7):1034-1039.

Kitayama, N., V. Vaccarino, M. Kutner, P. Weiss, and J. D. Bremner. 2005. Magnetic resonance imaging (MRI) measurement of hippocampal volume in posttraumatic stress disorder: A meta-analysis. *Journal of Affective Disorders* 88(1):79-86.

Kitterle, F. L. 1995. *Hemispheric communication: Mechanisms and models.* Hillsdale, NJ: Lawrence Erlbaum Associates.

Kleindienst, N., M. F. Limberger, U. W. Ebner-Priemer, J. Keibel-Mauchnik, A. Dyer, M. Berger, C. Schmahl, and M. Bohus. 2011. Dissociation predicts poor response to dialectial behavioral therapy in female patients with borderline personality disorder. *Journal of Personality Disorders* 25(4):432-447.

Klinnert, M., J. Campos, J. Sorce, R. Emde, and M. Svejda. 1983. Emotions as behavior regulators in infancy: Social referencing in infancy. In *Emotion: Theory, research and experience*, edited by R. P. H. Kellerman. New York: Academic Press. Pp. 57-86.

Knutson, J. F., S. M. Taber, A. J. Murray, N.-L. Valles, and G. Koeppl. 2010. The role of care neglect and supervisory neglect in childhood obesity in a disadvantaged sample. *Journal of Pediatric Psychology* 35(5):523-532.

Kolko, D. J. 2010. Posttraumatic stress symptoms in children and adolescents referred for child welfare investigation a national sample of in-home and out-of-home care. *Child Maltreatment* 15(1):48-63.

Kotch, J. B., T. Lewis, J. M. Hussey, D. English, R. Thompson, A. J. Litrownik, D. K. Runyan, S. I. Bangdiwala, B. Margolis, and H. Dubowitz. 2008. Importance of early neglect for childhood aggression. *Pediatrics* 121(4):725-731.

Kreppner, J. M., T. G. O'Connor, and M. Rutter. 2001. Can inattention/overactivity be an institutional deprivation syndrome? *Journal of Abnormal Child Psychology* 29(6):513-528.

Kreppner, J. M., M. Rutter, C. Beckett, J. Castle, E. Colvert, C. Groothues, A. Hawkins, T. G. O'Connor, S. Stevens, and E. J. Sonuga-Barke. 2007. Normality and impairment following profound early institutional deprivation: A longitudinal follow-up into early adolescence. *Developmental Psychology* 43(4):931-946.

Kurtz, P. D., J. M. Gaudin, Jr., J. S. Wodarski, and P. T. Howing. 1993. Maltreatment and the school-aged child: School performance consequences. *Child Abuse & Neglect* 17(5):581-589.

Lanius, R., M. Miller, E. Wolf, B. Brand, P. Frewen, E. Vermetten, and D. Spiegel. 2013. *Dissociative subtype of PTSD*. Washington, DC: U.S. Department of Veterans Affairs.

Lanktree, C. B., A. M. Gilbert, J. Briere, N. Taylor, K. Chen, C. A. Maida, and W. R. Saltzman. 2008. Multi-informant assessment of maltreated children: Convergent and discriminant validity of the TSCC and TSCYC. *Child Abuse & Neglect* 32(6):621-625.

Lansford, J. E., K. A. Dodge, G. S. Pettit, J. E. Bates, J. Crozier, and J. Kaplow. 2002. A 12-year prospective study of the long-term effects of early child physical maltreatment on psychological, behavioral, and academic problems in adolescence. *Archives of Pediatrics and Adolescent Medicine* 156(8):824-830.

Lansford, J. E., S. Miller-Johnson, L. J. Berlin, K. A. Dodge, J. E. Bates, and G. S. Pettit. 2007. Early physical abuse and later violent delinquency: A prospective longitudinal study. *Child Maltreatment* 12(3):233-245.

Lansford, J. E., M. M. Criss, K. A. Dodge, D. S. Shaw, G. S. Pettit, and J. E. Bates. 2009. Trajectories of physical discipline: Early childhood antecedents and developmental outcomes. *Child Development* 80(5):1385-1402.

Lansford, J. E., K. A. Dodge, G. S. Pettit, and J. E. Bates. 2010. Does physical abuse in early childhood predict substance use in adolescence and early adulthood? *Child Maltreatment* 15(2):190-194.

Larson, M. C., M. R. Gunnar, and L. Hertsgaard. 1991. The effects of morning naps, car trips, and maternal separation on adrenocortical activity in human infants. *Child Development* 62(2):362-372.

Lavenex, P., P. Banta Lavenex, and D. G. Amaral. 2007. Postnatal development of the primate hippocampal formation. *Developmental Neuroscience* 29(1-2):179-192.

Leiter, J., and M. C. Johnsen. 1997. Child maltreatment and school performance declines: An event-history analysis. *American Educational Research Journal* 34(3):563-589.

Levine, S., S. G. Wiener, and C. L. Coe. 1993. Temporal and social factors influencing behavioral and hormonal responses to separation in mother and infant squirrel monkeys. *Psychoneuroendocrinology* 18(4):297-306.

Lewis, E. E., M. Dozier, J. Ackerman, and S. Sepulveda-Kozakowski. 2007. The effect of placement instability on adopted children's inhibitory control abilities and oppositional behavior. *Developmental Psychology* 43(6):1415-1427.

Lewis-Morrarty, E., M. Dozier, K. Bernard, S. M. Terracciano, and S. V. Moore. 2012. Cognitive flexibility and theory of mind outcomes among foster children: Preschool follow-up results of a randomized clinical trial. *Journal of Adolescent Health* 51(2 Suppl.):S17-S22.

Libby, A. M., M. R. Sills, N. K. Thurston, and H. D. Orton. 2003. Costs of childhood physical abuse: Comparing inflicted and unintentional traumatic brain injuries. *Pediatrics* 112(1):58-65.

Lissau, I., and T. I. Sorensen. 1994. Parental neglect during childhood and increased risk of obesity in young adulthood. *Lancet* 343(8893):324-327.

Lodico, M. A., and R. J. DiClemente. 1994. The association between childhood sexual abuse and prevalence of HIV-related risk behaviors. *Clinical Pediatrics* 33(8):498-502.

Loman, M. M., K. L. Wiik, K. A. Frenn, S. D. Pollak, and M. R. Gunnar. 2009. Postinstitutionalized children's development: Growth, cognitive, and language outcomes. *Journal of Developmental and Behavioral Pediatrics* 30(5):426-434.

Loman, M. M., A. E. Johnson, A. Westerlund, S. D. Pollak, C. A. Nelson, and M. R. Gunnar. 2013. The effect of early deprivation on executive attention in middle childhood. *Journal of Child Psychology and Psychiatry* 54(1):37-45.

Luthar, S. S., D. Cicchetti, and B. Becker. 2000. The construct of resilience: A critical evaluation and guidelines for future work. *Child Development* 71(3):543-562.

Lynch, M., and D. Cicchetti. 1998. An ecological-transactional analysis of children and contexts: The longitudinal interplay among child maltreatment, community violence, and children's symptomatology. *Developmental Psychopathology* 10(2):235-257.

Lyons, S. J., J. R. Henly, and J. R. Schuerman. 2005. Informal support in maltreating families: Its effect on parenting practices. *Children and Youth Services Review* 27(1): 21-38.

Lyons-Ruth, K. 2008. Contributions of the mother-infant relationship to dissociative, borderline, and conduct symptoms in young adulthood. *Infant Mental Health Journal* 29(3):203-218.

Lyons-Ruth, K., L. Alpern, and B. Repacholi. 1993. Disorganized infant attachment classification and maternal psychosocial problems as predictors of hostile-aggressive behavior in the preschool classroom. *Child Development* 64(2):572-585.

Lyons-Ruth, K., J. F. Bureau, C. D. Riley, and A. F. Atlas-Corbett. 2009. Socially indiscriminate attachment behavior in the strange situation: Convergent and discriminant validity in relation to caregiving risk, later behavior problems, and attachment insecurity. *Development and Psychopathology* 21(2):355-372.

Macfie, J., D. Cicchetti, and S. L. Toth. 2001. Dissociation in maltreated versus nonmaltreated preschool-aged children. *Child Abuse & Neglect* 25(9):1253-1267.

Maheu, F. S., M. Dozier, A. E. Guyer, D. Mandell, E. Peloso, K. Poeth, J. Jenness, J. Y. Lau, J. P. Ackerman, D. S. Pine, and M. Ernst. 2010. A preliminary study of medial temporal lobe function in youths with a history of caregiver deprivation and emotional neglect. *Cognitive, Affective, and Behavioral Neuroscience* 10(1):34-49.

Main, M., and J. Solomon. 1990. Procedures for identifying infants as disorganized/disoriented during the Ainsworth Strange Situation. *Attachment in the Preschool Years: Theory, Research, and Intervention* 1:121-160.

Malatesta, C. Z., and C. E. Izard. 1984. The ontogenesis of human social signals: From biological imperative to symbol utilization. In *The psychobiology of affective development*, edited by N. A. Fox and R. J. Davidson. Hillsdale, NJ: Psychology Press. Pp. 161-206.

Manly, J. T., J. E. Kim, F. A. Rogosch, and D. Cicchetti. 2001. Dimensions of child maltreatment and children's adjustment: Contributions of developmental timing and subtype. *Development and Psychopathology* 13(4):759-782.

Marshall, P. J., N. A. Fox, and Bucharest Early Intervention Project Core Group. 2004. A comparison of the electroencephalogram between institutionalized and community children in Romania. *Journal of Cognitive Neuroscience* 16(8):1327-1338.

Marshall, P. J., B. C. Reeb, N. A. Fox, C. A. Nelson, and C. H. Zeanah. 2008. Effects of early intervention on EEG power and coherence in previously institutionalized children in Romania. *Developmental Psychopathology* 20(3):861-880.

Masten, A. S., and A. Tellegen. 2012. Resilience in developmental psychopathology: Contributions of the project competence longitudinal study. *Development and Psychopathology* 24(2):345-361.

Maughan, A., and D. Cicchetti. 2002. Impact of child maltreatment and interadult violence on children's emotion regulation abilities and socioemotional adjustment. *Child Development* 73(5):1525-1542.

Maxfield, M. G., and C. S. Widom. 1996. The cycle of violence: Revisited 6 years later. *Archives of Pediatrics & Adolescent Medicine* 150(4):390-395.

McCabe, K. M., R. L. Hough, M. Yeh, S. E. Lucchini, and A. Hazen. 2005. The relation between violence exposure and conduct problems among adolescents: A prospective study. *American Journal of Orthopsychiatry* 75(4):575-584.

McCurdy, K. 2005. The influence of support and stress on maternal attitudes. *Child Abuse & Neglect* 29(3):251-268.

McDermott, J. M., A. Westerlund, C. H. Zeanah, C. A. Nelson, and N. A. Fox. 2012. Early adversity and neural correlates of executive function: Implications for academic adjustment. *Developmental Cognitive Neuroscience* 2(Suppl. 1):S59-S66.

McEwen, B. S. 1998. Stress, adaptation, and disease. Allostasis and allostatic load. *Annals of the New York Academy of Sciences* 840:33-44.

McGloin, J. M., and C. S. Widom. 2001. Resilience among abused and neglected children grown up. *Development and Psychopathology* 13(4):1021-1038.

McGowan, P. O., A. Sasaki, T. C. T. Huang, A. Unterberger, M. Suderman, C. Ernst, M. J. Meaney, G. Turecki, and M. Szyf. 2008. Promoter-wide hypermethylation of the ribosomal RNA gene promoter in the suicide brain. *PLoS ONE* 3(5).

McGowan, P. O., A. Sasaki, A. C. D'Alessio, S. Dymov, B. Labonte, M. Szyf, G. Turecki, and M. J. Meaney. 2009. Epigenetic regulation of the glucocorticoid receptor in human brain associates with childhood abuse. *Nature Neuroscience* 12(3):342-348.

McGowan, P. O., M. Suderman, A. Sasaki, T. C. T. Huang, M. Hallett, M. J. Meaney, and M. Szyf. 2011. Broad epigenetic signature of maternal care in the brain of adult rats. *PLoS ONE* 6(2).

McLaughlin, K. A., N. A. Fox, C. H. Zeanah, M. A. Sheridan, P. Marshall, and C. A. Nelson. 2010. Delayed maturation in brain electrical activity partially explains the association between early environmental deprivation and symptoms of attention-deficit/hyperactivity disorder. *Biological Psychiatry* 68(4):329-336.

Meaney, M. J., and M. Szyf. 2005. Environmental programming of stress responses through DNA methylation: Life at the interface between a dynamic environment and a fixed genome. *Dialogues in Clinical Neuroscience* 7(2):103-123.

Mehta, M. A., N. I. Golembo, C. Nosarti, E. Colvert, A. Mota, S. C. R. Williams, M. Rutter, and E. J. S. Sonuga-Barke. 2009. Amygdala, hippocampal and corpus callosum size following severe early institutional deprivation: The English and Romanian adoptees study pilot. *Journal of Child Psychology and Psychiatry* 50(8):943-951.

Miller, E. K., and J. D. Cohen. 2001. An integrative theory of prefrontal cortex function. *Annual Review of Neuroscience* 24:167-202.

Milner, J. S. 2000. Social information processing and child physical abuse: Theory and research. *Motivation and Child Maltreatment* 46:39-84.

Moriceau, S., T. L. Roth, and R. M. Sullivan. 2010. Rodent model of infant attachment learning and stress. *Developmental Psychobiology* 52(7):651-660.

Mueller, S. C., F. S. Maheu, M. Dozier, E. Peloso, D. Mandell, E. Leibenluft, D. S. Pine, and M. Ernst. 2010. Early-life stress is associated with impairment in cognitive control in adolescence: An fMRI study. *Neuropsychologia* 48(10):3037-3044.

Murray-Close, D., G. Han, D. Cicchetti, N. R. Crick, and F. A. Rogosch. 2008. Neuroendocrine regulation and physical and relational aggression: The moderating roles of child maltreatment and gender. *Developmental Psychology* 44(4):1160-1176.

National Center for PTSD. 2013. *DSM-5 criteria for PTSD.* Washington, DC: U.S. Department of Veterans Affairs.

Natsuaki, M. N., D. Cicchetti, and F. A. Rogosch. 2009. Examining the developmental history of child maltreatment, peer relations, and externalizing problems among adolescents with symptoms of paranoid personality disorder. *Development and Psychopathology* 21(4):1181-1193.

Nelson, C. A. 2007. A neurobiological perspective on early human deprivation. *Child Development Perspectives* 1(1):13-18.

Nelson, C. A., III, C. H. Zeanah, and N. A. Fox. 2007a. The effects of early deprivation on brain-behavioral development: The Bucharest Early Intervention Project. In *Adolescent psychopathology and the developing brain: Integrating brain and prevention science*, edited by D. Romer and E. F. Walker. New York: Oxford University Press. Pp. 197-215.

Nelson, C. A., C. H. Zeanah, N. A. Fox, P. J. Marshall, A. T. Smyke, and D. Guthrie. 2007b. Cognitive recovery in socially deprived young children: The Bucharest Early Intervention Project. *Science* 318(5858):1937-1940.

Nelson, C. A., K. Bos, M. R. Gunnar, and E. J. S. Sonuga-Barke. 2011. V. The neurobiological toll of early human deprivation. *Monographs of the Society for Research in Child Development* 76(4):127-146.

New, M., and L. Berliner. 2000. Mental health service utilization by victims of crime. *Journal of Traumatic Stress* 13(4):693-707.

Nikulina, V., C. S. Widom, and S. Czaja. 2011. The role of childhood neglect and childhood poverty in predicting mental health, academic achievement and crime in adulthood. *American Journal of Community Psychology* 48(3-4):309-321.

Noll, J. G., P. K. Trickett, and F. W. Putnam. 2003. A prospective investigation of the impact of childhood sexual abuse on the development of sexuality. *Journal of Consulting and Clinical Psychology* 71(3):575-586.

Noll, J. G., M. H. Zeller, P. K. Trickett, and F. W. Putnam. 2007. Obesity risk for female victims of childhood sexual abuse: A prospective study. *Pediatrics* 120(1):e61-e67.

Noll, J. G., C. E. Shenk, and K. T. Putnam. 2009. Childhood sexual abuse and adolescent pregnancy: A meta-analytic update. *Journal of Pediatric Psychology* 34(4):366-378.

NRC (National Research Council). 1993. *Understanding child abuse and neglect.* Washington, DC: National Academy Press.

O'Connor, T. G., R. S. Marvin, M. Rutter, J. T. Olrick, P. A. Britner, C. Beckett, M. Brophy, J. Castle, E. Colvert, C. Croft, J. Dunn, C. Groothues, and J. Kreppner. 2003. Child-parent attachment following early institutional deprivation. *Development and Psychopathology* 15(1):19-38.

Offer, D., M. Kaiz, K. I. Howard, and E. S. Bennett. 2000. The altering of reported experiences. *Journal of the American Academy of Child and Adolescent Psychiatry* 39(6):735-742.

Ogawa, J. R., L. A. Sroufe, N. S. Weinfield, E. A. Carlson, and B. Egeland. 1997. Development and the fragmented self: Longitudinal study of dissociative symptomatology in a nonclinical sample. *Development and Psychopathology* 9(4):855-879.

Olivan, G. 2003. Catch-up growth assessment in long-term physically neglected and emotionally abused preschool age male children. *Child Abuse & Neglect* 27(1):103-108.

Olofsson, J. K., S. Nordin, H. Sequeira, and J. Polich. 2008. Affective picture processing: An integrative review of ERP findings. *Biological Psychology* 77(3):247-265.

Otto, T., and H. Eichenbaum. 1992. Neuronal activity in the hippocampus during delayed non-match to sample performance in rats: Evidence for hippocampal processing in recognition memory. *Hippocampus* 2(3):323-334.

Pears, K. C., H. K. Kim, and P. A. Fisher. 2008. Psychosocial and cognitive functioning of children with specific profiles of maltreatment. *Child Abuse & Neglect* 32(10):958-971.

Perez, C. M., and C. S. Widom. 1994. Childhood victimization and long-term intellectual and academic outcomes. *Child Abuse & Neglect* 18(8):617-633.

Pollak, S. D., and P. Sinha. 2002. Effects of early experience on children's recognition of facial displays of emotion. *Developmental Psychology* 38(5):784-791.

Pollak, S. D., and S. A. Tolley-Schell. 2003. Selective attention to facial emotion in physically abused children. *Journal of Abnormal Psychology* 112(3):323-338.

Pollak, S. D., D. Cicchetti, R. Klorman, and J. T. Brumaghim. 1997. Cognitive brain event-related potentials and emotion processing in maltreated children. *Child Development* 68(5):773-787.

Pollak, S. D., D. Cicchetti, K. Hornung, and A. Reed. 2000. Recognizing emotion in faces: Developmental effects of child abuse and neglect. *Developmental Psychology* 36(5):679-688.

Pollak, S. D., R. Klorman, J. E. Thatcher, and D. Cicchetti. 2001. P3b reflects maltreated children's reactions to facial displays of emotion. *Psychophysiology* 38(2):267-274.

Pomerleau, A., G. Malcuit, J.-F. Chicoine, R. Séguin, C. Belhumeur, P. Germain, I. Amyot, and G. Jéliu. 2005. Health status, cognitive and motor development of young children adopted from China, East Asia, and Russia across the first 6 months after adoption. *International Journal of Behavioral Development* 29(5):445-457.

Power, R. A., L. Lecky-Thompson, H. L. Fisher, S. Cohen-Woods, G. M. Hosang, R. Uher, G. Powell-Smith, R. Keers, M. Tropeano, A. Korszun, L. Jones, I. Jones, M. J. Owen, N. Craddock, I. W. Craig, A. E. Farmer, and P. McGuffin. 2013. The interaction between child maltreatment, adult stressful life events and the 5-HTTLPR in major depression. *Journal of Psychiatric Research* 47(8):1032-1035.

Price, J. M., and K. Glad. 2003. Hostile attributional tendencies in maltreated children. *Journal of Abnormal Child Psychology* 31(3):329-343.

Putnam, F. W. 1997. *Dissociation in children and adolescents: A developmental perspective.* New York: Guilford Press.

Richert, K. A., V. G. Carrion, A. Karchemskiy, and A. L. Reiss. 2006. Regional differences of the prefrontal cortex in pediatric PTSD: An MRI study. *Depression and Anxiety* 23(1):17-25.

Roeber, B. J., C. L. Tober, D. M. Bolt, and S. D. Pollak. 2012. Gross motor development in children adopted from orphanage settings. *Developmental Medicine and Child Neurology* 54(6):527-531.

Rogosch, F. A., D. Cicchetti, and J. L. Aber. 1995. The role of child maltreatment in early deviations in cognitive and affective processing abilities and later peer relationship problems. *Development and Psychopathology* 7(4):591-609.

Ross, L. T., and E. M. Hill. 2002. Childhood unpredictability, schemas for unpredictability, and risk taking. *Social Behavior and Personality: An International Journal* 30(5): 453-473.

Ross, M. 1989. Relation of implicit theories to the construction of personal histories. *Psychological Review* 96(2):341-357.

Rovi, S., P. H. Chen, and M. S. Johnson. 2004. The economic burden of hospitalizations associated with child abuse and neglect. *American Journal of Public Health* 94(4):586-590.

Rubia, K., A. B. Smith, J. Woolley, C. Nosarti, I. Heyman, E. Taylor, and M. Brammer. 2006. Progressive increase of frontostriatal brain activation from childhood to adulthood during event-related tasks of cognitive control. *Human Brain Mapping* 27(12):973-993.

Sanchez, M. M. 2006. The impact of early adverse care on HPA axis development: Nonhuman primate models. *Hormones and Behavior* 50(4):623-631.

Sapolsky, R. M., H. Uno, C. S. Rebert, and C. E. Finch. 1990. Hippocampal damage associated with prolonged glucocorticoid exposure in primates. *Journal of Neuroscience* 10(9):2897-2902.

Schatzberg, A. F., and S. Lindley. 2008. Glucocorticoid antagonists in neuropsychiatric [corrected] disorders. *European Journal of Pharmacology* 583(2-3):358-364.

Schmahl, C. G., E. Vermetten, B. M. Elzinga, and J. Douglas Bremner. 2003. Magnetic resonance imaging of hippocampal and amygdala volume in women with childhood abuse and borderline personality disorder. *Psychiatry Research* 122(3):193-198.

Schuengel, C., I. H. V. Marinus, M. J. Bakermans-Kranenburg, and M. Blom. 1998. Frightening maternal behaviour, unresolved loss, and disorganized infant attachment: A pilot-study. *Journal of Reproductive and Infant Psychology* 16(4):277-283.

Senn, T., M. P. Carey, and P. A. Vanable. 2008. Childhood and adolescent sexual abuse and subsequent sexual risk behavior: Evidence from controlled studies, methodological critique, and suggestions for research. *Clinical Psychology Review* 28(5):711-735.

Shackman, J. E., A. J. Shackman, and S. D. Pollak. 2007. Physical abuse amplifies attention to threat and increases anxiety in children. *Emotion* 7(4):838.

Shannon, C., M. Champoux, and S. J. Suomi. 1998. Rearing condition and plasma cortisol in rhesus monkey infants. *American Journal of Primatology* 46(4):311-321.

Shapiro, D. N., J. B. Kaplow, L. Amaya-Jackson, and K. A. Dodge. 2012. Behavioral markers of coping and psychiatric symptoms among sexually abused children. *Journal of Traumatic Stress* 25(2):157-163.

Sheridan, M. A., N. A. Fox, C. H. Zeanah, K. A. McLaughlin, and C. A. Nelson, III. 2012. Variation in neural development as a result of exposure to institutionalization early in childhood. *Proceedings of the National Academy of Sciences of the United States of America* 109(32):12927-12932.

Shields, A., and D. Cicchetti. 2001. Parental maltreatment and emotion dysregulation as risk factors for bullying and victimization in middle childhood. *Journal of Clinical Child Psychology* 30(3):349-363.

Shipman, K. L., and J. Zeman. 2001. Socialization of children's emotion regulation in mother-child dyads: A developmental psychopathology perspective. *Development and Psychopathology* 13(2):317-336.

Shonkoff, J. P., A. S. Garner, B. S. Siegel, M. I. Dobbins, M. F. Earls, A. S. Garner, L. McGuinn, J. Pascoe, and D. L. Wood. 2012. The lifelong effects of early childhood adversity and toxic stress. *Pediatrics* 129(1):e232-e246.

Silbert, M. H., and A. M. Pines. 1983. Early sexual exploitation as an influence in prostitution. *Social Work* 28(4):285-289.

Simpson, T. L., and W. R. Miller. 2002. Concomitance between childhood sexual and physical abuse and substance use problems. A review. *Clinical Psychology Review* 22(1):27-77.

Smith, C., and T. P. Thornberry. 1995. The relationship between childhood maltreatment and adolescent involvement in delinquency. *Criminology* 33(4):451-481.

Smith, C. A., T. O. Ireland, and T. P. Thornberry. 2005. Adolescent maltreatment and its impact on young adult antisocial behavior. *Child Abuse & Neglect* 29(10):1099-1119.

Smyke, A. T., A. Dumitrescu, and C. H. Zeanah. 2002. Attachment disturbances in young children. I: The continuum of caretaking casualty. *Journal of the American Academy of Child and Adolescent Psychiatry* 41(8):972-982.

Sowell, E. R., B. S. Peterson, P. M. Thompson, S. E. Welcome, A. L. Henkenius, and A. W. Toga. 2003. Mapping cortical change across the human life span. *Nature Neuroscience* 6(3):309-315.

Spann, M. N., L. C. Mayes, J. H. Kalmar, J. Guiney, F. Y. Womer, B. Pittman, C. M. Mazure, R. Sinha, and H. P. Blumberg. 2012. Childhood abuse and neglect and cognitive flexibility in adolescents. *Child Neuropsychology* 18(2):182-189.

Sperry, D. M., and C. S. Widom. 2013. Child abuse and neglect, social support, and psychopathology in adulthood: A prospective investigation. *Child Abuse & Neglect* 37(6): 415-425.

Spiegel, D., R. J. Loewenstein, R. Lewis-Fernández, V. Sar, D. Simeon, E. Vermetten, E. Cardeña, and P. F. Dell. 2011. Dissociative disorders in DSM-5. *Depression and Anxiety* 28(12):E17-E45.

Springs, F. E., and W. N. Friedrich. 1992. Health risk behaviors and medical sequelae of childhood sexual abuse. *Mayo Clinic Proceedings* 67(6):527-532.

Staudt, M. M. 2003. Mental health services utilization by maltreated children: Research findings and recommendations. *Child Maltreatment* 8(3):195-203.

Stein, D. J., K. C. Koenen, M. J. Friedman, E. Hill, K. A. McLaughlin, M. Petukhova, A. M. Ruscio, V. Shahly, D. Spiegel, G. Borges, B. Bunting, J. M. Caldas-de-Almeida, G. de Girolamo, K. Demyttenaere, S. Florescu, J. M. Haro, E. G. Karam, V. Kovess-Masfety, S. Lee, H. Matschinger, M. Mladenova, J. Posada-Villa, H. Tachimori, M. C. Viana, and R. C. Kessler. 2013. Dissociation in posttraumatic stress disorder: Evidence from the world mental health surveys. *Biological Psychiatry* 73(4):302-312.

Stoltz, J. A., K. Shannon, T. Kerr, R. Zhang, J. S. Montaner, and E. Wood. 2007. Associations between childhood maltreatment and sex work in a cohort of drug-using youth. *Social Science & Medicine* 65(6):1214-1221.

Stouthamer-Loeber, M., R. Loeber, D. L. Homish, and E. Wei. 2001. Maltreatment of boys and the development of disruptive and delinquent behavior. *Development and Psychopathology* 13(4):941-955.

Suomi, S. J. 1997. Early determinants of behaviour: Evidence from primate studies. *British Medical Bulletin* 53(1):170-184.

Swanston, H. Y., J. S. Tebbutt, B. I. O'Toole, and R. K. Oates. 1997. Sexually abused children 5 years after presentation: A case-control study. *Pediatrics* 100(4):600-608.

Szyf, M., and J. Bick. 2013. DNA methylation: A mechanism for embedding early life experiences in the genome. *Child Development* 84(1):49-57.

Teicher, M. H., S. L. Andersen, A. Polcari, C. M. Anderson, C. P. Navalta, and D. M. Kim. 2003. The neurobiological consequences of early stress and childhood maltreatment. *Neuroscience and Biobehavioral Reviews* 27(1-2):33-44.

Teicher, M. H., N. L. Dumont, Y. Ito, C. Vaituzis, J. N. Giedd, and S. L. Andersen. 2004. Childhood neglect is associated with reduced corpus callosum area. *Biological Psychiatry* 56(2):80-85.

Thompson, R. A., and C. A. Nelson. 2001. Developmental science and the media. Early brain development. *American Psychologist* 56(1):5-15.

Thompson, R., T. R. A. Wiley, T. Lewis, D. J. English, H. Dubowitz, A. J. Litrownik, P. Isbell, and S. Block. 2012. Links between traumatic experiences and expectations about the future in high risk youth. *Psychological Trauma: Theory, Research, Practice, and Policy* 4(3):293-302.

Thornberry, T. P., T. O. Ireland, and C. A. Smith. 2001. The importance of timing: The varying impact of childhood and adolescent maltreatment on multiple problem outcomes. *Development and Psychopathology* 13(4):957-979.

Thornberry, T. P., K. L. Henry, T. O. Ireland, and C. A. Smith. 2010. The causal impact of childhood-limited maltreatment and adolescent maltreatment on early adult adjustment. *Journal of Adolescent Health* 46(4):359-365.

Tolin, D. F., and E. B. Foa. 2006. Sex differences in trauma and posttraumatic stress disorder: A quantitative review of 25 years of research. *Psychological Bulletin* 132(6):959-992.

Tottenham, N., and M. A. Sheridan. 2010. A review of adversity, the amygdala and the hippocampus: A consideration of developmental timing. *Frontiers in Human Neuroscience* 3(68).

Tottenham, N., J. W. Tanaka, A. C. Leon, T. McCarry, M. Nurse, T. A. Hare, D. J. Marcus, A. Westerlund, B. Casey, and C. Nelson. 2009. The NimStim set of facial expressions: Judgments from untrained research participants. *Psychiatry Research* 168(3):242-249.

Tottenham, N., T. A. Hare, B. T. Quinn, T. W. McCarry, M. Nurse, T. Gilhooly, A. Millner, A. Galvan, M. C. Davidson, I. Eigsti, K. M. Thomas, P. J. Freed, E. S. Booma, M. R. Gunnar, M. Altemus, J. Aronson, and B. J. Casey. 2010. Prolonged institutional rearing is associated with atypically large amygdala volume and difficulties in emotion regulation. *Developmental Science* 13(1):46-61.

Tottenham, N., T. A. Hare, A. Millner, T. Gilhooly, J. D. Zevin, and B. J. Casey. 2011. Elevated amygdala response to faces following early deprivation. *Developmental Science* 14(2):190-204.

Trickett, P. K., J. G. Noll, A. Reiffman, and F. W. Putnam. 2001. Variants of intrafamilial sexual abuse experience: Implications for short- and long-term development. *Development and Psychopathology* 13(4):1001-1019.

Trickett, P. K., J. G. Noll, and F. W. Putnam. 2011. The impact of sexual abuse on female development: Lessons from a multigenerational, longitudinal research study. *Development and Psychopathology* 23(2):453-476.

Tronick, E. Z. 1989. Emotions and emotional communication in infants. *American Psychologist* 44(2):112-119.

Twardosz, S., and J. R. Lutzker. 2010. Child maltreatment and the developing brain: A review of neuroscience perspectives. *Aggression and Violent Behavior* 15(1):59-68.

van Ijzendoorn, M. H., and F. Juffer. 2006. The Emanuel Miller memorial lecture 2006: Adoption as intervention. Meta-analytic evidence for massive catch-up and plasticity in physical, socio-emotional, and cognitive development. *Journal of Child Psychology and Psychiatry* 47(12):1228-1245.

van Ijzendoorn, M. H., and C. Schuengel. 1996. The measurement of dissociation in normal and clinical populations: Meta-analytic validation of the Dissociative Experiences Scale (DES). *Clinical Psychology Review* 16(5):365-382.

van Tilburg, M. A., D. K. Runyan, A. J. Zolotor, J. C. Graham, H. Dubowitz, A. J. Litrownik, E. Flaherty, D. K. Chitkara, and W. E. Whitehead. 2010. Unexplained gastrointestinal symptoms after abuse in a prospective study of children at risk for abuse and neglect. *Annals of Family Medicine* 8(2):134-140.

Vanderwert, R. E., P. J. Marshall, C. A. Nelson, C. H. Zeanah, and N. A. Fox. 2010. Timing of intervention affects brain electrical activity in children exposed to severe psychosocial neglect. *PLoS ONE* 5(7):e11415.

Vorria, P., Z. Papaligoura, J. Sarafidou, M. Kopakaki, J. Dunn, M. H. van Ijzendoorn, and A. Kontopoulou. 2006. The development of adopted children after institutional care: A follow-up study. *Journal of Child Psychology and Psychiatry* 47(12):1246-1253.

Walker, E. A., A. Gelfand, W. J. Katon, M. P. Koss, M. Von Korff, D. Bernstein, and J. Russo. 1999. Adult health status of women with histories of childhood abuse and neglect. *American Journal of Medicine* 107(4):332-339.

Wang, C.-T., and J. Holton. 2007. *Total estimated cost of child abuse and neglect in the United States.* Chicago: Prevent Child Abuse America.

Watamura, S. E., A. M. Sebanc, and M. R. Gunnar. 2002. Rising cortisol at childcare: Relations with nap, rest, and temperament. *Developmental Psychobiology* 40(1):33-42.

Waters, H., A. Hyder, Y. Rajkotia, S. Basu, J. A. Rehwinkel, and A. Butchart. 2004. *The economic dimensions of interpersonal violence.* Geneva: Department of Injuries and Violence Prevention, World Health Organization.

Weaver, I. C., N. Cervoni, F. A. Champagne, A. C. D'Alessio, S. Sharma, J. R. Seckl, S. Dymov, M. Szyf, and M. J. Meaney. 2004. Epigenetic programming by maternal behavior. *Nature Neuroscience* 7(8):847-854.

Webb, E. 2013. Poverty, maltreatment and attention deficit hyperactivity disorder. *Archives of Disease in Childhood* 98(6):397-400.

Wechsler-Zimring, A., C. A. Kearney, H. Kaur, and T. Day. 2012. Posttraumatic stress disorder and removal from home as a primary, secondary, or disclaimed trauma in maltreated adolescents. *Journal of Family Violence* 27(8):813-818.

Weich, S., J. Patterson, R. Shaw, and S. Stewart-Brown. 2009. Family relationships in childhood and common psychiatric disorders in later life: Systematic review of prospective studies. *British Journal of Psychiatry* 194(5):392-398.

Weierich, M. R., and M. K. Nock. 2008. Posttraumatic stress symptoms mediate the relationship between childhood sexual abuse and nonsuicidal self-injury. *International Journal of Emergency Mental Health* 10(2):156-158.

Wellman, C. L. 2001. Dendritic reorganization in pyramidal neurons in medial prefrontal cortex after chronic corticosterone administration. *Journal of Neurobiology* 49(3):245-253.

Wherry, J. N., D. A. Neil, and T. N. Taylor. 2009. Pathological dissociation as measured by the child dissociative checklist. *Journal of Child Sexual Abuse* 18(1):93-102.

Widom, C. S. 1988. Sampling biases and implications for child abuse research. *American Journal of Orthopsychiatry* 58(2):260-270.

Widom, C. S. 1989. The cycle of violence. *Science* 244(4901):160-166.

Widom, C. S. 1998. Childhood victimization: Early adversity and subsequent psychopathology. *Adversity, Stress, and Psychopathology* 81-95.

Widom, C. S. 1999. Posttraumatic stress disorder in abused and neglected children grown up. *American Journal of Psychiatry* 156(8):1223-1229.

Widom, C. S., and L. M. Brzustowicz. 2006. MAOA and the "cycle of violence": Childhood abuse and neglect, MAOA genotype, and risk for violent and antisocial behavior. *Biological Psychiatry* 60(7):684-689.

Widom, C. S., and J. B. Kuhns. 1996. Childhood victimization and subsequent risk for promiscuity, prostitution, and teenage pregnancy: A prospective study. *American Journal of Public Health* 86(11):1607-1612.

Widom, C. S., and M. G. Maxfield. 2001. *An update on the "cycle of violence."* Washington, DC: U.S. Department of Justice, Office of Justice Programs, National Institute of Justice.

Widom, C. S., T. Ireland, and P. J. Glynn. 1995. Alcohol abuse in abused and neglected children followed-up: Are they at increased risk? *Journal of Studies on Alcohol* 56(2):207-217.

Widom, C. S., B. L. Weiler, and L. B. Cottler. 1999. Childhood victimization and drug abuse: A comparison of prospective and retrospective findings. *Journal of Consulting and Clinical Psychology* 67(6):867-880.

Widom, C. S., N. R. Marmorstein, and H. Raskin White. 2006. Childhood victimization and illicit drug use in middle adulthood. *Psychology of Addictive Behaviors* 20(4):394-403.

Widom, C. S., K. DuMont, and S. J. Czaja. 2007a. A prospective investigation of major depressive disorder and comorbidity in abused and neglected children grown up. *Archives of General Psychiatry* 64(1):49-56.

Widom, C. S., H. R. White, S. J. Czaja, and N. R. Marmorstein. 2007b. Long-term effects of child abuse and neglect on alcohol use and excessive drinking in middle adulthood. *Journal of Studies on Alcohol and Drugs* 68(3):317-326.

Widom, C. S., S. J. Czaja, and J. Paris. 2009. A prospective investigation of borderline personality disorder in abused and neglected children followed up into adulthood. *Journal of Personality Disorders* 23(5):433-446.

Widom, C. S., S. J. Czaja, T. Bentley, and M. S. Johnson. 2012. A prospective investigation of physical health outcomes in abused and neglected children: New findings from a 30-year follow-up. *American Journal of Public Health* 102(6):1135-1144.

Wilson, H. W., and C. S. Widom. 2008. An examination of risky sexual behavior and HIV in victims of child abuse and neglect: A 30-year follow-up. *Health Psychology* 27(2):149-158.

Wilson, H. W., and C. S. Widom. 2010. The role of youth problem behaviors in the path from child abuse and neglect to prostitution: A prospective examination. *Journal of Research on Adolescence* 20(1):210-236.

Wolf, E. J., C. A. Lunney, M. W. Miller, P. A. Resick, M. J. Friedman, and P. P. Schnurr. 2012. The dissociative subtype of PTSD: A replication and extension. *Depression and Anxiety* 29(8):679-688.

Wolfe, D. A., C. Wekerle, K. Scott, A.-L. Straatman, and C. Grasley. 2004. Predicting abuse in adolescent dating relationships over 1 year: The role of child maltreatment and trauma. *Journal of Abnormal Psychology* 113(3):406-415.

Woon, F. L., and D. W. Hedges. 2008. Hippocampal and amygdala volumes in children and adults with childhood maltreatment-related posttraumatic stress disorder: A meta-analysis. *Hippocampus* 18(8):729-736.

Yates, T. M., E. A. Carlson, and B. Egeland. 2008. A prospective study of child maltreatment and self-injurious behavior in a community sample. *Development and Psychopathology* 20(2):651-671.

Yehuda, R., S. L. Halligan, and L. M. Bierer. 2002. Cortisol levels in adult offspring of holocaust survivors: Relation to PTSD symptom severity in the parent and child. *Psychoneuroendocrinology* 27(1-2):171-180.

Zagar, A. K., R. J. Zagar, B. Bartikowski, and K. G. Busch. 2009. Cost comparisons of raising a child from birth to 17 years among samples of abused, delinquent, violent, and homicidal youth using victimization and justice system estimates. *Psychological Reports* 104(1):309-338.

Zanarini, M. C., C. S. Laudate, F. R. Frankenburg, D. B. Reich, and G. Fitzmaurice. 2011. Predictors of self-mutilation in patients with borderline personality disorder: A 10-year follow-up study. *Journal of Psychiatric Research* 45(6):823-828.

Zeanah, C. H., and M. M. Gleason. 2010. *Reactive attachment disorder: A review for DSM-V.* Washington, DC: APA.

Zeanah, C. H., A. T. Smyke, and A. Dumitrescu. 2002. Attachment disturbances in young children. II: Indiscriminate behavior and institutional care. *Journal of the American Academy of Child and Adolescent Psychiatry* 41(8):983-989.

Zeanah, C. H., C. A. Nelson, N. A. Fox, A. T. Smyke, P. Marshall, S. W. Parker, and S. Koga. 2003. Designing research to study the effects of institutionalization on brain and behavioral development: The Bucharest Early Intervention Project. *Developmental Psychopathology* 15(4):885-907.

Zeanah, C. H., M. Scheeringa, N. W. Boris, S. S. Heller, A. T. Smyke, and J. Trapani. 2004. Reactive attachment disorder in maltreated toddlers. *Child Abuse & Neglect* 28(8):877-888.

Zeanah, C. H., H. L. Egger, A. T. Smyke, C. A. Nelson, N. A. Fox, P. J. Marshall, and D. Guthrie. 2009. Institutional rearing and psychiatric disorders in Romanian preschool children. *American Journal of Psychiatry* 166(7):777-785.

Zingraff, M. T., J. Leiter, K. A. Myers, and M. C. Johnsen. 1993. Child maltreatment and youthful problem behavior. *Criminology* 31(2):173-202.

5

The Child Welfare System

Since 1993, a great deal of attention has been focused on policy, practice, and program initiatives aimed at improving both the delivery of child welfare services and the outcomes for children who come in contact with the public child welfare system—the system that implements, funds, or arranges for many of the programs and services provided when child abuse and neglect is suspected or has actually occurred. As described by Sanders (2012) at a workshop held for this study and elucidated by the discussion of research needs in Chapter 6, there is a need for further study of systemic factors that impact the response to child abuse and neglect. In keeping with the committee's statement of task, this chapter considers system-level issues and legislative, practice, and policy reforms as context for the discussion of interventions and evidence-based practices and of their implementation and dissemination in the following chapter. An understanding of these issues can illuminate what happens to children after their risk for child abuse and neglect has been determined, including dispositions and outcomes for children and families, as well as how the system that serves them functions. The chapter begins with an overview of the child welfare system. Following this overview, examined in turn are major policy shifts in child welfare since the 1993 National Research Council (NRC) report was issued, research on key policy and practice reforms, and issues that remain to be addressed. The final section presents conclusions.

OVERVIEW OF THE CHILD WELFARE SYSTEM

Public child welfare agencies provide four main sets of services—child protection investigation, family-centered services and supports, foster care, and adoption. Child welfare agencies need to have some availability 24 hours a day, 7 days a week, to respond to child abuse and neglect reports. They are also expected to meet the needs of diverse populations that come to their attention, despite the families' different histories, needs, resources, cultures, and expectations (McCroskey and Meezan, 1998).

For situations involving child abuse and neglect, children come into contact with the designated state or local (county-based) child welfare agency when a call is made to report child abuse and neglect, and the child protective services agency decides whether to accept the report and investigate it, and then decides on a course of action related to the outcome of that investigation.

Children found to be abused or neglected may remain in their own home, but those assessed as not being safe in their own home are placed in out-of-home care. Initially, such care is almost always considered to be temporary, providing an opportunity for change in the behavior, social supports, and living environment of the parents and/or the children's behavior or health status such that is safe to reunify the children with their families. According to data from the 2007-2008 round of Child and Family Service Reviews, which cover 32 states, reasons for a child welfare agency's opening a case were neglect (37 percent), parental substance abuse (15 percent), physical abuse (13 percent), child's behavior (7 percent), other (5 percent), domestic violence (4 percent), sexual abuse (4 percent), juvenile justice system (4 percent), abandonment (3 percent), medical neglect (3 percent), health of parent (3 percent), health of child (2 percent), emotional maltreatment (1 percent), and substance abuse of the child (0.4 percent) (ACF, 2012b) (see Figure 5-1). Figure 5-2 depicts a child's journey through the child welfare system, while Box 5-1 describes the child welfare system for American Indian children.

Scope of Child Welfare Placement

Each year, more than 3 million referrals for child abuse and neglect are received (3.4 million in 2011) that involve around 6 million individual children (6.2 million in 2011) (ACF, 2012c). In 1998, 560,000 children were in foster care (ACF, 2000). By September 30, 2011, the number of children in foster care had declined to 400,540 (ACF, 2012a). Approximately 3 of 5 referrals to child protective services agencies are screened in for investigation or assessment, and from 1 in 4 to 1 in 5 (25.2 percent in 2007, 20.0 percent in 2011) of these investigations lead to a finding that

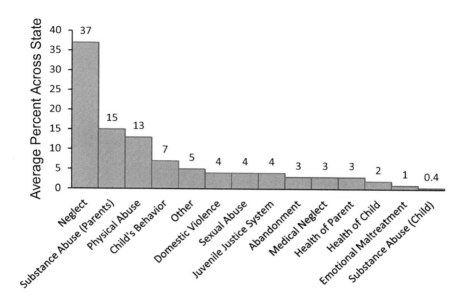

FIGURE 5-1 Case-level data: Primary reason for case opening in 32 states.
SOURCE: ACF, 2012b.

at least one child was a victim of child abuse or neglect, resulting in an estimated number of 794,000 unique child victims in 2007 and 681,000 in 2011 (ACF, 2007, 2012c). Neglect is by far the major type of maltreatment, with more than four-fifths (78.5 percent) of victims being neglected in 2011, while 17.6 percent were physically abused and 9.1 percent were sexually abused (ACF, 2012c).

Although the public perception may be that most substantiated child abuse and neglect reports result in placement of the child in out-of-home care (and perhaps siblings as well, who may or may not have been abused), this is not in fact the case. The number of child victims (and child non-victims) placed in foster care represents a relatively small percentage of substantiated reports and can best be estimated from the National Survey of Child and Adolescent Well-Being (NSCAW). In the first NSCAW cohort, 82.3 percent of the children remained in their home after investigation (Horwitz et al., 2011) (compared with 79.3 percent based on federal data in 2007 [ACF, 2007]).

Whether any given abused or neglected child is placed in foster care varies substantially. Children under 1 year old are most likely to be placed (ACF, 2012a). Among black children in this age group, the risk of placement is particularly high. Once children are in foster care, placement trajectories

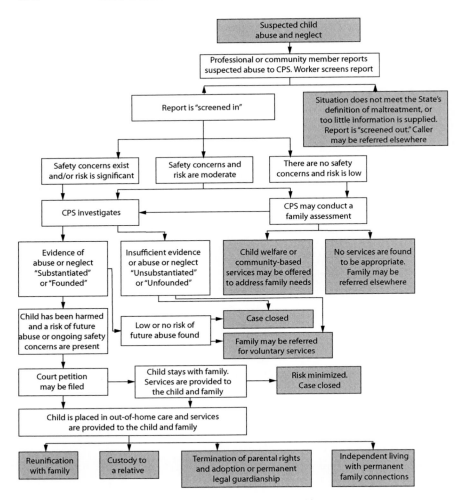

FIGURE 5-2 A child's journey through the child welfare system.
SOURCE: CWIG, 2013b, p. 9.

vary considerably. Although group and other forms of congregate care have been linked to negative developmental sequelae (Barth, 2005; Berger et al., 2009), 22 percent of all children and 48 percent of all teenagers are placed in some type of group facility upon admission to out-of-home care.

Caregiver changes, which also are associated with negative developmental sequelae (Aarons et al., 2010; Barth et al., 2007; Newton et al., 2000), affect more than half of all children who are placed, with roughly 30 percent of foster children experiencing three or more placements (Landsverk

---

BOX 5-1
The Child Welfare System for American Indian Children

A child abuse and neglect report relating to an American Indian child may be investigated by the child's tribe, the Bureau of Indian Affairs, or a state or county agency (Cross, 2012; see also CWIG, 2012b). Child abuse and neglect reports may also be investigated by multiple actors, with tribes being involved in 65 percent of investigations (23 percent as sole investigators), states in 42 percent, counties in 21 percent, the Bureau of Indian Affairs in 19 percent, and a consortium of tribes in 9 percent (Earle, 2000).

The aim of the Indian Child Welfare Act (ICWA),* which was passed in 1978, is to preserve tribal authority over decisions to place American Indian children in out-of-home care. According to the ICWA, tribes with active courts maintain exclusive jurisdiction for American Indian children residing on the reservation, and states and tribes share jurisdiction for children who do not live on reservations but are members of federally recognized tribes or are eligible for tribal membership with a biological parent who is a tribal member. State courts conducting involuntary child welfare proceedings concerning children subject to the ICWA must notify the appropriate tribe, which has the right to intervene in the case. The ICWA requires that American Indian children placed in foster care be placed close to home, with preference for placement with a member of the child's extended family; a foster home licensed, approved, or specified by the tribe; an American Indian foster home licensed or approved by a nontribal authority; or an institution approved by the tribe. American Indian children placed for adoption should be placed with a member of the child's extended family, a member of the child's tribe, or another American Indian family.

---

*P.L. 95-068.

---

and Wulczyn, 2013). About 60 percent of all placed children are reunified with their family; 20 percent are adopted; and the remainder leave for other reasons, including aging out (6 percent). Frequently unaccounted for, however, is the significant variation among and within states with respect to how long children remain in foster care. The median length of stay ranges from 5 to 24 months at the state level and from 2 to 35 months at the county level. Finally, about 1 in 5 children will return to care within 2 years of exit; for some populations, the reentry rate is as high as 35 percent (Wulczyn et al., 2007, 2011).

Aging out of foster care is strongly related to age at entry, as shown in Figure 5-3. Infants are the least likely to age out. Based on the Multistate Foster Care Data Archive (FCDA), fewer than 25 of 2,500 infants (less than 1 percent) remained in placement for their entire childhood. At the other end of the age continuum, about 50 percent of 17-year-olds aged out

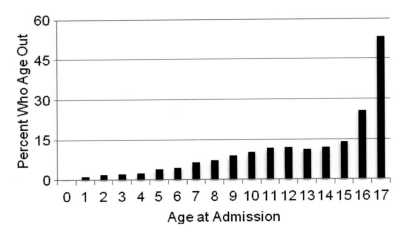

FIGURE 5-3 Probability of aging out of foster care by age at admission.
SOURCE: Data from Wulczyn, 2012.

directly from foster care. Between these two extremes, less than 15 percent
of any single age group aged out, except for 16-year-olds.

As noted, the youngest children, particularly those under the age of 1
year, have the greatest risk of placement. For that age group, placement
rates were never below 10 per 1,000 and reached 12 per 1,000 in 2006.
Among children aged 6 and above, the incidence of placement hovered close
to 2 per 1,000, also with a peak in 2006.

The stark age-graded disparity in placement rates is seen clearly in
Figure 5-4. The height of these bars depicts the magnitude of the difference
in placement rates for infants relative to three other age groups. Compared with 1- to 5-year-olds, infants are about 3.5 times more likely to be
placed. The disparity between infant placement rates and the rates for 6- to
12-year-olds averaged 6 placements per 1,000 between 2003 and 2010.

Type of Placement

Because of how much time foster children spend in living arrangements
other than those provided by their parents, the settings in which they are
placed make a difference. In general, states offer three main types of placement. Family-based care, which is preferred, consists of regular foster family
care and relative (kinship) care. Children placed in family foster care may
live with other foster children, but the number of unrelated foster children
allowed in the home is regulated. More important, the foster parents are in

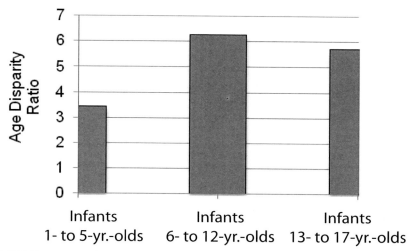

FIGURE 5-4 Age disparity ratios for infants relative to children of other ages.
SOURCE: Data from Wulczyn, 2012.

most cases psychological strangers to the child. Relative foster care involves foster parents who are related to the child either biologically or through fictive kin relationships. Over the past 15 years, kinship care has become the preferred practice option, and its use has increased as a result. The last general placement type is group care. States support a wide variety of group or congregate care settings, from smaller group homes with, for example, six unrelated youth residents to larger campus-based residential treatment facilities. States vary considerably in the range of group care settings, with some states using classification systems that differentiate 10 or more group-based settings depending on the level of care needed.

The data in Figure 5-5 show, by age at admission, how children spent the majority of their time with regard to placement setting in 2003 and 2010. "Predominant placement setting" refers to the setting where children spent more than half their time in foster care. The mixed care type refers to situations in which no one placement type accounted for more than half the time spent in care. The overwhelming majority of children under the age of 13 spent most of their time in placement in a family setting. Nearly 96 percent of infants admitted between 2003 and 2010 spent the majority of their time in a family setting. For older children, group care was the most common care type, with about 38 percent of adolescents spending the majority of their time in foster care in some type of group care setting.

Data also suggest that the use of family-based care is on the rise. As shown in Figure 5-6, the data suggest that the use of both regular and

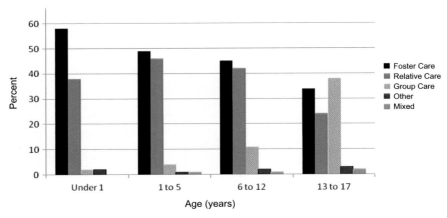

FIGURE 5-5 Predominant placement type.
SOURCE: Data from Wulczyn, 2012.

kinship foster care increased between 2003 and 2010, whereas the use of group care declined.

The deleterious impact on children of multiple placements in foster care has been a salient topic in child welfare policy and programmatic debates for decades. Legislative initiatives to promote permanency for foster children (e.g., the Adoption Assistance and Child Welfare Act, the Adoption and Safe Families Act) have led to increased emphasis on greater placement stability. The U.S. Department of Health and Human Services (HHS) now monitors the number of movements recorded for children in foster care as part of the national outcomes standards (ACF, 2002).

Although stable placements are preferred, children do move between

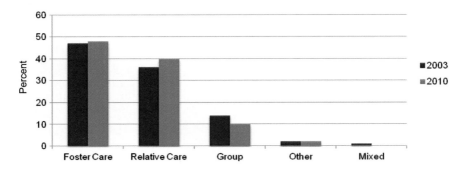

FIGURE 5-6 Change in predominant placement settings, 2003-2010.
SOURCE: Data from Wulczyn, 2012.

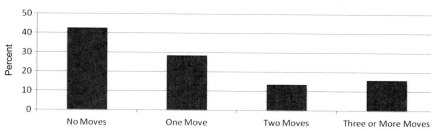

FIGURE 5-7 Average number of moves per child, 2003-2010.
SOURCE: Data from Wulczyn, 2012.

placement settings (see Figure 5-7). Grouped by how many moves they experienced, the largest group of children (43 percent) experienced but one placement (i.e., no moves). About 28 percent of children experienced two placements, while 30 percent experienced three or more placements.

The clinical literature documents the negative effects of placement instability on children. Multiple placements are alleged to affect children's attachment to primary caregivers, an important early developmental milestone (e.g., Fahlberg, 1991; Lieberman, 1987; Provence, 1989; Stovall and Dozier, 1998). Empirical evidence from other strands of research suggests that multiple placements lead to psychopathology and other problematic outcomes in children, such as externalizing behavior problems (Kurtz et al., 1993; Newton et al., 2000; Widom, 1991).

Despite what is known about the likely impact of placement moves, relatively little research exists on placement stability. An early review of that literature (Proch and Taber, 1985) indicates that the majority of foster children do not experience more than two placements while in foster care. The limited subsequent research focuses on placement disruption rates and factors associated with movement. Generally, researchers report that between one-third and two-thirds of traditional foster care placements are disrupted within the first 1-2 years (e.g., Berrick et al., 1998; Palmer, 1996; Staff and Fein, 1995). Research on treatment foster care has documented a wider range for rates of disruption, from 17 to 70 percent (Redding et al., 2000; Smith et al., 2001; Staff and Fein, 1995). Although kinship foster homes tend to be more stable than traditional foster homes (Courtney and Needell, 1997), some evidence suggests that kinship placements also may be disrupted frequently, reflecting the vulnerability of the child and the family (Terling-Watt, 2001). Findings from Cochrane Collaboration systematic review of kinship care for children who have experienced child abuse and neglect (Winokur et al., 2009) suggest that children in kinship foster care experience better behavioral development, mental health functioning, and placement stability than children in nonkinship foster care. Although no difference in reunification rates was found, children in nonkinship foster care were more likely to be adopted, while children in kinship foster care were more likely to be in guardianship. Children in nonkinship foster care also were more likely to utilize mental health services.

Several studies identify factors associated with placement disruption. Early research by Pardeck and colleagues (Pardeck, 1984, 1985; Pardeck et al., 1985) suggests that such child characteristics as older age and behavioral or emotional problems are associated with increased rates of disruption. These findings are corroborated by more recent research (e.g., Palmer, 1996; Smith et al., 2001; Staff and Fein, 1995; Walsh and Walsh, 1990). Findings concerning the relationship of placement disruption to child race and gender are mixed (Palmer, 1996; Smith et al., 2001).

Another study on placement stability examined the link between turnover among child welfare caseworkers and the achievement of permanence for children in Milwaukee County. The authors found that children who experienced caseworker turnover had more placements (Flower et al., 2005).

Many studies investigate the attributes of children and their circumstances in an effort to explain variation in the number of movements. Relatively little work focuses on the movement patterns themselves, and few studies (James et al., 2004; Usher et al., 1999) examine combinations of moves to understand whether the patterns have meaning for child welfare policy and practice.

The timing of moves is also important (see Figure 5-8). Movement early in the placement experience may magnify a child's sense of instability; movement late in the placement experience may signal changes in the child's status, the caregiver's capacity, or both. Because movement and length of stay are so closely intertwined, however, care must be taken in isolating when movement is most common.

Although placement stability is desirable, placement changes are sometimes necessary. For example, children placed in a group care setting may transfer to a family setting if the reasons for placement in group care are no longer material to further progress. Similarly, when caseworkers find a willing and able relative, transfer out of foster care to relative care may be in the long-term best interest of the child. Thus, the number of moves is not the only metric by which to judge whether stability has been achieved. Movement between levels of care or up and down the care continuum provides another view of what happens while children are placed away from home.

The data do suggest that changes in the level of care are common. About 60 percent of children who started off in family foster care and were then transferred to a group care setting went on to experience a third placement, which half of the time involved a return to family care.

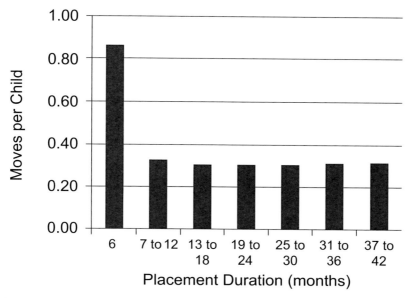

FIGURE 5-8 Period-specific movement rates, 2003-2010.
SOURCE: Data from Wulczyn, 2012.

Exit from Foster Care

For the past 30 years, child welfare policy and practice have focused on reducing the time spent in foster care. The goal of reduced time in care aligns with the notion that foster care is a temporary alternative to care provided by parents. Figure 5-9 shows the cumulative probability of exit for reunification, by age at first admission to foster care. The cumulative probability indicates the likelihood of exit with the passage of time. Referring to Figure 5-9, for example, about 40 percent of infants placed will have been discharged back to their parents within 5 years. Among 13- to 17-year-olds, the figure is closer to 50 percent; for children between the ages of 1 and 12 at the time of admission, the cumulative probability of reunification falls to between 55 and 60 percent.[1]

The data in Figure 5-9 also suggest that after 2 years, the cumulative probability does not change dramatically, regardless of the age at admission.

---

[1]The cumulative probabilities are based only on those cohorts for which at least 3 years of data are available: 2003, 2004, and 2005. The cumulative probability of reunification within 6 months is based on the experience of the 2003 through 2009 admission cohorts. Thus, for the first interval (i.e., 6 months), seven estimates are averaged together, while for the last interval, only three estimates are available.

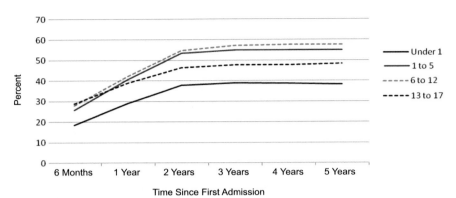

FIGURE 5-9 Cumulative probability of reunification by age at first admission to foster care.
SOURCE: Data from Wulczyn, 2012.

In large measure, this pattern is attributable to the fact as the likelihood of reunification drops off, the likelihood of some other exit to permanency increases. The drop-off in reunification after 2 years is compensated for by an increase in exits to relatives and adoptions.

Reentry to Foster Care

Reentry to foster care refers to children who return to placement after having been discharged from foster care. Although reentry to foster care may be preceded by repeated child abuse and neglect, few studies actually follow that sequence of events. From a policy and practice perspective, there are three types of permanency: reunification, guardianship, and adoption. Of those types, reentry to foster care following reunification or guardianship is easy to track with administrative data. Tracking reentry to foster care following adoption is more difficult. When children are adopted, in keeping with the idea that a new family has been formed, states typically establish a new identity for the child, including new client and case identifiers. In the process of creating a new identity, connections between the old and the new are often severed.

Even among children who exit to permanency for reasons unrelated to adoption, following reentry is difficult with respect to the amount of time needed to observe the full extent of the process. For example, some children admitted to foster care will be reunited with their families after 2 years in placement. Among those children, some will return to care, but not for 2 or more years after reunification. When the time segments are added together, it can take more than 5 years to establish the likelihood of reentry.

Although statistical methods are available to address these concerns, those methods do not alleviate completely the time needed to understand the full extent of reentry.

Child Abuse and Neglect in Out-of-Home Care

While the impact of placement on access to ameliorative services is clearly beneficial, as has been robustly shown in the case of access to mental health services, it is also important to consider the potential negative consequences of placement in foster care. This section examines this issue briefly with regard to what is known about child abuse and neglect in foster care. This subject is difficult to address because of the nature of abuse and neglect that occurs while a child is under the official care of the state, the court, and the child welfare system as a result of abuse and neglect suffered in the child's biological home—a kind of double jeopardy. It is also a difficult subject to examine empirically because there are three quite disparate sources of information to consider: (1) "official" data generated by child welfare systems and reported by states to the federal government through the Child and Family Service Reviews (CFSRs) and the National Child Abuse and Neglect Data System (NCANDS); (2) findings from investigative and advocacy organizations, such as newspapers and advocacy groups; and (3) data and findings generated by researchers.

When children are placed in out-of-home care, the state assumes responsibility for their care, including their safety. The Adoption and Safe Families Act[2] states that child safety is the primary consideration in determining services, placement, and permanency. The federal CFSRs require that child welfare agencies reduce the incidence of abuse and neglect of children in out-of-home care. In 2010, states reported that abuse and neglect rates for children in foster care ranged from 0.00 to 2.33 percent, with a median of 0.35 percent (ACF, 2010).

There are reasons to believe that this source generates underestimates of the true rate of abuse and neglect experienced by children while in foster care. First, the definition used by the CFSRs—"Of all children who were in foster care during the year, what percentage were the subject of substantiated or indicated maltreatment by a foster parent or facility staff member?" (ACF, 2011)—is very limited. It does not include abuse or neglect by other adults or youth in the home, or abuse and neglect that was experienced by the child while in care but that might have been prevented by actions of the adult caregivers in the home. Second, investigative sources such as newspaper articles offer clear evidence that some child welfare systems, or other agencies designated to respond to such reports, do not thoroughly

---

[2]P.L. 105-89.

investigate allegations of abuse or neglect of children in foster care or keep good records of these investigations (Cleveland, 2013; Kaufman and Jones, 2003). Investigative reporting has quite different rules of evidence from those used in formal research studies, and may also be biased toward negative examples (e.g., the most egregious service systems) and fail to consider the full range of child welfare systems. Yet these examples raise serious question about the possible underestimation of child abuse and neglect in foster care, although they do not provide research evidence on the size of this underestimation.

Unfortunately, research on abuse and neglect in out-of-home care is sparse (Benedict et al., 1994; Poertner et al., 1999; Zuravin et al., 1993). Nonetheless, it demonstrates some differences in the type of abuse reported and the substantiation rate for reports as compared with abuse and neglect reports in general. Some studies indicate that reports received while a child is in foster care may pertain to abuse or neglect that occurred prior to entering foster care (Tittle et al., 2001, 2008). Poertner and colleagues (1999) report on the results of a study of a large state public child welfare agency using existing management information systems that found a rate of abuse and neglect in foster care ranging from a low of 1.7 percent to a high of 2.3 percent over a 5-year period. However, this study suffers from the same problems seen in the CFSR reports and does little to resolve the large differences in rates between research-based work and newspaper investigations. The conclusion to be drawn is that this research literature is thin, and a well-designed national study that can address the problem is needed.

Finally, the committee notes that efforts to prevent abuse and neglect in foster care include (1) training and services for foster families and facility staff members; (2) increased interaction among the caseworker, the caregiver, and the youth; and (3) more stringent background check requirements for those who provide foster care. The Child Welfare League of America has established best practice guidelines for how child welfare agencies should prevent abuse and neglect and respond to abuse and neglect reports for youth in foster care (Child Welfare League of America, 2003).

State-to-State Variation

Although federal child welfare policy creates a national context for the operation of foster care programs, it is important to remember that states have considerable leeway as to the form and structure of their local child welfare systems. Most states operate what are called state-supervised, state-administered systems; however, 11 states devolve authority for administering the child welfare system to counties. Almost all states use private foster care providers to some extent; in some localities, all foster care is in the hands of private, nongovernmental agencies. As important, states differ with respect to the types of child abuse and neglect brought to the public agency's attention. Thus considerable variation exists among and within states in the use of foster care as a response to child abuse and neglect.

As a result of these many sources of variation in state and local child welfare systems, state-to-state comparisons of children's experiences in child welfare systems may obscure important and consequential differences in child and case characteristics. Only rarely are data collected to a level of detail sufficient to permit examination of the fate of equivalent cases across states and policies, beyond simple comparisons of cases matched by race and age. With this type of data, analysis using emerging quasiexperimental methods may be able to examine more complex interactions between state and local policies and children's experiences in child welfare systems.

States vary as well in the duration of out-of-home care. Figure 5-10 shows the duration for three states to illustrate the magnitude of the differences. First, it is important to highlight the similarities. In each of these three states, infants remain in care longer than children of other ages; older children (13- to 17-year-olds) remain for the least amount of time. That said, the state differences are stark. In state A, the median duration of care for infants is in excess of 30 months; in state B, the figure for the same group of children is under 10 months; and in state C, the figure is just over 20 months. State variation also is considerable for other indicators—use of group care, placement stability, and reentry.

It should be noted that variability within states is as significant as that among states. To a large extent, states are a reflection of their largest county or counties, and what is true in medium-sized counties can be quite different from what is true in larger counties. Because of the variability among states, one must be careful in drawing inferences about state-level outcomes

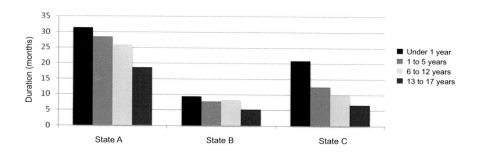

FIGURE 5-10 Variation among states in median duration (in months) of first admission to out-of-home care, by age.
SOURCE: Data from Wulczyn, 2012.

from a national picture; likewise, local (e.g., county) outcomes may be quite different from state-level outcomes.

Finally, a note about the possible impact of state differences with respect to their administrative structure (i.e., county- versus state-administered systems) is in order. No published research examines whether state administrative structure is in some way related to the performance of child welfare systems. In an unpublished exploratory study looking at length of stay in foster care, Wulczyn and colleagues (2011) used administrative structure as a model covariate and found no significant relationship between duration of care and administrative structure, given other variables in the model. More to the point, states differ in so many ways—spending on foster care, poverty rates, policy, use of private agencies—that it is difficult to predict whether administrative structure makes a unique contribution to the system's underlying performance. This is an important area for study given the cost of operating county-administered systems.

> *Finding:* Contrary to popular belief, most investigated reports of child abuse and neglect do not result in out-of-home placement; only about 20 percent of investigated cases result in the removal of a child from his or her home.

> *Finding:* Risk of placement and length of stay in out-of-home care can vary considerably based on such factors as the child's age and the family's race, socioeconomic status, and state of residence.

> *Finding:* Significant variation has been found among and within states in the length of time children remain in foster care. However, this variable frequently is omitted in studies on out-of-home placement. Little research has assessed the factors accounting for this variation to support the development of placement, placement prevention, and reunification practices so as to avoid or shorten placements.

> *Finding:* Children placed in kinship foster care have been shown to experience better behavioral development, mental health functioning, and placement stability than children placed in other forms of care, and can achieve permanency through guardianship (as supported by the Guardianship Assistance Program in the Fostering Connections to Success Act of 2008). As a result, evidence suggests that placement with kin has in the last 15 years become an increasingly preferred option for child welfare systems.

> *Finding:* Evidence suggests that placement instability can lead to a variety of negative consequences for children in the child welfare system.

However, relatively little research has been conducted on this issue, especially with regard to the impact of multiple placements, including research on the separate effects of movement patterns, the timing of moves, and movement between levels of care. Further, definitions of placement instability vary across states, and little research has been done to elucidate the meaning of these varying definitions.

Finding: Current research is inadequate to permit an accurate assessment of rates of reentry into foster care, particularly with regard to tracking reentry after adoption and following children longitudinally for a length of time sufficient to observe the full extent of reentry.

Finding: The experiences of children involved in the child welfare system vary considerably among and within states. These variations are due largely to differences in the form and structure of states' local child welfare systems, as well as differences in how child abuse and neglect are defined, reported, and responded to by public agencies. Research is insufficient to determine whether differences in state administrative structures (county- versus state-administered systems, extent of privatization) relate to the performance of child welfare systems.

MAJOR POLICY SHIFTS IN CHILD WELFARE SINCE 1993

Public child welfare services occur in the context of the prescribed federal child welfare outcomes of safety, permanency, and well-being that were codified in the Adoption and Safe Families Act. The three principal outcomes—safety (being safe from further child abuse and neglect), permanency (stability when in child welfare care and achieving permanency through reunification, adoption, or guardianship), and well-being (often characterized as child well-being, focused primarily on physical health; behavioral, emotional, and social functioning; and education)—frame the mission for child welfare services in response to child abuse and neglect. Historically, child welfare agencies have focused on the first two outcomes as their primary mandate and the areas in which they have clear expertise. They have been ambivalent about fully embracing the third element because the expertise for providing both preventive and ameliorative services targeting child well-being usually resides in other child-serving systems, such as child physical and mental health, developmental, and educational services. Nonetheless, child welfare policy, practice, and research recently have demonstrated a more robust focus on child well-being, as indicated by both the title of the landmark national child welfare study National Survey on Child and Adolescent Well-Being and multiple initiatives from the Administration

on Children, Youth and Families (ACYF) under the leadership of Commis-
sioner Bryan Samuels since 2009.

Child welfare services also are intended to embrace a "systems of
care" perspective that federal child welfare oversight has recommended for
adoption by state and local agencies (Children's Bureau, 2012). Systems of
care, drawn from wraparound services in the children's mental health field,
is a service delivery approach intended to build partnerships for creating
an integrated process that can meet families' multiple needs. It is based on
principles of interagency collaboration; individualized, strengths-based care
practices; cultural competence; community-based services; accountability;
and full participation and partnerships with families and youth at all levels
of the system. To be effective, systems of care need to build an infrastructure that will result in positive outcomes for children, youth, and families
(CWIG, 2008).

Since 1993, child welfare systems have undergone a number of changes
in policy, service delivery, and system design so as to better meet safety,
permanency, and well-being goals. Some of these changes are due to the
implementation of new federal[3] and state legislation (see Chapter 8) and to
replications of innovative program models (see Chapter 6) that have been
widely disseminated after garnering some positive program evaluations.

Improvements and service changes also have occurred as a result of
efforts to address service gaps identified in class action lawsuits, frequently
filed by national entities such as Children's Rights or the Youth Law Center, or in response to deficiencies identified in the federal CFSRs that assess
states' delivery of child welfare services. These changes have signaled the
desire to implement programs and services that better target the needs of
children in their own homes, that address service and decision-making
disparities that result in the overrepresentation of children of color in the
child welfare system, and that address strategies for engaging families more
effectively and actively in the development of their own plan of services.
The focus of child welfare services may also change after a horrific and
highly visible death due to child abuse and neglect—sometimes causing
the decision-making pendulum to swing toward placing children in out-of-
home care, while at another point in time the same assessment might have
resulted in a child's staying with his or her family.

Numerous policy and programmatic initiatives have been designed to
keep children from entering the child welfare service system (e.g., differential or alternative response—see the discussion on p. 198); to keep children
from being placed in out-of-home care (family-based interventions such as
family preservation services and family group conference decision making);
to place children with kin (e.g., subsidized guardianship and increased at-

---

[3]For example, see P.L. 103-66, P.L. 105-89, and P.L. 110-351.

tention to finding relatives that might become placement options); and to move children on to more permanent placement more quickly through family reunification, subsidized guardianship with kin, or adoption. Expedited time frames for permanency were made more explicit through the imposition of placement time limits designed to achieve permanency once a child has entered out-of-home care, along with incentives to states to increase adoptions, under the Adoption and Safe Families Act of 1997.[4] During the 20-year period since the 1993 NRC report was issued, increased attention has been focused on the development of decision-making tools for assessing immediate risk, safety, and family and child functioning to support the formulation of a plan of care (see the discussion of risk, safety, and needs assessment later in this chapter).

To understand the outcomes of abused and neglected children in the child welfare system, it is important to understand the legislative and system-level reforms that drive child welfare services. The key reforms are described in the following subsections.

Legislative Reforms

Legislative reforms driving child welfare services include provisions for family preservation and family support programs, the Adoption and Safe Families Act, the Fostering Connections to Success and Increasing Adoptions Act, the Child and Family Services Improvement and Innovation Act, and Title IV-E waivers.

Family Preservation and Family Support

The release of the 1993 NRC report occurred close to the passage of the Family Preservation and Family Support provisions of P.L. 103-66, amending the Social Security Act to create Title IV-B Part 2. The hope was that states would use these new funds to focus on prevention through community-based family support programs designed to strengthen and stabilize families through parent training, drop-in centers and early screening, and family preservation programs targeting families at risk or in crisis, thus helping to keep children out of out-of-home care and to support more timely reunification.

Not only was this funding very limited, however, but as with many child welfare services, states varied widely in how they carried out these efforts, how the funds were allocated across the state, whether specific program models (e.g., Homebuilders) were implemented, and which particular populations were targeted (e.g., urban/rural, older/younger, preplacement

---

[4]P.L. 105-89.

interventions/reunification). The 1993 legislation required the Secretary of HHS to evaluate the effectiveness of Family Preservation and Family Support Programs, which would also help better identify the evidence base for these efforts. But variations in implementation made evaluation difficult, and the federal evaluations were equivocal, especially with respect to outcomes of foster care placement (ASPE, 2008a).

Although attention to programs specifically called Family Preservation and Family Support has waned, a commitment to working together with families in their own homes and assisting with parenting and other interventions has continued, using different terms and program names (see below and Chapter 6).

Adoption and Safe Families Act

Enacted in 1997, the Adoption and Safe Families Act[5] reauthorized the Family Preservation and Family Support Programs, retitled Safe and Stable Families; codified the expectations of child welfare outcomes related to safety, permanency, and well-being; and required that safety be assessed at every decision point in case planning and judicial review. The legislation also emphasized the role of substance abuse in child abuse and neglect, stressed children's health and safety and clarified "reasonable efforts" emphasizing children's health and safety, and required states to specify situations in which services to prevent foster care placement and reunification are not required. The Adoption and Safe Families Act also set specific timelines for making decisions about permanent placement, requiring that states initiate termination of parental rights after a child has been in foster care for 15 of the previous 22 months. When parental rights are terminated, the parents no longer have a legal relationship with their child, allowing the child to be placed for adoption (CWIG, 2013a). States also became eligible for bonuses for increasing the number of children adopted. HHS was required to establish new outcome measures with which to monitor and improve states' performance, which resulted in creation of the CFSRs. Finally, the act reauthorized the option of using child welfare funding more flexibility through Title IV-E waivers (discussed below), first created in 1994.

Fostering Connections to Success and Increasing Adoptions Act

Enacted in 2008, the Fostering Connections to Success and Increasing Adoptions Act[6] amended Title IV-E and Title IV-B of the Social Security Act

---

[5]P.L. 105-89.
[6]P.L. 110-351.

to connect and support relative caregivers, improve outcomes for children in foster care, provide for tribal foster care and adoption access, improve incentives for adoption, and extend Medicaid eligibility to children in kinship guardian assistance settings. The act also required agencies to find relatives and make greater efforts to keep siblings together, and sought to ensure better coordination among education, health, dental, mental health, and child welfare services. In addition, Title IV-E assistance was extended to older youth who are in care by age 16, and the development of a youth-directed transition plan for such cases was encouraged. The act also emphasized connection to families for children in foster care or at risk of placement by providing states with grants to find families, support kinship placements through subsidized guardianship, and support family group conferencing and kinship navigators so that youth could remain more connected to family and perhaps find family with whom to stay.

Child and Family Services Improvement and Innovation Act of 2011[7]

This legislation reauthorized the Safe and Stable Families Program and further amended Title IV-B by focusing on the well-being of children, addressing the emotional trauma of children who experience the child welfare system, providing special attention to the needs of young children (under 5), and requiring states to monitor the use of psychotropic medications for children in foster care. This legislation also reauthorized the availability of Title IV-E waivers (see below) through 2014.

Title IV-E Waivers

Title IV-E waivers, first authorized in 1994 under P.L. 103-432 and reauthorized under the Adoption and Safe Families Act, expired in 2006, but were reauthorized again in 2011 under the Child and Family Services Improvement and Innovation Act (described above). They allow states to waive certain Title IV-B and Title IV-E requirements that govern foster care, adoption, kinship guardianship assistance, and other programs to create demonstration programs that are cost neutral. States can redistribute the use of funding to keep children from entering out-of-home care and to offer and access more comprehensive services. Between fiscal year (FY) 1994 and FY 2006, 23 states implemented one or more waivers to target service strategies including subsidized guardianship and kinship permanence, flexible funding to local child welfare agencies, managed care systems, services for caregivers with substance abuse disorders, intensive services including expedited reunification, and adoption and postpermanency services (Patel

---

[7]P.L. 112-34.

et al., 2012). These initiatives required extensive evaluations, several of which used random assignment in experimental designs (Testa, 2010), and the findings from these programs helped set the stage for the reauthorization of both the authority and provisions related to kinship guardianship assistance that were included in the Fostering Connections Act.

The new 2011 waiver authority, which enables the secretary of HHS to authorize up to 10 demonstration projects each year during FY 2012-2014, has more explicit goals than the previous waiver programs, including increasing permanency for youth; reducing time in foster care; promoting positive outcomes for children, youth, and families in their homes; and preventing child abuse and neglect and the reentry of infants, children, and youth into foster care. The legislation also contains a stipulation that the federal waiver application review cannot consider whether the waiver will use an experimental design for the application, an interesting turn since many view the use of random assignment in the earlier waivers as a positive process (Testa, 2012). The new waiver authority specifies that funds can be used to establish programs designed to provide permanency and prevent children from entering foster care. These programs include intensive family finding, kinship navigator, and family counseling programs; comprehensive family-based substance abuse treatment; programs designed to identify and address domestic violence; and youth mentoring programs. The new waiver authority also establishes as priorities the production of positive well-being outcomes, with attention to addressing trauma; enhancement of the social and emotional well-being of children and youth; contributions to the evidence base for improving the lives of children and families; and leveraging of the involvement of other resources and partners. In FY 2012, the Children's Bureau funded nine new waivers. (Summaries of these new programs can be found at http://www.acf.hhs.gov/programs/cb/programs/child-welfare-waivers#summaries [accessed March 6, 2014].) It will be important to continue to follow these efforts, especially with regard to the intent to reduce child abuse and neglect and implement evidence-based programs.

SYSTEM-LEVEL REFORMS INTENDED TO IMPROVE PRACTICE AND OUTCOMES

Beyond specific federal legislation that has paved the way for practice reforms, states and localities have adopted a number of system-level reforms most likely intended to improve child and family outcomes.

Safety, Risk, and Needs Assessment

Assessment in child welfare involves at least three distinct processes: safety assessment, in which the social worker determines whether a child is currently safe in his or her home or out-of-home placement; risk assessment, in which the social worker assesses the likelihood that the child will experience a recurrence of abuse and neglect in the future; and needs assessment of child and family functioning, which is used to develop case plans. Assessment may occur at multiple points during the child's engagement with the child welfare system, including determination of the response to an initial report of abuse or neglect, placement decisions, and case closure (D'andrade et al., 2008).

All three types of assessment are critical decision aids designed to complement case workers' clinical judgment in determining the best course of action for each child and case. Two approaches to assessment have been pursued within the field of child abuse and neglect: actuarial, which has been used to determine risk, and consensus-based, which has been used to determine safety, risk, and needs. Actuarial risk instruments use statistical methods to calculate the probability that a child will experience a recurrence of abuse or neglect in the future, based on risk factors identified with recurrence of abuse and neglect in the empirical literature. Consensus-based instruments are created based on theories of child abuse and neglect etiology, empirical research, and expert opinion on relevant case characteristics.

Actuarial risk assessment instruments clearly have the greatest potential to estimate the recurrence of child abuse and neglect reliably and accurately, and child welfare agencies in the majority of U.S. states use such tools (Coohey et al., 2013; Schwalbe, 2008). This type of risk assessment, however, does not indicate which clinical factors are most important to address and certainly does not indicate which services are most likely to be effective. The Structured Decision Making (SDM)© approach is an example of an effort to integrate actuarial risk assessment and consensus-based assessment of child and family needs into child welfare practice (Kim et al., 2008). In the SDM model, a case worker uses a consensus-based safety assessment at points throughout the case to determine whether a child can safely remain in his or her home, as well as an actuarial risk assessment to determine the level of risk (high, medium, or low) that a child will experience a recurrence of abuse or neglect in the long term. These assessments of risk and safety are complemented by a consensus-based family strengths and needs assessment, which is used to identify relevant services. This approach was developed and is trademarked by the National Center for Crime and Delinquency (CWIG, 2013c; NCCD, 2013).

In their research using SDM©, Shlonsky and Wagner (2005) identify the process of evidence-based practice as the key to linking the predictive power of actuarial risk assessment with the choice of effective services based on structured needs assessment. Building on their work, Schwalbe (2008) suggests further theoretical refinement of the link between actuarial risk assessment and the identification of needs for the purposes of case planning, arguing that the distinction is not between risk factors and needs but between static and dynamic risks. Empirical testing of these theoretical models will be critical to understanding the best practices to support caseworkers' decision making about safety, risk, and interventions. As states, localities, and tribes implement such efforts, it will also be important to ensure that they are integrated with other practice efforts and that staff have the necessary competencies to make these clinical judgments, suggesting the continuing need for evaluation and implementation research.

Differential Response

An innovation over the past 20 years, one that is encouraged by the 2010 reauthorization of the Child Abuse Prevention and Treatment Act, is differential or alternative response, also referred to as dual-track, multi-track, or multiple-response systems (QIC-DR, 2011). The several differing names are just one indication that this innovation has been implemented quite differently across states. The term "differential response" is used here to denote the various processes by which child welfare agencies have implemented a differential way of responding to child abuse and neglect cases based on the severity of the alleged abuse or neglect and the child's needs (Casey Family Programs, 2012). An overview of differential response is available from the Quality Improvement Center on Differential Response,[8] funded by the Children's Bureau.

Differential response offers multiple pathways for addressing the needs of children and families referred to child welfare services. In its simplest form, child abuse and neglect referrals are screened and, based on level of risk and other criteria, referred to either an assessment pathway or a traditional investigation pathway. Low- or moderate-risk families are often assigned to the assessment pathway, whereby workers assess the strengths and needs of families and offer services to address those needs, engaging families in the planning of services (QIC-DR, 2011). No formal determination is made regarding the alleged abuse or neglect, and families may decide to accept or refuse services (QIC-DR, 2011). Families are assigned to the traditional investigation pathway when they are at moderate to high risk; the child abuse and neglect type is sexual abuse, serious physical abuse, or other abuse and neglect types designated by the state (e.g., serious neglect in some states); and when other state-specific criteria are met (e.g., age of the child, precipitating factors) (Merkel-Holguin et al., 2006).

Differential response systems allow workers to reassign families from the assessment pathway to investigation if higher risk is discovered, and

---

[8] See http://www.ucdenver.edu/academics/colleges/medicalschool/departments/pediatrics/subs/can/DR/Pages/DiffResp.aspx (accessed January 27, 2014).

in some states workers may reassign families from the investigation to the assessment pathway (Merkel-Holguin et al., 2006; QIC-DR, 2012). This approach is intended to provide an engaging service array for low- or moderate-risk families, supporting the well-being of children and families while still protecting child safety and avoiding future involvement with child protection systems (QIC-DR, 2011).

Tremendous growth has occurred in the implementation of differential response systems over the two decades since the first two states piloted the approach in 1993 (QIC-DR, 2011). Currently, differential response systems have been implemented in 21 states, the District of Columbia, and four tribes (QIC-DR, 2012). Another state (Maryland) enacted legislation requiring a study of differential response, and currently has a bill in the state legislature proposing the establishment of a differential response system beginning in 2013 (NCSL, 2012). In addition, some states and localities have implemented this approach without legislation to guide them (QIC-DR, 2012). Three-quarters of the above 21 states and the District of Columbia have implemented differential response statewide, and the remaining states have implemented it regionally in pilot sites (QIC-DR, 2012). More states (n = 12) are planning or considering the implementation of differential response (QIC-DR, 2012), including one state (Florida) that previously discontinued the approach (QIC-DR, 2011). A few states (Arizona, Arkansas, West Virginia) have discontinued the use of differential response (QIC-DR, 2012).

Privatization

Also known as "outsourcing," "public-private partnership," or "community-based care," child welfare privatization involves an arrangement in which private agencies assume responsibility for public child welfare functions. Privatization is a cross-cutting issue because of the variety of child welfare services that can be outsourced, including case management, family preservation and support, contracting, referral, foster care, and adoptions. In Florida, all child protection functions have been outsourced except for child protection investigation (Armstrong et al., 2008), although in most instances, states that have pursued privatization of their case management functions have not privatized child protection functions. The private-sector provision of child welfare services has a long history, even predating the rise of public child welfare agencies, entailing an array of family services and child welfare and residential agencies, many of which were under sectarian auspices. With the growth of the public child welfare system, many states contracted with private agencies for specific services, and public funding has become an increasing source of revenue for private agencies over the past 30 years (Collins-Camargo et al., 2011). In recent years, however, states have begun to pursue contracting out not just child welfare services but also their case management functions.

To understand the evolving roles of private agencies in the provision of public services, HHS's Office of the Assistant Secretary for Planning and Evaluation undertook a series of studies to understand privatization efforts, their rationale, and their implications (ASPE, 2009). The major focus was on the privatization of the case management functions—how it affects placement, placement stability, decision making, court efforts, staffing, and all of the processes needed to meet the needs of abused and neglected children in the child welfare system (ASPE, 2008b).

Models of Family and Parent Engagement

Since the 1993 NRC report was published, child welfare systems have expanded their efforts to engage families, especially parents (including fathers), more fully as part of the service planning and intervention process. Findings of the CFSRs indicated that agencies had difficulty involving parents and children in case planning, and 46 states addressed this issue in their Program Improvement Plans. The findings of the CFSRs suggested that agencies had difficulty with family engagement because of (CWIG, 2012a)

- Staff lacking the skills needed for family engagement in case planning (42 states);
- Staff attitudes and behaviors (25 states);
- Organizational issues (e.g., high workloads) (21 states);
- Parent attitudes, behaviors, or conditions that impede active involvement in case planning (17 states);
- Difficulties created by court-related requirements (14 states); and
- System issues and documentation requirements precluding the production of a written case plan in a family-friendly format (17 states) (CWIG, 2012a, pp. 7-8).

Safe and stable families legislation and community-based child abuse prevention efforts have been among the forces that have promoted a number of family engagement models (see Center for the Study of Social Policy, Kempe Centre Family Group Decision-making, Friends National Resource Center, for information on different models). Family group decision making is one key model, found in 29 states (CWIG, 2012a, p. 8). This model has been broadly disseminated and vigorously promoted since the late 1990s by the American Humane Association's Child Division (now housed at the Kempe Center). Parent engagement models such as Parents Anonymous (discussed below in the section on models of parent and family engagement) also have long-standing connections with child protection programs in addressing child abuse and neglect through promotion of a self-help and parent leadership model.

RESEARCH ON KEY POLICY AND PRACTICE REFORMS

The years since the 1993 NRC report was issued have seen improved access to and use of empirical data that are now having a greater influence on decision making. As will be described, focus on the use of administrative and case data to inform child welfare practices has increased. As states and localities use these data, agencies begin to examine differences in decision making among workers and to develop services that are more responsive to the age of the child and the characteristics of the parents (e.g., mothers experiencing depression or parents who abuse substances or have disabilities). Reforms also are being driven by the findings of the federally funded NSCAW, which provide a fuller picture than was previously available of the characteristics of children, families, and workers involved in the child welfare system.

The NSCAW, mandated under the Personal Responsibility and Work Opportunity Reconciliation Act of 1996, Sec. 429A,[9] has been under way since 1997, with two cohorts of children being enrolled. Data are drawn from first-hand reports from children, parents, and other caregivers, as well as reports from caseworkers and teachers and data from administrative records. The NSCAW is a nationally representative, longitudinal survey of children and families who have been the subject of investigation by child protective services. The study examines child and family well-being outcomes in detail and seeks to relate those outcomes to experience with the child welfare system and to family characteristics, the community environment, and other factors (OPRE, 2013). It is the first longitudinal study in the child welfare field to collect information directly from children and families. The Cohort 1 phase of the NSCAW collected information 5 to 7 years following investigation by child protective services. Because of budget restraints, the Cohort 2 phase is collecting data only over the course of 3 years, and additional funds for further study are not available.

Another data source that provides useful information at the national level is the FCDA.[10] Containing the records of more than 2 million chil-

---

[9]P.L. 104-193.

[10]As a resource for social scientific research, the archive was designed deliberately to capture children's experiences in foster care using a life-course, social ecological lens, making it possible to overlay those experiences onto age-graded trajectories that provide a basis for understanding whether placement happens and when in the life course it is most likely to happen. From the socioecological perspective, it is known that where children live exerts a strong influence on what happens to them over the life course. All of the state data in the FCDA are available at the county level, which includes a link to relevant time-series census

dren, the FCDA is the oldest reliable source of data on foster care, dating back as far as 1976. For the 25 states that contribute data to the archive today, the FCDA maintains a harmonized record of placement through each revision to the state's data. The discussion below uses information on the experiences of abused and neglected children in the child welfare system drawn from FCDA data for 2003 to 2010, when coverage within the archive reached as high as 70 percent of all foster children in the United States, depending on the question posed. The FCDA is the closest thing to a record of exactly what happened to 2 million children placed away from home in the United States.

A more accurate picture of the experiences of abused and neglected children in the child welfare system has allowed researchers to better evaluate the effectiveness of programs and services. As will be discussed in Chapter 6, child welfare agencies, along with other service providers, now have a robust array of proven model programs on which to draw in designing service practices. However, more research is needed to devise strategies for replicating these models across the varied settings and localities in which children and families receive care.

Title IV-E Waivers

As discussed previously, Title IV-E waivers have been used to target service strategies, including subsidized guardianship and kinship permanence; flexible funding to local child welfare agencies; managed care systems; services for caregivers with substance abuse disorders; intensive services, including expedited reunification; and adoption and post-permanency services (Patel et al., 2012). Many of these initiatives required extensive evaluation, in several cases using random assignment in experimental designs.

In Illinois, the first 10 years of a subsidized guardianship demonstration that used random assignment and an experimental evaluation design saw the state's foster care population shrink from 51,000 children in 1997 to 16,000 in 2007. The subsidized guardianship waiver allowed the state to use millions of dollars in IV-E reimbursements for child welfare services and system improvements that it otherwise would not have been able to accomplish (Testa, 2010). The strong evidence resulting from the demonstration's experimental evaluation design encouraged five additional states to apply for waivers to replicate the Illinois strategy, and as previously noted, the findings from these programs resulted in reauthorization in the Fostering Connections Act to use Title IV-E dollars to fund guardianship subsidies.

---

data. In some states, the geographic data are available at the block group level, a vantage point from which one may assess close up where placement as a response to child abuse and neglect fits into the community narrative.

Several states that used Title IV-E waivers only to allow more flexible use of funds, without a specific program focus, had less clear outcomes. Absent an experimental evaluation design, determining whether changes are due to the waiver or to broader social, economic, and demographic influences is more difficult (HHS 2005 synthesis of findings from IV-E flexible funding child welfare waiver demonstrations).

Differential Response

The literature examining differential response has uncovered some key considerations for the design and implementation of differential response systems. Examples are shown in Boxes 5-2 and 5-3. Box 5-2 presents core components of differential response, developed by Merkel-Holguin and colleagues (2006), while Box 5-3 presents core values to be included in the noninvestigation pathway of differential response, derived by Kaplan and Merkel-Holguin (2008).

The growth in the use of differential response systems has been accompanied by evaluations in some states, as well as the establishment of the federally funded National Quality Improvement Center for Differential

---

BOX 5-2
Core Elements of Differential Response

- The use of two or more discrete responses of intervention;
- The creation of multiple responses for reports of maltreatment that are *screened in and accepted for* response;
- The determination of the response assignment by the presence of imminent danger, level of risk, and existing legal requirements;
- The capacity to re-assign families to a different pathway in response to findings from initial investigation or assessment (e.g., a family in the alternative response pathway could be re-assigned to the investigation pathway if the level of risk of the child is found to be higher than originally thought);
- The establishment of multiple responses is codified in statute, policy, and/ or protocols;
- Families in the assessment pathway may refuse services without consequence as long as child safety is not compromised;
- No formal determination of child abuse and neglect is made for families in an assessment pathway, and services are offered to such families without any such determination; and
- No listing of a person in an assessment pathway as a child abuse and neglect perpetrator in the state's central registry of child abuse and neglect.

SOURCE: Merkel-Holguin et al., 2006, pp. 10-11.

BOX 5-3
Core Values for a Differential Response
Non-investigative Pathway

- Family engagement versus an adversarial approach;
- Services versus surveillance;
- Labeling as "in need of services/support" versus "perpetrator";
- Being encouraging with families versus threatening;
- Identification of needs versus punishment; and
- A continuum of response versus "one size fits all."

SOURCE: Kaplan and Merkel-Holguin, 2008, p. 7.

Response in Child Protective Services (QIC-DR). Evaluations of differential response systems have been undertaken with varying levels of rigor (QIC-DR, 2011). To the committee's knowledge, just three randomized controlled trials (RCTs) of the approach have been conducted, including studies in Ohio (Loman and Siegel, 2012), Minnesota (Siegel and Loman, 2006), and one county in New York (Ruppel et al., 2011). In each RCT, families that met the criteria for the assessment pathway were randomly assigned to receive either the assessment pathway or traditional investigation services, allowing comparison of outcomes for similar groups of families. Random assignment yielded equivalent groups in one study (Loman and Siegel, 2012) and groups that were similar on all measured characteristics except history of child protective services/previous case, which the researchers statistically controlled for, in the other two studies (Ruppel et al., 2011; Siegel and Loman, 2006). Administrative data were used for most measures, minimizing problems with attrition but also limiting the quality of measurement of outcomes related to developmental well-being.

In addition to the RCTs, seven quasiexperimental studies have evaluated differential response systems using comparison groups of matched sites or families, supplemented in two states by pre-post data comparisons (QIC-DR, 2011). Another 10 states have only monitored administrative data as they implemented their differential response systems (QIC-DR, 2011).

Results from the most rigorous evaluations—three RCTs of differential response—indicate better outcomes for families on an assessment pathway compared with investigated families. Overall, these studies suggest that differential response maintains or increases safety of children, increases access to services, and increases family satisfaction with services. Findings include the following:

- Child safety was maintained. Evaluators found that children in families following the assessment pathway were as safe as or safer than investigated families as measured by administrative data. The assessment pathway families were the basis for similar (Ruppel et al., 2011) or significantly lower numbers of subsequent screened-in child abuse and neglect reports (Loman and Siegel, 2012; Siegel and Loman, 2006) compared with traditionally investigated families. Because this finding is based on administrative data rather than direct measures of safety, however, it must be interpreted carefully, because the differential response process could plausibly result in less involvement of any agency with the children, who could then be less likely to be rereported even though they were being reabused.
- Fewer removals from home occurred. Children in families receiving assessments were also less likely to be removed from home (Loman and Siegel, 2012; Siegel and Loman, 2006) than those in families subject to the investigation pathway.
- Access to services increased. Among families responding to follow-up surveys, those receiving assessments reported increased access to services compared with investigated families (Loman and Siegel, 2012; Ruppel et al., 2011; Siegel and Loman, 2006).
- Families were more satisfied. Families receiving assessments reported higher levels of satisfaction than investigated families (Ruppel et al., 2011; Siegel and Loman, 2006).

Quasiexperimental studies and natural experiments have yielded similar results, including similar or increased levels of safety (Loman and Siegel, 2004; QIC-DR, 2011), increased access to services (QIC-DR, 2011), and increased cooperation and satisfaction (Loman and Siegel, 2004; QIC-DR, 2011) for families in the assessment pathway compared with those in the investigation pathway. However, several studies have found no positive impact on removals from home (e.g., Loman and Siegel, 2004), and one of the three RCTs did not report a finding on removals (Ruppel et al., 2011).

In addition to positive outcomes for families, evidence suggests that differential response systems cost less in the long term. In a cost-benefit analysis, differential response was identified as an evidence-based policy associated with improved outcomes that has a positive benefit-to-cost ratio ($8.88), thus being highly likely to have a net positive value and save taxpayers money (Lee et al., 2012). This analysis was based on the three RCTs discussed above, as the analysts opted to use only studies of high rigor. Results of the examination of costs in individual studies are, however, mixed. In one study (Siegel and Loman, 2006), the researchers reported that the initial average costs for the assessment group were higher, but over the longer term, the average cost per assessment family ($3,688) was lower than the cost per investigated family ($4,967). In another study (Loman et al., 2010), also included in the cost-benefit analysis (Lee et al., 2012), the researchers found that on average, overall costs were somewhat higher for assessment families ($1,325) than for investigated families ($1,233).

Results from existing RCTs are promising, and consistent with findings from less rigorous evaluations. However, the number of rigorous evaluations of differential response systems is low. More rigorous evaluations are needed to understand what factors guide successful implementation and ensure desired outcomes and to learn the extent to which the differential response approach works within different contexts. Knowledge also is needed of how different definitions of abuse and neglect, varied criteria for the assessment pathway, unique approaches to service provision, and adequate funding for services contribute to outcomes. Perhaps most critically, there is a need for studies that do not rely solely on administrative data. Fortunately, three additional RCTs and a cross-site evaluation are under way to add to the evidence base (QIC-DR, 2011). As more rigorous studies emerge, additional cost-benefit analyses will be needed as well, including examination of costs associated with different differential response models. At the same time, states should initiate or continue with state-specific evaluations to understand the ongoing impact of their differential response systems.

Privatization

Privatization efforts have undergone limited evaluation, and most applicable studies have methodological shortcomings that limit the generalizability of their results. Evaluation studies included mainly quasiexperimental designs or qualitative analyses of implementation processes. The committee was unable to identify any RCTs of the privatization of child welfare services. A quasiexperimental study (Yampolskaya et al., 2004) analyzed longitudinal administrative data in Florida to compare outcomes for 4 counties using community-based care with those for 33 counties using traditional public care. Results of this study suggested that the performance of counties using community-based care was similar to that of counties not using this approach; however, this study had several methodological limitations, and thus its results should be interpreted with caution.

Three qualitative studies have focused on barriers to implementation. Yang and van Landingham (2012) conducted a qualitative case study of contract monitoring in Florida. Barillas (2011) conducted a historical review of three states (Florida, Kansas, Texas) in an effort to examine the implementation of outsourced case management. And Flaherty and colleagues (2008) examined implementation processes by conducting focus groups with participants from 12 states. Two common themes emerged from these implementation studies: the key role of politics in privatization and the critical importance of strategic planning before crafting legislation that forces outsourcing. Because government outsourcing often occurs as a reaction to a tragic event, political pressures can lead to ignoring strategic planning and creating overly aggressive implementation schedules and procedures. Yang and van Landingham (2012) suggest that states contemplating whether to outsource services should consider several key questions, including Is privatization economically desirable? Is it administratively feasible? Is it socially and democratically controllable? Is it politically viable? Is it legally appropriate? Identification of measurable performance indicators should also be a key part of the strategic planning process (Flaherty et al., 2008; Yampolskaya et al., 2004). Finally, time and learning play important roles in the successful implementation of privatization; unfortunately, political environments often do not allow the time necessary for systems to mature and management capacities to fully develop (Yang and van Landingham, 2012).

Empirical evidence on the benefits of privatization is limited. Because the focus of recent studies is largely on implementation, further research is required to better understand the effectiveness of specific privatization efforts. The heterogeneity of the field complicates evaluation, as the scope of privatization efforts ranges from very limited performance-based contracts to large, statewide initiatives. Single case studies such as those reviewed above have limited generalizability and would benefit from replication. Future research also should include cost-benefit analyses of privatization. Privatization of the differential response assessment pathway is one area ripe for evaluation. One quasiexperimental study evaluating a differential response program that entails privatizing the assessment pathway through family resource centers (Siegel et al., 2010) yielded promising results, but a more rigorous design and comparison with a publicly provided assessment pathway are needed. Future studies with experimental designs and more robust measurement of effects could examine differences in outcomes and costs between a privatized assessment pathway and public provision of this pathway.

A critical concern identified in several privatization efforts relates to staffing issues. When Kansas privatized foster care, family preservation, and adoption in the mid-1990s, for example, the public agency caseworkers did not choose to move to the private agency, and there have been similar experiences in other states and localities (ASPE, 2008b; Flower et al., 2005). Furthermore, for staff in the private agencies, the need to recompete contracts results in job uncertainty. The Center for Public Policy Priorities

(2005) found that private and public agencies faced similar concerns related to the ability to access adequate services, caseload, and staff turnover (McCown, 2005). That same report notes that improved case outcomes through privatization will not be achieved without adequate social, health, and mental health resources in communities, as well as sufficient numbers of qualified staff and foster and adoptive homes—the same factors that would improve outcomes in the public delivery of services.

Models of Family and Parent Engagement

Family group decision making (FGDM), one of the key models of family engagement, has been examined through many small qualitative and quantitative studies across the globe (Pennell and Burford, 2000), and these authors are now undertaking a systematic review. The model is currently being tested in an RCT as part of a 2011-2014 Family Connections grant from the Children's Bureau. No Place Like Home is a collaboration among the Kempe Center, Casey Family Programs, and three child welfare jurisdictions. The California Evidence-Based Clearinghouse for Child Welfare rates FGDM as Promising Research Evidence (3 on the Scientific Rating Scale), and notes that it has several distinctive features:

> FGDM promotes the involvement of family groups in decision making about children who need protection or care. Child welfare agencies initiate it in making critical decisions regarding the child. Features of the specific FGDM model include a trained coordinator/facilitator who is independent of the case, bringing together the family and agency staff to create and carry-out a safety plan. The intent is for the family group to undergo a process that leads to a case decision that the statutory authorities agree to support if it adequately addresses the agency concerns. The child welfare agency will also organize other service providers to assist in implementing the plan.[11]

Other models of family engagement include child protection mediation, family group conferencing, family team meetings, the permanency teaming process, and the family unity meeting model (American Humane, n.d.). Additional rigorous research on these models is needed, as is examination of a range of parent and child outcomes with respect to safety, permanency, and well-being. Cost analysis, looking at both long- and short-term costs, also is important.

Parents Anonymous (founded in 1969), a parent engagement model, addresses child abuse and neglect through promotion of a self-help and

---

[11]See http://www.cebc4cw.org/program/family-group-decision-making/detailed (accessed January 27, 2014).

parent leadership model. Despite its more than 40-year history, Parents Anonymous is identified as a Promising Practice by the California Evidence-Based Clearinghouse for Child Welfare because of the lack of rigorous studies. A 2010 study funded by the Department of Justice and published in *Child Welfare* found that, measured using standardized scales, all parents showed improvements in some child abuse and neglect outcomes, risk factors, and protective factors. Parents starting out with particularly serious needs showed statistically significant improvement on every scale. Results indicated that participation in Parents Anonymous contributes to reductions in child abuse and neglect (Polinsky et al., 2010).

Family Support Programs, developed through the Family Preservation and Family Support provisions of P.L. 103-66 discussed earlier, underwent extensive evaluation during the first few years of implementation (Layzer et al., 2001). That evaluation, a meta-analysis of the programs, found that

- Family Support services generally were small-scale efforts with modest budgets and produced small but significant effects across a range of outcomes for parents and children.
- A range of Family Support Program models addressed a host of problems, from child abuse and neglect to school failure and delinquency. Those models with the largest effects had been tested in single sites.
- Among the hundreds of Family Support Programs nationwide, effects were unevenly distributed across program models. The core services were primarily parent education, and programs using professional staff and delivering parent education and support through group meetings had the strongest effects on parenting behavior and on outcomes for children.
  - o Programs targeting a specific type of family rather than all low-income families in a neighborhood were found to be more effective. This finding is in contrast to philosophies that emphasize nontargeted services.
  - o Family Support Programs focused on teen mothers with very young children and on families with children with special needs or behavioral problems had the strongest positive effects on both children and families.
  - o Parent groups led by professional staff were important for parents of children with special needs, and organized parent-child activities were important for teenage parents.

Such findings, along with the implementation and replication of an array of Family Support Programs targeting early parenting over the past 15 years, have not only built the evidence base for Family Support efforts but also set the stage in 2010 for inclusion of the Maternal and Infant and Early Childhood Home Visitation Program in the Affordable Care Act and other efforts to implement early parent-child interventions. Current evidence regarding the efficacy of these efforts in reducing subsequent child abuse and neglect, and particularly in targeting child welfare populations, is mixed.[12] (See Chapter 6 for additional detail.)

In Los Angeles County, a partnership among the public child welfare agency and diverse community agencies has yielded promising outcomes by developing stronger relationships to engage public child welfare agencies; allied public agencies; and community-based networks that offer family-centered services, economic assistance, and capacity building. Findings indicate that the Prevention Initiative Demonstration Project could make a significant contribution to the prevention of child abuse and neglect as well as its recurrence, and that both clinical and community support services are required (McCroskey et al., 2012).

FOCUS ON WELL-BEING OUTCOMES

Several recent developments signal a renewed focus on the prescribed federal child welfare outcome of child well-being. These developments include the Initiative to Improve Access to Needs-Driven, Evidence-Based/Evidence-Informed Mental and Behavioral Health Services in Child Welfare (HHS-2012-ACF-ACYF-CA-0279) and Regional Partnership Grants to Increase the Well-Being of, and to Improve the Permanency Outcomes for, Children Affected by Substance Abuse (HHS-2012-ACF-ACYF-CU-0321), buttressed by policy documents such as the Information Memorandum issued by the Administration for Children and Families (ACF)/ACYF on April 17, 2012, on "Promoting Social and Emotional Well-Being for Children and Youth Receiving Child Welfare Services" (Log No: ACYF-CB-IM-12-04). This increase in attention to child well-being can also be linked to a recent significant decrease in the number of children entering foster care, with 2011 seeing the lowest number of foster care placements in the 15 years since the Adoption and Safe Families Act was enacted. This decline has allowed child welfare agencies to consider how to use potential savings in funding for out-of-home care to increase resources for prevention services and services to address child well-being. These shifts are exemplified and supported by the recent ACF/ACYF initiative to award up to 30 state-level Title IV-E waivers over the next 3 years (9 were recently awarded).

---

[12]Many Family Support interventions have shifted enrollment guidelines to focus on first-time or new parents or families who have not had prior contact with the public child welfare system. The evidence on the efficacy of those home-based interventions not engaging child welfare-involved families is discussed in the section on prevention strategies in Chapter 6.

Recent findings from analyses of the NSCAW data commissioned by the Annie E. Casey Foundation (Landsverk et al., 2009) support this increased focus on child well-being, not only for children placed in foster care but also for children in families investigated for child abuse who have not been placed:

- Children involved with child welfare systems (including both those placed and those not placed in foster care) showed marked elevations on measures of risk for behavioral and developmental problems compared with population norms. For example, such children are about four times as likely as the normative population to score within the clinical range of the Child Behavior Checklist, and about twice as likely to score in the clinical range on measures of intelligence, language, adaptive behavior, and school achievement (Landsverk et al., 2009).

- Children placed in foster care following a protective services investigation and those not placed showed marked similarities on measures of risk for behavioral and developmental problems. At the time of the NSCAW Wave 1 interviews, children placed were somewhat more likely than those remaining at home to score in the clinical range on measures of behavior and adaptive behavior; significant differences between the two groups were not seen on the other measures of child risks and needs. In addition, other studies have shown that children placed in foster care have elevated levels of internalizing problems, increased behavior problems, poorer school performance and educational attainment, higher levels of cortisol in their blood stream, and poorer mental and physical health (Berger et al., 2009; Dozier et al., 2006; Fisher et al., 2000; Gunnar and Fisher, 2006; Gunnar et al., 2007; Lawrence et al., 2006; see also Chapter 4).

The researchers divided the children who remained at home after a protective services investigation into four groups based on (1) whether the allegation was substantiated (or, in jurisdictions where substantiation is not recorded, whether the allegation was classified as "high risk") and (2) whether the child(ren) and family involved received services from the child welfare system after investigation. Children in these four in-home groups showed remarkable similarities on measures of behavioral and developmental functioning; in fact, there were no statistically significant differences among the four subgroups on any of these measures.

Children served by the child welfare system, whether in out-of-home care or not, also have similar health characteristics. According to Schneiderman's analysis of NSCAW data and other research, children's chances of being diagnosed with a health problem are greater the longer they remain in foster care and the more visits are made by the agency, and young children (under age 6) in foster care are more likely to be diagnosed with a health problem or a developmental delay than their older counterparts or the general population (Berkoff et al., 2006; Leslie et al., 2005; Stahmer et al., 2005; Sullivan and van Zyl, 2008). Chronic medical conditions, occurring at a high rate among children in out-of-home care (27.9 percent), are more likely among children under age 2 than among older children, and the rate does not vary across placement type (Ringeisen et al., 2008). Among children who have been in foster care for 1 year, 30 percent have chronic conditions—20 percent having one such condition, 3.8 percent having two, and 3.1 having three or more (Jee et al., 2006).

> *Finding:* Public child welfare services occur in the context of the prescribed federal child welfare outcomes of safety, permanency, and well-being that were codified in the Adoption and Safe Families Act. Historically, child welfare agencies have focused on safety and permanency as their primary mandate and the areas in which they have clear expertise. However, child welfare policy, practice, and research recently have demonstrated a more robust focus on child well-being.

> *Finding:* The implementation of differential response systems has greatly expanded in the past two decades across a number of states and localities. Program characteristics of differential response vary, as have approaches to its evaluation, which have varied in design and rigor. Such evaluations have generally shown positive results when families involved in differential response have been compared with those to which traditional child welfare approaches have been applied, particularly with regard to such metrics as child safety, access to services, and family satisfaction. However, there has been a lack of rigorous evaluations needed to understand what factors guide successful implementation of differential response and ensure desired outcomes, as well as the extent to which the approach works within different contexts. Also, many current evaluations are limited by relying solely on administrative data.

> *Finding:* Rigorous evaluations of the privatization of child welfare functions have been limited and have focused mainly on implementation issues. Thus there is limited evidence to support an understanding of the effectiveness and cost-effectiveness of specific privatization efforts and of mechanisms for the effective replication of successful case studies.

> *Finding:* In the past two decades, child welfare systems have expanded their efforts to engage families and parents in their planning and in-

tervention processes. Many promising models, such as family group decision making, have been promulgated, but analysis of these models has been limited to focused, small-scale studies, with little examination of a range of parent and child outcomes regarding safety, permanency, and well-being, as well as short- and long-term cost-effectiveness.

ISSUES THAT REMAIN TO BE ADDRESSED

A number of important issues concerning the child welfare system remain to be addressed by research. These issues include disproportionality and disparity by race/ethnicity, region, and socioeconomic status; interaction between the child welfare system and related systems and services; and a number of systemic issues.

Disproportionality and Disparity

Contact with the child welfare system by children of color in the United States has been a focal point of attention for quite some time (Hill, 2006; Rosner and Markowitz, 1997). With respect to black children in particular, Billingsley and Giavonnoni (1972) wrote about the tragic effects of racism on black children and used the child welfare system as their primary example. Similarly, the modern-day treatment of American Indian children within the child welfare system is burdened by a history of racist practices by the U.S. government, in which American Indian children were removed from their families and communities in a concerted effort to promote their assimilation into mainstream American society by breaking their ties to their tribes (Jones et al., 2000).

Although it depends on the specific indicator of interest (i.e., incidence rate or length of stay) and on the region of the country one examines, children of color generally have greater involvement with the foster care system than white children. According to an analysis of 2010 data from the Adoption and Foster Care Analysis and Reporting System (AFCARS)[13] and U.S. census data, American Indian children were disproportionately represented within foster care by an index of 2.1 and black children by an index of 2.0 nationwide, with significant variation among states (Summers et al., 2012). Explanations for these disparities tend to focus on differing needs, racial bias, and policy effects (Fluke et al., 2011; Hines et al., 2004; Osterling et al., 2008), a framework that mimics how the Institute of

---

[13]AFCARS is a federally mandated reporting system for all state and tribal Title IV-B/IV-E agencies responsible for the placement, care, or supervision of children in foster care and adoption (45 CFR 1355.40). Case-level data on all children in foster care and adopted with Title IV-E agency involvement are reported to the Children's Bureau of HHS twice a year.

Medicine differentiates the sources of health disparities (IOM, 2003). On nearly all measures of risk for involvement with foster care—poverty, family structure, unemployment, and adult education levels—children of color face significantly higher risks.

Child abuse and neglect is the main entry point into the child welfare system, and a significant body of research points to higher rates of reported child abuse and neglect among children of color, especially black children, while evidence suggests that these children experience abuse and neglect at higher rates as well (Drake and Johnson-Reid, 2010; Drake et al., 2009; Sedlak et al., 2010). Research also suggests that, along the various decision points that determine whether a child will be placed (i.e., investigation, disposition, and service choice), black children have a greater likelihood of moving forward in the system than either Hispanic or white children (Needell et al., 2003; Rivaux et al., 2008), perhaps because they are less likely to be offered in-home services (GAO, 2007; Marts et al., 2008). There is a marked lack of research on the mechanisms of disparate treatment of American Indian and Asian children in the child welfare system (Hill, 2006).

The overrepresentation of children of color within the foster care population is a function of differences in entry and exit rates. Measured as disparity in entry rates, the gap between placement rates for white and black or Latino children measures how much more likely placement is for the latter children. Disparity ratios for black and white, black and Latino, and Latino and white children are presented in Figure 5-11.

The data in Figure 5-12 provide deeper background on the reasons why disparity rates have changed. Displayed are the changes in disparity ratios between 2000 and 2009 for each pair of comparisons, controlling for the level of urbanicity. "Urban" refers to each state's largest county based on a count of foster children; "secondary urban" refers to counties that, according to the census designation, have urban populations smaller than that of the one largest county; and "rural" includes all other counties not included in the other two categories. These data show that changes in disparity are highly idiosyncratic with respect to geography. In large urban counties, black/white and black/Hispanic disparity ratios fell dramatically, whereas the Hispanic/white disparity increased. In secondary urban and rural counties, disparity ratios increased except for the Hispanic/white disparity in rural counties. All told, the changes in large urban counties, where most black children live, were large enough to offset the increases observed in the other parts of states.

There has been a surprising lack of research with which to better understand disproportionality, the term (along with disparity) most often used to characterize the difference in black and white child welfare experiences. As discussed in Chapter 2 of this report, disproportionality has a variety

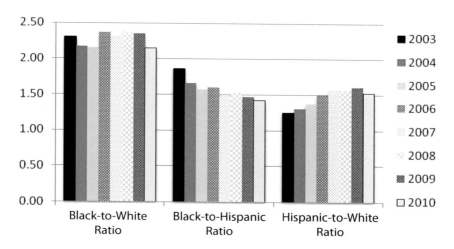

FIGURE 5-11 Change in entry rate disparity ratios, 2003-2010.
SOURCE: Data from Wulczyn, 2012.

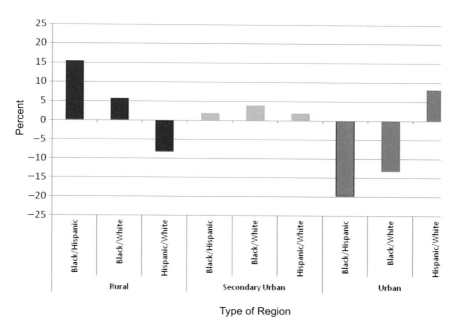

FIGURE 5-12 Change in entry rate disparity ratios by type of region and race/ethnicity, 2000-2009.
SOURCE: Data from Wulczyn, 2012.

of causes. One of the gaps in the disproportionality literature relates to the fact that relatively few studies have looked directly at ecological variation. For example, differences in the likelihood of entry into foster care often are described in relation to poverty, but only a handful of studies actually examine foster care placement across a range of spatial units (e.g., counties, neighborhoods, or census tracts) and social contexts (Freisthler et al., 2007; Lery, 2009; Wulczyn, 1986). As a consequence, even though placement rates are higher on average in poor areas, little is known about how placement rates vary with respect to poverty rates and other social conditions. Because the issue has not been studied, the field is essentially blind to the reasons why some high-poverty areas place many more children per thousand than other areas with equally high poverty rates (Garbarino and Crouter, 1978). A recent study by Wulczyn and colleagues (2013) highlights the need to look more closely at these issues.

Missing from disproportionality analyses and other research, then, is the important work needed to understand why observed levels of disproportionality differ from place to place. In this regard, a Government Accountability Office (GAO) (2007) report serves as a ready example. The GAO found state disproportionality ratios that ranged from 0.44 in Hawaii (i.e., underrepresentation of blacks) to 6.06 in Utah, yet the GAO did not test whether the observed variation in disproportionality accorded with state poverty rates and the presence of bias, even though poverty and bias were used to explain why black children were overrepresented in the child welfare system.

Put more succinctly, research to date has concentrated on analyses that feature race and ethnicity as independent variables in models that treat involvement in the child welfare system (e.g., placement, reporting, or substantiation) as the dependent variable. These models often include other child and family characteristics, such as poverty level or family structure, but the purpose of including those characteristics is limited to understanding whether the effect of a child's race or ethnicity remains intact when other covariates are included in the model. What the research does not do is assess black/white differences in models that treat those differences as the dependent variable. Disproportionality is nearly 14 times greater in Utah than in Hawaii. Is this because poverty levels are so much greater in Utah than in Hawaii? Or is it because racial bias is so much more pronounced in Utah than anywhere else? The answer to both questions requires a shift from an approach that treats race effects as independent variables to one that examines the level of disparity across units of aggregation (e.g., organizations, administrative units, neighborhoods, or counties). Without such analysis, it is much more difficult to say how service units (e.g., states, counties, offices, agencies, or workers) that exhibit greater levels of bias are linked to greater disparity.

Interaction Between the Child Welfare System
and Related Systems and Services

The past two decades have seen a growing emphasis on coordination and collaboration across the legal and social service systems that serve abused and neglected children and vulnerable families. A related development has been increased federal emphasis on the implementation of evidence-based practices (Haskins and Baron, 2011). A by-product of these efforts is an increasing emphasis on evaluation, which is often multidisciplinary. This section details the important relationships between the child welfare system and providers of mental health and substance abuse services as well as court systems, and explores opportunities to support cross-system collaboration and interdisciplinary research.

Child Welfare and Mental Health Services

A rich literature on the use of mental health care by children involved with the child welfare system has developed over the past 20 years (Horwitz et al., 2010; Landsverk et al., 2002). The research has evolved from regional studies to more recent findings from the NSCAW, with a national probability sample that includes a sample of all children in families investigated by child protective services, a 36-month cohort design, and standardized measures of the need for and use of mental health services (Haskins et al., 2007; Webb et al., 2010). The NSCAW is the first national study to allow examination of whether entry into any child welfare service increases use of subsequent mental health care and whether there is continuity in mental health care after involvement with child welfare ends. Child welfare researchers also have developed methods for understanding the complex longitudinal service pathways of children as their biological and nonbiological caregivers facilitate access to mental health care.

The child welfare system as a gateway to mental health services Because all children in foster care are categorically eligible for Medicaid, an examination of statistics on the use of mental health services among child and adolescent Medicaid populations highlights the increased needs for mental health services of children involved in the child welfare system. While children in foster care represent only 3.7 percent of nondisabled children enrolled in Medicaid, they account for 12.3 percent of expenditures for this group. Use of mental health services is 8 to 15 times greater for children enrolled in foster care than for other low-income, high-risk children enrolled in Medicaid. Children in foster care also are much more likely to use psychotropic medications and are prescribed such medications at a 2 to 3 times higher rate than other children who qualify for Medicaid (dosReis et al., 2001; Green, 2005; Harman et al., 2000). NSCAW data have now confirmed that the child welfare system functions as a gateway into the child mental health care system, and this increased access to mental health care is associated with high levels of continuity of mental health care even when children leave foster care.

Leslie and colleagues (2005) used NSCAW 18-month cohort data on youth aged 2-14 at study enrollment and examined use of mental health care at three time points: entry into investigation by child protective services, opening of a service case by the child welfare system, and entry into out-of-home care. A significant increase in the use of mental health services occurred immediately after the initial contact with child welfare, varying by level of child welfare involvement and leveling off by 3 months after the initial contact. The models indicated that children involved in child welfare at all three time points were more likely to receive mental health services after that involvement was initiated by an investigation, with rates of use directly related to level of involvement. Thus those in in-home care who received no further child welfare services after investigation were one-third as likely to use mental health services as those who were placed out of home, and those in in-home care receiving child welfare services after investigation were half as likely to use mental health services as those placed in out-of-home care. Based on these findings, the authors conclude that child welfare functions as a gateway into the mental health care system, with the size of the gateway increasing as the child enters more deeply into the child welfare system. Figure 5-13 shows this finding graphically.

As noted, NSCAW data have also been used to determine whether this increased use of mental health care by children involved in child welfare continues after involvement stops. Landsverk and colleagues (2010) examined the use of mental health services by youth after exiting from out-of-home care. The authors believed that because the movement into out-of-home care was found to be by far the largest gateway into the mental health system, examining continuity or discontinuity of mental health services after exit from out-of-home care would provide the strongest test of the offset hypothesis. Their findings were consistent across multiple tests using different longitudinal cohorts and varying statistical techniques for analyzing longitudinal mental health services. No tests showed that children reunified with their parents after out-of-home care subsequently used specialty mental health care less than children who remained in out-of-home care. In fact, one comparison demonstrated statistically significant greater use of such care for reunified children compared with children remaining in out-of-home care. In addition, the results suggested relatively high continuity of use of specialty mental health services in both groups of children. These findings are displayed graphically in Figure 5-14.

These findings strongly suggest that children's involvement with the

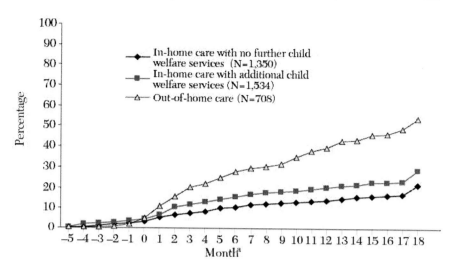

FIGURE 5-13 Cumulative percentage of mental health service use by level of child welfare involvement for a cohort of children investigated for possible child abuse or neglect (N = 3,592, weighted percents).

[a]Percentages are weighted. Time frame is from 5 months before the initial contact with child welfare to 18 months after the contact; time zero is contact date with child welfare.

SOURCE: Leslie et al., 2005 (reprinted with the permission of *Scientific American*).

child welfare system is positively associated with this high-risk population's increased access to mental health care and that involvement with the child welfare system also is associated with high levels of continuity of mental health care. The association of increased access to and high continuity of mental health care with child welfare involvement also has been reported by Horwitz and colleagues (2010), who used different approaches to the NSCAW longitudinal study, making the evidence even stronger. To use the metaphor of a service system functioning as a gateway into another service system, the gateway into mental health care provided by the child welfare system clearly does not swing both ways. This finding lends support to the idea that the child welfare system can be positively conceptualized as a gateway system from a public health perspective (Garrison, 2004). If one thinks of the child protection system as a kind of surveillance system for risky parenting behaviors and the related heightened risk for the onset of emotional and behavioral problems in children, one can also think of the child welfare system as a gateway into other service systems that can address the higher rates of problems in children involved with the child

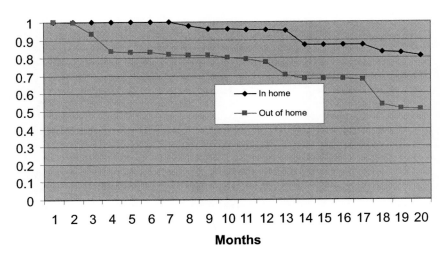

FIGURE 5-14 Survival curves for use of mental health services (N = 453).
SOURCE: Landsverk et al., 2010 (reprinted with the permission of Oxford University Press).

welfare system, especially given that continuity of mental health care is not contingent upon remaining in out-of-home care.

Quality of the mental health services received by children in the child welfare system While it has been shown that the child welfare system provides increased access to mental health care, it is important as well to assess whether children are receiving sufficient and appropriate forms of care to fully understand whether their needs are being met. That is, one must consider not only access and continuity but also the quality of the services being received. Access to ineffective or inappropriate mental health care provides no greater benefit to children than no access at all. Indeed, Bickman's research on the impact of the systems of care model (Bickman, 1996; Bickman and Heflinger, 1995; Bickman et al., 1997) suggests that better access to care may not be associated with better outcomes for youth receiving care from public mental health systems.

Mental health care also may be inappropriate. For example, despite the clear evidence pointing to high rates of externalizing behavior problems in children involved with the child welfare system (see Chapter 4), much of the mental health care offered in public service systems is provided directly to children, whereas research evidence supports the use of parent training models designed to change parents' response to the problematic behaviors exhibited by their children. Recently, Chamberlain and Fisher from the

Oregon Social Learning Center demonstrated promising outcomes from the use of multidimensional treatment foster care (Chamberlain, 2003; Chamberlain and Reid, 1991; Fisher and Kim, 2007; Fisher et al., 2005), while Chamberlain and colleagues have shown promising outcomes with relative and nonrelative foster parents with a modified version of this approach (Chamberlain et al., 2008a,b). This research is taking evidence-based mental health interventions directly into child welfare settings and shows great promise for enhancing child well-being by strengthening the response of substitute and biological parents to the behavioral problems of children and adolescents.

The National Child Traumatic Stress Network The National Child Traumatic Stress Network (NCTSN) was authorized in 2000 by the U.S. Congress as part of the Children's Health Act. The original 17 centers have grown to more than 150 funded and affiliated centers located in diverse communities as well as within academic institutions in more than 40 states. The NCTSN is funded by the Substance Abuse and Mental Health Services Administration (SAMHSA) with HHS. Cumulatively funded since 2001 at more than $377 million and with an FY 2013 budget of $46 million, the NCTSN represents a well-established, multidisciplinary, trauma treatment services-based network with significant potential as a national child abuse and neglect/family trauma research infrastructure. Local NCTSN centers frequently have extensive partnerships with service organizations in their neighborhoods and are well positioned for community-based research.

The NCTSN consists of three types of funded centers and a wider range of affiliated centers, many of which were previously funded centers. The National Center for Child Traumatic Stress, collocated at Duke University and the University of Southern California, Los Angeles, has national partnerships with major professional and service organizations (the American Psychological Association, the National Council of Family Court Judges, Zero-to-Three, the Red Cross, and the Child Welfare League of America) and can coordinate multicenter studies.[14] Its role is to develop and integrate the network structure, provide technical assistance to NCTSN centers, oversee resource development and product dissemination, and coordinate national educational and training efforts. Treatment and Services Adaptation Centers (Category II Centers) usually are academically affiliated and provide national expertise on specific types of traumatic events (e.g., child abuse and neglect, disaster, school crises) and/or work with specific populations (e.g., minorities, Native Americans, or immigrant groups) and/or systems (military, juvenile justice, child welfare). These centers develop and adapt existing evidence-based treatments for specific traumas, populations,

---

[14]See http://www.nctsn.org/about-us/strategic-partnerships (accessed January 27, 2014).

and systems. The Community Treatment and Services Centers (Category III) implement and evaluate the treatment and services developed by the Category II Centers in their local communities. They also collaborate with other NCTSN centers on clinical issues, new approaches to service, and postgrant sustainability initiatives.

The NCTSN has a long track record of high-quality program evaluation and a core data system with detailed trauma histories on more than 14,000 children and adolescents. Forty percent of this sample have experienced four or more types of traumatic events and are at high risk for costly long-term outcomes. The majority of children, however, show improvement with treatment. Although the SAMHSA NCTSN grants do not include research funds, all NCTSN centers contribute data on their clients, services, and outcomes to a core dataset. Utilizing other funding, some NCTSN Category II Centers are conducting formal clinical trials and other trauma-related research.

Child Welfare and the Courts

Since the Adoption Assistance and Child Welfare Act of 1980 was enacted, the juvenile/family courts hearing abuse and neglect cases (often referred to as dependency courts) have played an increasingly active role in the child welfare system process. Once a child has been removed from home, if the child welfare agency is to have that child's placement eligible for Title IV-E funding, certain "findings" must be made by the court and clearly recorded. These include findings that the child's continuing to live in his/her home is contrary to the child's welfare and that "reasonable efforts" have been made both to avoid placement and to speed reunification. Moreover, the 1980 law established a requirement for periodic judicial involvement as cases progress. Coupled with the Child Abuse Prevention and Treatment Act (CAPTA) requirement dating back to 1974 that every child in these cases must have an appointed lawyer, guardian ad litem, or court-appointed special advocate, these requirements have meant that in the past 40 years, the child welfare process has become far more guided by legal and judicial requirements than was previously the case.

Since the advent of the HHS-supported federal Court Improvement Program (CIP), interactions and coordination at the statewide level between the child welfare agency and the state's high court administration have greatly increased. The state CIP, authorized under section 438 of the Social Security Act and established by the Omnibus Budget Reconciliation Act of 1993, provides annual grants to all 50 states, the District of Columbia, and Puerto Rico to improve dependency court proceedings in child welfare cases. Funds are awarded to the highest court in the state to assess foster care and adoption laws and judicial processes and to develop and implement plans for system improvement. Coordination activities between child welfare agencies and the courts include joint agency-court training, linked agency-court data systems, one judge/one family models, time-specific docketing, and formalized relationships with the child welfare agency.[15] Although each jurisdiction is required to conduct assessments, some have engaged in more intensive efforts that support the development of research infrastructure across the courts and the child welfare system. A national evaluation of the State CIP found that more than one-third of the states augmented their statewide management information systems; eight states targeted research and evaluations of court activities and reforms with CIP funds, addressing kinship placement, minority overrepresentation, large-scale reviews, or statistical analyses (National Evaluation of the Court Improvement Program, 2007). Technical assistance to support system reform efforts and research/evaluation between courts and child welfare agencies is provided by the National Council of Juvenile and Family Court Judges and the National Center on State Courts (Fiermonte and Sidote Salyers, 2005).

Over the years, many state CIP programs collaborated with tribes as required by the legislation and provided support for cross-trainings, ICWA conferences, and implementation of best practices. However, tribes were not eligible to apply directly for CIP funding. The Child and Family Services Improvement and Innovation Act of 2011,[16] discussed earlier, created a new tribal CIP. Through this discretionary grant program, eligible tribes and tribal consortia[17] will receive funds to enhance and improve tribal courts' ability to handle child welfare cases. The law allocates $1 million annually for FY 2012-2016 for competitive grants.[18] Activities include conducting assessments of tribal court child welfare proceedings; creating or revising child welfare or family code; enhancing court orders; addressing the handling of ICWA cases; providing training for judges, attorneys, and legal personnel in child welfare cases; and building infrastructure for the collection of court data or improving case management systems.[19] Seven grants were awarded for FY 2012.[20] As with the state CIP, the tribal CIP calls for third-party evaluations of project activities.

---

[15]See http://www.acf.hhs.gov/programs/cb/resource/court-improvement-program (accessed January 27, 2014).

[16]P.L. 112-34.

[17]Eligible applicants are the highest courts of Indian tribes or tribal consortia that (1) are operating an approved Title IV-E Foster Care and Adoption Assistance Program, (2) have been awarded a tribal implementation grant (indicating that they are seeking to implement a Title IV-E plan), or (3) have a court responsible for proceedings related to foster care or adoption.

[18]ACF Tribal Consultation Response: Tribal Consultation for the Tribal Court Improvement Program.

[19]See http://www.acf.hhs.gov/grants/open/foa/view/HHS-2012-ACF-ACYF-CS-0323 (accessed January 27, 2014).

[20]See https://www.acf.hhs.gov/programs/cb/resource/discretionary-grant-awards-2012 (accessed January 27, 2014).

The state-level involvement demonstrated by the state CIPs has been replicated at the local level, particularly with courts designated "model courts" by the National Council of Juvenile and Family Court Judges (NCJFCJ). HHS also has for many years supported a National Child Welfare Resource Center on Legal and Judicial Issues through the American Bar Association's Center on Children and the Law. During the past few years, the courts, through the work of the Resource Center and both NCJFCJ and the National Center for State Courts, have addressed such issues as how the courts can more effectively address such topics as child safety, racial disproportionality, and measurement of child well-being.

Despite these legal and judicial advances, one cannot state unequivocally that specific court reforms in child welfare cases are evidence-based practices. Greater support for program evaluation is needed to focus on how various court actions and reforms are related to child and family outcomes. For example, does providing higher-quality legal representation for parents accused of child abuse and neglect lead to better outcomes for both the child and family? How does the quality of legal representation for children, or for the child welfare agency, affect case outcomes? Do special types of court hearings (e.g., addressing mental health/trauma) help improve access to needed services?

Integration of Child Abuse and Substance Abuse Programs and Services

Another area of interagency collaboration and integration of programs and services with a rigorous evaluation component concerns the co-occurrence of child abuse and neglect and substance abuse and the associated risk or reality of out-of-home placement. The Child and Family Services Improvement Act of 2006 reauthorized the Promoting Safe and Stable Families program and provided funding over a 5-year period to implement a targeted program of grants to Regional Partnerships aimed at improving permanency outcomes for children affected by methamphetamine or other substance abuse. This legislation was enacted to address parental substance abuse as a key factor underlying the abuse or neglect experienced by many children in the child welfare system. In FY 2007, 53 Regional Partnership Grants were awarded to strengthen cross-system collaboration and service integration through a number of strategies, including family treatment drug courts, increased staffing to address shortages in both child welfare services and substance abuse treatment systems, reconciliation of conflicting time frames across legal and treatment systems to achieve outcomes, and use of evidence-based practices and delivery of trauma-informed services. The Child and Family Services Improvement and Innovation Act continues this collaborative emphasis and includes a targeted grants program (section 437(f) of the Social Security Act) for Regional Partnership Grants to Improve the Well-Being of Children Affected by Substance Abuse.[21] In FY 2012, the Children's Bureau awarded 17 grants to grantees with demonstrated collaborative infrastructure in place across child welfare, substance abuse treatment and mental health agencies, and the courts.[22] Along with tracking performance indicators that form the basis of the annual Report to Congress, grantees are required to implement evidence-based (or evidence-informed) and trauma-informed services/activities and to conduct rigorous impact evaluations of child and family outcomes.

Child Welfare: Systemic Issues

Casey Family Programs' (2012) analysis of evidence-informed interventions to address common forms of child abuse and neglect identified many promising practices that need further testing and limited interventions that could be directly implemented by public child welfare agencies. In many instances, the need for specialized expertise or more intensive services for many of the evidence-based practices requires contracting out the services. PolicyLab of The Children's Hospital of Philadelphia found that to implement the delivery of the two-tiered intervention of parent-child interaction therapy and child-adult relationship enhancement, it was necessary to build organizational/agency capacity, including collocation of behavioral health services with the foster care agency, training of local mental health providers, and identification of public Medicaid and child welfare dollars to support service delivery (Social Work Policy Institute, 2012a). As noted in Chapter 7, as well as in numerous other publications, child welfare agencies face many issues related to high caseloads, poorly trained staff, limited supervision, and a culture that does not necessarily support autonomy, quality practice, and critical thinking (GAO, 2003; Zlotnik et al., 2005).

Child welfare agencies face challenges regarding instability of leadership and funding streams, as well as workforce issues related to staff retention, competency, and supervision. Notable efforts to improve service delivery in child welfare agencies have included child welfare performance assessment and continuous quality improvement initiatives, as well as training and technical assistance strategies; however, more systematic evaluation and implementation of such efforts are needed.

---

[21]The original grant program focused principally on the prevalence of methamphetamine use and its relation to child abuse and neglect.

[22]Note that this is another area in which the Children's Bureau requires rigorous local evaluation and participation of grantees in a national evaluation. Reports to Congress on the current regional grants can be found on the Child Welfare Information Gateway at http://www.childwelfare.gov (accessed January 27, 2014).

Leadership

Among the many issues that can impact child abuse and neglect outcomes is the lack of stability of child welfare reforms. Leadership of child welfare agencies changes, perhaps as often as every 18 months, and new leaders bring new visions, new key staff, and new plans. Changes often occur when political leaders change, as the child welfare director responsible for child protection and other child welfare services may be a political appointee or hold a senior position under a political appointee. Because of this changing environment, the leadership qualities of middle managers in child welfare programs are also a concern. Indeed, one of the essential elements of the federally funded National Child Welfare Workforce Institute is the Leadership Academy for Middle Managers (www.ncwwi.org). Research has indicated that involving all levels of staff in leadership and planning efforts can help change the climate and culture of child welfare agencies.

Funding

Both federal and state funding of child protective services is subject to the current fiscal crisis and constraints on public support for human services. When funding is tight, money to support caseworker staff who conduct mandated investigations may be saved or even increased; however, some of the support programs that help improve child and family outcomes are cut or curtailed. This situation is especially problematic for prevention services and evidence-based practices that must follow a specific protocol and are predicated on being carried out by highly skilled staff. As noted in Chapter 8, the Child Abuse Prevention and Treatment Act's appropriation has never come close to matching its authorization level, and child welfare agencies provide services by cobbling together local and state funds, along with funds from CAPTA, Titles IV-B and IV-E, and Title XX (Social Services Block Grant) of the Social Security Act, along with Temporary Assistance for Needy Families (TANF) and Medicaid funding. While the entitlement funds are not subject to appropriations, the Title IV-B and IV-E and Medicaid dollars are more oriented to children receiving foster care and adoption services—hence the appeal to many states, as previously discussed, to pursue Title IV-E waivers.

Front-Line Workforce and Supervision

Since the 1993 NRC report was published, an increasing body of research has focused on recruitment and retention of child welfare workers—those who serve as the key point of contact between children and families and the child welfare system. It is increasingly understood that competent and committed workers with support from supervisors and with attention to the organizational culture and climate are critical to quality service delivery (GAO, 2003; Glisson and Hemmelgarn, 1997; Mor Barak et al., 2009; Social Work Policy Institute, 2011) and to the implementation of evidence-based programs (see Chapter 6).

Attention to workforce issues is essential in decision making related to child protection. For example, substantiation is closely tied to definitions of child abuse and neglect, the training and caseloads of the child protective services workforce, and the type and volume of reports received. As stated earlier in Chapter 2, the utilization of substantiation is questionable in practice. All states and territories have specific requirements for the initial response by agencies receiving reports of child abuse and neglect. In most states, a screening process is used to determine whether a report will be accepted, a process that includes a review of the report against the state's definitions of child abuse and neglect. All states require that child protective services initiate an investigation in a timely manner, usually within 72 hours, and even sooner when there is reasonable cause to believe that the child is in imminent danger (CWIG, 2009). The outcomes of these assessments are dependent on the knowledge, skills, and caseload of the investigative workers, along with the supervision and support they receive from those above them. Reflecting workforce concerns, the 2010 reauthorization of the Child Abuse Prevention and Treatment Act[23] includes a provision (Sec. 106(d)) that requires states "to include data on numbers of [child protective services] personnel, average caseloads, education and training requirements, demographic information, and workload requirements" in the plans they present to the federal agency.

In examining the connection among staff turnover, rates of reabuse, and child welfare system functioning, a California study found that counties with low rates of reabuse also had the lowest turnover rates and best-paid staff, as well as compliance with recognized practice standards (http://www.cpshr.us/workforceplanning/documents/06.02_Relation_Staff.pdf [accessed March 6, 2014]). A systematic review identified several personal and organizational factors that impact retention of child welfare staff (with recruitment considered an independent variable of retention). In addition, using a targeted strategy to educate social workers for child welfare careers is an effective strategy for bringing workers into the system, as well as linking them to the knowledge and skills required to do the work (Ellett et al., 2003; Zlotnik, 2009; Zlotnik et al., 2005). Research on retention indicates the following salient factors (see Figure 5-15):

---

[23]P.L. 111-320.

- Personal factors
  o commitment to child welfare,
  o personal experience (age and being bilingual),
  o previous experience,
  o wanting to work with children and families, and
  o goodness of fit.
- Organizational factors
  o quality supervision,
  o attributes of supervisors (e.g., skills in mentoring, high level of practice knowledge),
  o manageable workload,
  o peer support,
  o feeling valued,
  o opportunities for advancement,
  o safety and resource availability, and
  o salary and benefits.

Negative factors that decrease staff retention include the attributes of burnout, including emotional exhaustion, depersonalization, and lack of personal accomplishment; a negative organizational environment that can lead to or reinforce personal burnout factors; imbalance in work and family life; and lack of commitment that might be viewed as having no "goodness of fit." Although a systemic review by the American Public Human Service Association (2005) found that states reported training as the most frequent strategy used to address retention, the review uncovered no studies examining the link between in-service training and retention. The most studied retention strategy was Title IV-E-supported education for master's in social work (MSW) and/or bachelor's in social work (BSW) students. Retained workers who have benefited from the specialized child welfare education and placement efforts cite self-efficacy, commitment to the agency, feeling valued, and special job title/position for those with social work degrees as important factors in their retention. Research indicates that those who participate in these programs tend to remain on the job longer. Other research has found that these IV-E graduates also facilitate better service outcomes for the children they work with and have a better understanding of the children and families served in the system (Zlotnik et al., 2005).

Although the systematic review of the American Public Human Service Association (2005) found that providing support for social workers to obtain BSW and MSW degrees to pursue child welfare careers is an effective strategy, the major funding source for its implementation is Title IV-E entitlement. Thus the focus is more on the administration of foster care than specifically on educating social workers to be child protective service

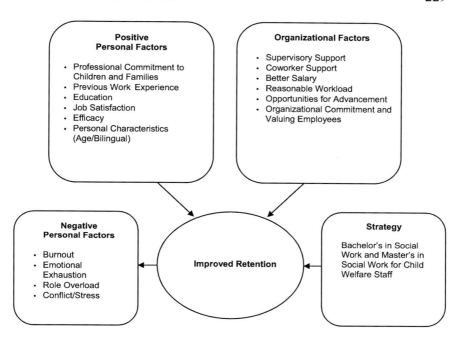

FIGURE 5-15 Strategies and conditions that influence the retention of staff in public child welfare.
SOURCE: Adapted with permission from Zlotnik et al., 2005.

investigators or on developing the clinical skills needed for protective service intervention (Social Work Policy Institute, 2012b).

Several states and counties have implemented some of the organizational change strategies that have been found to be evidence based and effective for addressing retention of child welfare staff. For example, Glisson and colleagues (2006) implemented the availability, responsiveness, and continuity (ARC) organizational intervention strategy in a combined child welfare and juvenile justice system in a southeastern state. They found that 39 percent of employees in case management teams that received the ARC intervention quit their jobs during the 1-year period following the intervention, compared with 65 percent of caseworkers in the control group during the same time period. The study also found that the ARC intervention improved the organizational climate, with caseworkers who participated in the entire intervention reporting lower levels of depersonalization, emotional exhaustion, role conflict, and role overload than their peers in the control group. Analysis of NSCAW data has linked engaged organizational climates in child welfare systems to greater psychosocial improvements for children served by those systems compared with children served by case-workers in less engaged organizational climates (Glisson, 2010; Glisson and Green, 2011). This is an area in which more research is needed, especially to understand the mechanisms of the links between practice outcomes and workforce issues. Furthermore, it should be recognized that, looking across all of the processes involved, child protection work is a multidisciplinary field, and evidence-based strategies are necessary to ensure competent, qualified staff in medicine, social work, nursing, early childhood, law, and other subject areas.

Need for Continuous Quality Improvement

Public child welfare agencies often must face negative media attention, which in turn puts pressure on politicians to take some form of action (Chenot, 2011). Exposés of child protection efforts following a high-profile death of a child can result in the firing of both agency heads and front-line workers. Child welfare agencies appear to be unable as yet to take the same approach used by hospitals—fully examining internally what went wrong and creating a learning organization to learn from those mistakes. Instead, highly visible changes are made that have repercussions for staff at all levels. Rzepnicki and colleagues (2010) suggest that child welfare agencies need to learn more about the practices of high-reliability organization and incorporate them into the delivery of child welfare services. Agencies seeking accreditation must carry out a program improvement process, but little information is available about the extent to which these efforts are well developed and implemented (Zayas et al., 2013). One of the changes since the 1993 NRC report has been the targeted effort in a number of states, working with the Council on Accreditation (http://www.coanet.org/programs/public-agency-accreditation [accessed March 6, 2014]), to use accreditation as a way to address workforce standards, caseload, supervision, and quality improvement and monitoring of services. The Children's Bureau also has increased attention to continuous quality improvement by asking one of the resource centers to conduct an environmental scan of states to identify the processes they are using (http://www.acf.hhs.gov/programs/cb/news/continuous-quality-improvement [accessed March 6, 2014]), as well as by issuing an information memorandum in August 2012 (ACYF-CB-IM-12-07) to outline some expectations for continuous quality improvement efforts.

According to Zlotnik (2010, p. 328): "The barriers to establishing research, evaluation, and quality improvement departments in public child welfare agencies have prompted public administrators to seek out this expertise and to encourage its development by establishing and supporting partnerships with universities. These research partnerships also emerge from a more general desire to forge tighter linkages between universities and child welfare departments in the training of students and staff for public service careers." Lawrence and colleagues (2012) also note that it is difficult to design evaluations in child welfare agencies because of workforce turnover and organizational issues that impact workers' intent to leave.

Performance Assessment of Child Welfare Agencies

Another key change since 1993 is that in 2000, the Children's Bureau created the CFSR effort, which assesses how states are performing with respect to safety, permanency, and well-being outcomes; looks at how children and families are being served; and provides a process for improving performance. In the first round of the reviews (2001 to 2004), no state was found to be in substantial compliance, and the greatest gap in services was in serving children in their own homes. All states were required to implement Program Improvement Plans. The second round of reviews took place between 2007 and 2010.

The CFSRs measure seven outcomes and seven systemic factors. The outcomes measured include whether children under the care of the state are protected from abuse and neglect, whether children have permanency and stability in their living conditions, whether the continuity of family relationships and connections is preserved for children, whether families have enhanced capacity to provide for their children's needs, and whether children receive adequate services to meet their physical and mental health needs. The systemic factors measured by the reviews include the effectiveness of the state's systems for child welfare information, case review, and quality assurance; training of child welfare staff, parents, and other stakeholders; the array of services that support children and families; the agency's responsiveness to the community; and foster and adoptive parent licensing, recruitment, and retention.

Results of the first 2 years of the second round of CFSRs, covering 32 states, indicated that foster care was more likely than in-home services to achieve outcomes and that services to mothers were stronger than services to fathers in relationship to the systemic factors that were assessed. With regard to safety, 22 percent of the cases had unaddressed safety concerns, including child abuse and neglect reports that were inappropriately screened out, child abuse and neglect allegations that were never formally reported or investigated, delays in accepting an allegation for investigation, and allegations that were not substantiated despite evidence that would support substantiation. With regard to permanency, findings indicated that concurrent planning—the pursuit of primary and secondary permanency options simultaneously from the child's entry into the child welfare system (CWIG, 2012c)—was not implemented consistently or effectively. The reviews also found that petitions for termination of parental rights were not necessarily filed in a timely fashion (as defined by the Adoption and Safe Families Act). With regard to well-being, some challenges were identified: educational services were not well coordinated; dental services were not necessarily available in the community; and mental and behavioral health services in the community were insufficient to meet the need or were assessed but not addressed, or delays were incurred because of waiting lists (ACF, 2012b). More information on the results of the CFSRs is available at http://www. acf.hhs.gov/programs/cb/resource/cfsr-compiled-results-2001-2010 (accessed March 6, 2014).

Training and Technical Assistance Strategies: Filling a Gap

Since the 1993 NRC report was issued, the Children's Bureau has broadened its training and technical assistance strategy to work with states, counties, and tribes to improve child welfare practice and has convened states and tribes (including representatives from multiple agencies—child welfare, mental health, judicial, health, education) around critical issues (e.g., child fatality review, psychotropic medication, child welfare evaluation, workforce issues, prevention network). A complex network of close to 50 entities—including national resource centers, quality improvement centers, implementation centers, clearinghouses and information resources, institutes, and providers of services to grantees—is now engaged in the training and technical assistance endeavor (http://www.acf.hhs.gov/programs/cb/ assistance [accessed March 6, 2014]). Many states also seek consultation from a broad range of fee-for-service experts, and Casey Family Programs, working with the top leadership in many states, has developed a strategic consulting effort to improve outcomes. In the face of all of this effort to achieve change, individual programs have been evaluated, but there has been no known analysis of how all of these efforts work synergistically to improve the lives and outcomes of children who experience child abuse and neglect.

Finding: Research to date has not provided a clear understanding of differences in the experiences of children in the child welfare system based on race, socioeconomic status, and culture.

Finding: Children involved with the child welfare system often come into contact with a number of other systems, such as the courts or various service providers. Cohesive interaction between the child welfare system and these other, related systems is critical for the well-being of at-risk children. The interaction of these various systems also provides an opportunity for conducting interdisciplinary child abuse and neglect research that entails exploring systemic improvement through collaboration, aggregating data from multiple sources where abused and neglected children are seen, and understanding the relationship among cross-disciplinary outcomes.

Finding: The child welfare system functions as a gateway into the child mental health care system, and this increased access to mental health care is associated with high levels of continuity of mental health care even when children leave foster care. However, this improved access to care is not necessarily associated with improved child well-being outcomes, as the quality or type of care received may not adequately address a child's needs. There has been a lack of rigorous research on the effectiveness, quality, and scope of care received by children in the child welfare system.

Finding: Evidence has shown that rates of use of mental health referral services among children in the child welfare system are influenced by both clinical factors and nonclinical factors, such as the type of child abuse or neglect experienced, racial/ethnic background, age, and type of placement. However, most research in the area has taken an epidemiologic approach that entails simply reporting rates of need for service and rates of service utilization. Limited analysis has addressed the relationship between need and use, the role of the many different influences on service utilization, and the efficacy of actual interventions and their outcomes.

Finding: The Court Improvement Program, integration of the provision of child abuse and substance use services, and the National Traumatic Stress Network represent notable efforts to improve collaborative service provision for abused and neglected children and to create multidisciplinary research infrastructures.

Finding: The delivery of effective, evidence-based services by child welfare agencies requires an administrative, leadership, and workforce capacity that is often lacking. Barriers to sufficient organizational capacity include issues related to reduced funding; high caseloads; poorly trained staff, especially staff who are not trained to address the social and emotional needs of the children who come in contact with the child protective services system; and limited staff supervision.

Finding: While certain organizational change strategies have been found to be evidence based and effective for improving workforce retention in child welfare, more research in this area is needed, especially to link practice outcomes and workforce issues.

Finding: The evidence base is insufficient on effective strategies for bringing in the interdisciplinary knowledge necessary to carry out all the diverse functions of a child welfare agency, including experience in medicine, social work, nursing, early childhood, law, and other subject areas.

Finding: Child welfare agencies need to employ more effective quality improvement strategies. While agencies currently engage in a program improvement process, little evidence is available on the extent to which these processes are well developed, implemented, and sustained. These processes need to be thoroughly examined to determine the most successful strategies for quality improvement.

CONCLUSIONS

The societal response to child abuse and neglect is a complex one. Even before the passage of CAPTA (see Chapter 8), the public child welfare system was supported by the federal government and by states to respond to child abuse and neglect, with roles that ranged from responding to reports; to working with children and families; to strategizing on assessment, intervention, placement, and case disposition. This chapter has provided an overview of the children who come into contact with this complex child welfare system and framed the system's policies and practices as ever changing to best focus on children's safety, permanency, and well-being. Despite some progress, much remains to be done, and research is needed to connect what is found to work with the structures and processes that need to be addressed to implement evidence-based policy and practice in complex systems.

Improved access to empirical data from sources such as the NSCAW and the FCDA has led to a greater understanding of the experiences of children who come in contact with the child welfare system, which can help guide decision making and service delivery. However, further research is needed to fully understand important issues such as the impact of multiple foster care placements, especially the separate effects of movement patterns, the timing of moves, and movement between levels of care; differences in the experiences of children in the child welfare system based on race, socioeconomic status, and culture; and the impact of varying state administrative structures on the performance of the child welfare system.

Improved access to data also has enabled a more comprehensive examination of the impact of various child welfare system initiatives designed to improve performance with regard to the core goals of safety, permanency, and well-being. While a growing body of evaluations has shown the benefits of strategies such as differential response, family and parent engagement, and the use of practice models, there is a need for more rigorous evaluations and an even greater need to evaluate strategies used to implement successful models across varying settings. As the focus of child welfare system initiatives continues to evolve based on changes to laws and administrative policies and responses to tragic events, the developing evidence base needs to be used to promote the implementation of programs and service delivery strategies that have proven effectiveness.

While research on the effectiveness of programs and the science of implementation offers insight into successful strategies for child welfare agencies to replicate, the potential benefits of such research cannot be realized without the institutional capacity to implement programs and service delivery strategies. Achieving this capacity requires reconsideration of the competency and commitment of front-line staff, a link between training and education and service delivery, a greater focus on leadership and organization, and greater alignment of the policies and practice imperatives that are presented to child welfare managers. In light of the many aspects of the causes and consequences of child abuse and neglect (see Chapters 3 and 4, respectively), it is necessary to integrate the multidisciplinary experience needed for child welfare service delivery and to coordinate with the various other systems and service providers that encounter abused and neglected children.

To meet the above research needs in the varying contexts of individual agencies and in the face of the difficulties associated with conducting research in large, complex systems, a research enterprise needs to be built within child welfare agencies. Doing so would allow for examination of the experiences of children in the child welfare system in relation to the implementation of programs in specific settings, as well as the promotion of strategies to improve institutional performance.

REFERENCES

Aarons, G. A., S. James, A. R. Monn, R. Raghavan, R. S. Wells, and L. K. Leslie. 2010. Behavior problems and placement change in a national child welfare sample: A prospective study. *Journal of the American Academy of Child and Adolescent Psychiatry* 49(1):70-80.

ACF (Administration for Children and Families). 2000. *Child welfare outcomes 1998: Annual report.* Washington, DC: U.S. Department of Health and Human Services, Children's Bureau.

ACF. 2002. *Child welfare outcomes 1999: Annual report. Safety, permanency, well-being.* Washington, DC: Administration for Children and Families.

ACF. 2007. *Child maltreatment, 2007 report.* Washington, DC: U.S. Department of Health and Human Services, ACF.

ACF. 2010. *Child welfare outcomes 2007-2010: Report to Congress.* Washington, DC: U.S. Department of Health and Human Services, Children's Bureau.

ACF. 2011. *Child welfare outcomes 2003-2006: Report to Congress.* Washington, DC: U.S. Department of Health and Human Services, Children's Bureau.

ACF. 2012a. *The AFCARS report: Preliminary FY 2011 estimates as of July 2012. No. 19.* Washington, DC: U.S. Department of Health and Human Services, Children's Bureau.

ACF. 2012b. *Results of the 2007 and 2008 child and family services reviews.* http://www.acf. hhs.gov/programs/cb/resource/07-08-cfsr-results (accessed April 22, 2013).

ACF. 2012c. *Child maltreatment, 2011 report.* Washington, DC: U.S. Deparment of Health and Human Services, Children's Bureau. http://www.acf.hhs.gov/sites/default/files/cb/ cm11.pdf (accessed August 6, 2013).

American Humane. n.d. *Quick reference guide: Various approaches and models to engage the family group in child welfare decision making.* http://www.americanhumane.org/assets/ pdfs/children/fgdm/quick-reference.pdf (accessed August 26, 2013).

American Public Human Services Association. 2005. *Report from the 2004 Child Welfare Workforce Survey: State agency findings.* Washington, DC: American Public Health Human Services Association.

Armstrong, M. I., A. C. Vargo, N. Jordan, T. King-Miller, C. Sowell, and S. Yampolskaya. 2008. *Report to the legislature—evaluation of the department of children and families community-based care initiative fiscal year 2006-2007.* Tallahassee: Florida Department of Children and Families.

ASPE (Assistant Secretary for Planning and Evaluation). 2008a. *Evaluation of family preservation and reunification programs: Overview.* http://aspe.hhs.gov/hsp/evalfampres94/ (accessed May 3, 2013).

ASPE. 2008b. *Evolving roles of public and private agencies in privatized child welfare systems.* Washington, DC: U.S. Department of Health and Human Services.

ASPE. 2009. *Child welfare privatization initiatives. Assessing their implications for the child welfare field and the federal child welfare programs.* http://aspe.hhs.gov/hsp/07/CWPI/ (accessed July 10, 2013).

Barillas, K. H. 2011. State capacity: The missing piece in child welfare privatization. *Child Welfare* 90(3):111-127.

Barth, R. P. 2005. Residential care: From here to eternity. *International Journal of Social Welfare* 14(3):158-162.

Barth, R. P., E. C. Lloyd, R. L. Green, S. James, L. K. Leslie, and J. Landsverk. 2007. Predictors of placement moves among children with and without emotional and behavioral disorders. *Journal of Emotional and Behavioral Disorders* 15(1):46-55.

Benedict, M. I., S. Zuravin, D. Brandt, and H. Abbey. 1994. Types and frequency of child maltreatment by family foster-care providers in an urban-population. *Child Abuse & Neglect* 18(7):577-585.

Berger, L. M., S. K. Bruch, E. I. Johnson, S. James, and D. Rubin. 2009. Estimating the "impact" of out-of-home placement on child well-being: Approaching the problem of selection bias. *Child Development* 80(6):1856-1876.

Berkoff, M. C., L. K. Leslie, and A. C. Stahmer. 2006. Accuracy of caregiver identification of developmental delays among young children involved with child welfare. *Journal of Developmental & Behavioral Pediatrics* 27(4):310-318.

Berrick, J. D., B. Needell, R. P. Barth, and M. Jonson-Reid. 1998. *The tender years: Toward developmentally sensitive child welfare services for very young children.* New York: Oxford University Press.

Bickman, L. 1996. Implications of a children's mental health managed care demonstration evaluation. *Journal of Mental Health Administration* 23(1):107-117.

Bickman, L., and C. A. Heflinger. 1995. Seeking success by reducing implementation and evaluation failures. In *Children's mental health services: Research, policy, and evaluation,* Vol. 1, edited by L. Bickman and D. J. Rog. Newbury Park, CA: Sage Publications. Pp. 171-205.

Bickman, L., W. T. Summerfelt, J. Firth, and S. Douglas. 1997. The stark county evaluation project: Baseline results of a randomized experiment. In *Evaluating mental health services: How do programs for children "work" in the real world?*, edited by D. Northrup and C. Nixon. Newbury Park, CA: Sage Publications. Pp. 231-258.

Billingsley, A., and J. M. Giovannoni. 1972. *Children of the storm: Black children and American child welfare.* New York: Harcourt, Brace and Jovanovich.

Casey Family Programs. 2012. *Comparison of experiences in differential response (DR) implementation: 10 child welfare jurisdictions implementing DR.* Seattle, WA: Casey Family Programs.

Chamberlain, P. 2003. The Oregon multidimensional treatment foster care model: Features, outcomes, and progress in dissemination. *Cognitive and Behavioral Practice* 10(4): 303-312.

Chamberlain, P., and J. B. Reid. 1991. Using a specialized foster care community treatment model for children and adolescents leaving the state mental hospital. *Journal of Community Psychology* 19(3):266-276.

Chamberlain, P., J. Price, L. D. Leve, H. Laurent, J. A. Landsverk, and J. B. Reid. 2008a. Prevention of behavior problems for children in foster care: Outcomes and mediation effects. *Prevention Science* 9(1):17-27.

Chamberlain, P., J. Price, J. Reid, and J. Landsverk. 2008b. Cascading implementation of a foster and kinship parent intervention. *Child Welfare* 87(5):27-48.

Chenot, D. 2011. The vicious cycle. Recurrent interactions among the media, politicians, the public, and child welfare services organizations. *Journal of Public Child Welfare* 5(2-3): 167-184.

Child Welfare League of America 2003. *CWLA best practice guidelines: Child abuse and neglect in foster care.* Washington, DC: Child Welfare League of America.

Children's Bureau. 2012. *Promising approaches.* http://www.acf.hhs.gov/programs/cb/resource/promising-approaches (accessed November 27, 2012).

Cleveland, C. 2013. Who will protect state's children? Chattanooga Times Free Press (Tennessee), May 2, 2013, E1.

Collins-Camargo, C., B. McBeath, and K. Ensign. 2011. Privatization and performance-based contracting in child welfare: Recent trends and implications for social service administrators. *Administration in Social Work* 35(5):494-516.

Coohey, C., K. Johnson, L. M. Renner, and S. D. Easton. 2013. Actuarial risk assessment in child protective services: Construction methodology and performance criteria. *Children and Youth Services Review* 35(1):151-161.

Courtney, M. E., and B. Needell. 1997. Outcomes of kinship care: Lessons from California. *Child Welfare Research Review* 2:130-150.

Cross, T. 2012. *An overview of child maltreatment data in American Indian/Alaska Native communities.* Presentation to the Committee on Child Maltreatment Research, Policy, and Practice for the Next Decade, December 10, Washington, DC. http://iom.edu/~/media/Files/Activity%20Files/Children/Child%20Maltreatment/cross.pdf (accessed August 7, 2013).

CWIG (Child Welfare Information Gateway). 2008. *Systems of care.* Washington, DC: U.S. Department of Health and Human Services, Children's Bureau.

CWIG. 2009. *Making and screening reports of child abuse and neglect: Summary of state laws.* Washington, DC: U.S. Department of Health and Human Services, Children's Bureau.

CWIG. 2012a. *Engaging families in case planning.* Washington, DC: U.S. Department of Health and Human Services, Children's Bureau.

CWIG. 2012b. *Tribal-state relations.* Washington, DC: U.S. Department of Health and Human Services, Children's Bureau.

CWIG. 2012c. *Concurrent planning: What the evidence shows.* Washington, DC: U.S. Department of Health and Human Services, Children's Bureau. https://www.childwelfare. gov/pubs/issue_briefs/concurrent_evidence/concurrent_evidence.pdf (accessed August 16, 2013).

CWIG. 2013a. *Grounds for involuntary termination of parental rights.* Washington, DC: U.S. Department of Health and Human Services, Children's Bureau.

CWIG. 2013b. *How the child welfare system works.* Washington, DC: U.S. Department of Health and Human Services, Children's Bureau.

CWIG. 2013c. *Structured decision making.* https://www.childwelfare.gov/systemwide/ assessment/approaches/decision.cfm (accessed June 14, 2013).

D'andrade, A., M. J. Austin, and A. Benton. 2008. Risk and safety assessment in child welfare: Instrument comparisons. *Journal of Evidence-Based Social Work* 5(1-2):31-56.

dosReis, S., J. M. Zito, D. J. Safer, and K. L. Soeken. 2001. Mental health services for youths in foster care and disabled youths. *American Journal of Public Health* 91(7):1094-1099.

Dozier, M., M. Manni, M. K. Gordon, E. Peloso, M. R. Gunnar, K. C. Stovall-McClough, D. Eldreth, and S. Levine. 2006. Foster children's diurnal production of cortisol: An exploratory study. *Child Maltreatment* 11(2):189-197.

Drake, B., and M. Johnson-Reid. 2010. NIS interpretations: Race and the national incidence studies of child abuse and neglect. *Children and Youth Services Review* 33(1):309-316.

Drake, B., S. L. Lee, and M. Jonson-Reid. 2009. Race and child maltreatment reporting: Are blacks overrepresented? *Children and Youth Services Review* 31(3):309-316.

Earle, K. 2000. *Child abuse and neglect: An examination of American Indian data.* Seattle, WA: Casey Family Programs.

Ellett, A. J., C. D. Ellett, and J. K. Rugutt. 2003. *A study of personal and organizational factors contributing to employee retention and turnover in child welfare in Georgia: Final report.* Athens, GA: University of Georgia School of Social Work.

Fahlberg, V. I. 1991. *A child's journey through placement.* Indianapolis, IN: Perspectives Press.

Fiermonte, C., and N. Sidote Salyers. 2005. *Improving outcomes together: Court and child welfare collaboration.* Urbana-Champaign: Children and Family Research Center, School of Social Work, University of Illinois at Urbana-Champaign.

Fisher, P. A., and H. K. Kim. 2007. Intervention effects on foster preschoolers' attachment-related behaviors from a randomized trial. *Prevention Science* 8(2):161-170.

Fisher, P. A., M. R. Gunnar, P. Chamberlain, and J. B. Reid. 2000. Preventive intervention for maltreated preschool children: Impact on children's behavior, neuroendocrine activity, and foster parent functioning. *Journal of the American Academy of Child & Adolescent Psychiatry* 39(11):1356-1364.

Fisher, P. A., B. Burraston, and K. Pears. 2005. The early intervention foster care program: Permanent placement outcomes from a randomized trial. *Child Maltreatment* 10(1):61-71.

Flaherty, C., C. Collins-Camargo, and E. Lee. 2008. Privatization of child welfare services: Lessons learned from experienced states regarding site readiness assessment and planning. *Children and Youth Services Review* 30(7):809-820.

Flower, C., J. McDonal, and M. Sumski. 2005. *Review of turnover in Milwaukee county private agency child welfare ongoing case management staff.* Milwaukee, WI: Bureau of Milwaukee Child Welfare.

Fluke, J., B. J. Harden, M. Jenkins, and A. Ruehrdanz. 2011. A research synthesis on child welfare disproportionality and disparities. In *Disparities and disproportionality in child welfare: Analysis of the research.* Denver, CO: American Humane Association and the Annie E. Casey Foundation. Pp. 1-93.

Freisthler, B., P. J. Gruenewald, L. G. Remer, B. Lery, and B. Needell. 2007. Exploring the spatial dynamics of alcohol outlets and Child Protective Services referrals, substantiations, and foster care entries. *Child Maltreatment* 12(2):114-124.

GAO (Government Accountability Office). 2003. *Child welfare: HHS could play a greater role in helping child welfare agencies recruit and retain staff.* Washington, DC: GAO.

GAO. 2007. *African American children in foster care: Additional HHS assistance needed to help states reduce the proportion in care.* Washington, DC: GAO.

Garbarino, J., and A. Crouter. 1978. Defining the community context for parent-child relations: The correlates of child maltreatment. *Child Development* 49(3):604-616.

Garrison, M. 2004. Reforming child protection: A public health perspective. *Virginia Journal of Social Policy and the Law* 12:590.

Glisson, C. 2010. Organizational climate and service outcomes in child welfare settings. In *Child welfare and child well-being: New perspectives from the national survey of child and adolescent well-being,* edited by M. B. Webb, K. Dowd, B. J. Harden, J. Landsverk, and M. Testa. New York: Oxford University Press. Pp. 380-408.

Glisson, C., and P. Green. 2011. Organizational climate, services, and outcomes in child welfare systems. *Child Abuse & Neglect* 35(8):582-591.

Glisson, C., and A. Hemmelgarn. 1997. The effects of organizational climate and interorganizational coordination on the quality and outcomes of children's service systems. *Child Abuse & Neglect* 22(5):401-421.

Glisson, C., D. Dukes, and P. Green. 2006. The effects of the ARC organizational intervention on caseworker turnover, climate, and culture in children's service systems. *Child Abuse & Neglect* 30(8):855-880.

Green, H. 2005. *Mental health of children and young people in Great Britain, 2004.* Palgrave Macmillan Basingstoke.

Gunnar, M. R., and P. A. Fisher. 2006. Bringing basic research on early experience and stress neurobiology to bear on preventive interventions for neglected and maltreated children. *Development and Psychopathology* 18(3):651-677.

Gunnar, M. R., M. H. Van Dulmen, T. Achenbach, E. Ames, E. Ames, M. Berry, R. Barth, G. Bohlin, L. Janols, and M. Bohman. 2007. Behavior problems in postinstitutionalized internationally adopted children. *Development and Psychopathology* 19(1):129.

Harman, J. S., G. E. Childs, and K. J. Kelleher. 2000. Mental health care utilization and expenditures by children in foster care. *Archives of Pediatrics & Adolescent Medicine* 154(11):1114.

Haskins, R., and J. Baron. 2011. *Building the connection between policy and evidence: The Obama evidence-based initiatives.* London: NESTA.

Haskins, R., F. Wulczyn, and M. B. Webb, eds. 2007. *Child protection: Using research to improve policy and practice.* Washington, DC: Brookings Institution Press.

Hill, R. B. 2006. *Synthesis of research on disproportionality in child welfare: An update.* Washington, DC: Casey-Center for the Study of Social Policy (CSSP) Alliance for Racial Equity in the Child Welfare System. http://www.cssp.org/reform/child-welfare/other-resources/synthesis-of-research-on-disproportionality-robert-hill.pdf (accessed June 11, 2013).

Hines, A. M. , K. Lemon, P. Wyatt, and J. Merdinger. 2004. Factors related to the disproportionate involvement of children of color in the child welfare system: A review and emerging themes. *Children and Youth Services Review* 26(6):507-527.

Horwitz, S. M., M. S. Hurlburt, and Z. Zhang. 2010. Patterns and predictors of mental health services use by children in contact with the child welfare system. In *Child welfare and child wellbeing: New perspectives from the National Survey of Child and Adolescent Well-Being,* edited by M. B. Webb, K. Dowd, B. J. Harden, J. A. Landsverk, and M. F. Testa. New York: Oxford University Press. Pp. 279-329.

Horwitz, S. M., M. S. Hurlburt, S. D. Cohen, J. Zhang, and J. Landsverk. 2011. Predictors of placement for children who initially remained in their homes after an investigation for child abuse and neglect. *Child Abuse & Neglect* 35(3):188-198.

IOM (Institute of Medicine). 2003. *Unequal treatment: Confronting racial and ethnic disparities in health care.* Washington, DC: The National Academies Press.

James, S., J. Landsverk, and D. J. Slymen. 2004. Placement movement in out-of-home care: Patterns and predictors. *Children and Youth Services Review* 26(2):185-206.

Jee, S. H., R. P. Barth, M. A. Szilagyi, P. G. Szilagyi, M. Aida, and M. M. Davis. 2006. Factors associated with chronic conditions among children in foster care. *Journal of Health Care for the Poor and Underserved* 17(2):328-341.

Jones, B. J., J. A. Gillette, D. Painte, and S. Paulson. 2000. *Indian Child Welfare Act: A pilot study of compliance in North Dakota.* Washington, DC: Casey Family Programs. http://www.nicwa.org/resources/research/?p=Research_Docs_170 (accessed June 24, 2013).

Kaplan, C., and L. Merkel-Holguin. 2008. Another look at the National Study on Differential Response in Child Welfare. *Protecting Children* 23(1-2):5-21.

Kaufman, L., and R. L. Jones. 2003. Trenton finds abuse high in foster care. *The New York Times,* April 16.

Kim, A. K., D. Brooks, H. Kim, and J. Nissly. 2008. *Structured Decision Making® and child welfare service delivery project.* Berkeley: University of California at Berkeley, California Social Work Education Center (http://www.csulb.edu/projects/ccwrl/Brooks.pdf (accessed August 27, 2013).

Kurtz, P. D., J. M. Gaudin, P. T. Howing, and J. S. Wodarski. 1993. The consequences of physical abuse and neglect on the school age child: Mediating factors. *Children and Youth Services Review* 15(2):85-104.

Landsverk, J., and F. Wulczyn. 2013 (unpublished). *Child placement as a response to child abuse and neglect.* Paper commissioned by the Committee on Child Maltreatment Research, Policy, and Practice for the Next Decade, IOM, Washington, DC.

Landsverk, J. A., A. F. Garland, and L. K. Leslie. 2002. Mental health services for children reported to Child Protective Services. In *ASPAC handbook on child maltreatment,* edited by J. E. B. Myers, H. C. T., L. Berliner, C. Jenny, J. Briere, and T. Reid. Thousand Oaks, CA: Sage Publications. Pp. 487-507.

Landsverk, J., M. Hurlburt, S. Horwitz, J. Rolls Reutz, and J. Zhang. 2009. *Children and familes involved in child welfare and remaining in home after investigation for child abuse and neglect: Findings from the National Survey of Child Adolescent Well-Being (NSCAW).* Baltimore, MD: Annie E. Casey Foundation.

Landsverk, J., M. Hurlburt, L. Leslie, J. Rolls-Reutz, and J. Zhang. 2010. Exits from out-of-home care and continuity of mental health services use. In *Child welfare and child well-being: New perspectives from the National Survey of Child and Adolescent Well-Being* edited by M. B. Webb, K. Dowd, B. J. Harden, J. Landsverk, and M. F. Testa. New York: Oxford University Press. Pp. 330-350.

Lawrence, C. K., J. Strolin-Goltzman, J. Caringi, N. Claiborne, M. McCarthy, E. Butts, and K. O'Connell. 2012. Evaluation in child welfare organizations. *Administration in Social Work* 37(1):3-13.

Lawrence, C. R., E. A. Carlson, and B. Egeland. 2006. The impact of foster care on development. *Development and Psychopathology* 18(1):57-76.

Layzer, J. I., B. D. Goodson, L. Bernstein, and C. Price. 2001. *National evaluation of family support programs. Final report,* Vol. A. Cambridge, MA: Abt Associates.

Lee, S., S. Aos, E. Drake, A. Pennucci, M. Miller, and L. Anderson. 2012. Return on investment: Evidence-based options to improve statewide outcomes technical appendix. Olympia: Washington State Institute for Public Policy http://www.wsipp.wa.gov/Reports/322 (accessed August 25, 2013).

Lery, B. 2009. Neighborhood structure and foster care entry risk: The role of spatial scale in defining neighborhoods. *Children and Youth Services Review* 31(3):331-337.

Leslie, L. K., M. S. Hurlburt, S. James, J. Landsverk, D. J. Slymen, and J. Zhang. 2005. Relationshiop between entry into child welfare and mental health service use. *Psychiatric Services* 56(8):981-987.

Lieberman, A. 1987. Separation in infancy and toddlerhood: Contributions of attachment theory and psychoanalysis. *The Psychology of Separation and Loss: Perspectives on Development, Life Transitions, and Clinical Practice* 109-135.

Loman, L. A., and G. L. Siegel. 2004. *Differential response in Missouri after five years: Final report.* St. Louis, MO: Institute of Applied Research.

Loman, L. A., and G. L. Siegel. 2012. *Ohio alternative response evaluation extension: Interim report.* St. Louis, MO: Institute of Applied Research.

Loman, L. A., C. S. Filonow, and G. Siegel. 2010. *Ohio alternative response evaluation: Final report with technical appendix.* St. Louis, MO: Institute of Applied Research.

Marts, E. J., E. K. O. Lee, R. Mcroy, and J. McCroskey. 2008. Point of engagement: Reducing disproportionality and improving child and family outcomes. *Child Welfare* 87(2):335-358.

McCown, F. S. 2005. *Privatization of Child Protective Services.* Austin, TX: Center for Public Policy Priorities. http://library.cppp.org/files/4/privatization_pb.pdf (accessed August 27, 2013).

McCroskey, J., and W. Meezan. 1998. Family-centered services: Approaches and effectiveness. *The Future of Children* 8(1):54-71.

McCroskey, J., P. Pecora, T. Franke, C. Christie, and J. Lorthridge. 2012. Can public child welfare help to prevent child maltreatment? Promising findings from Los Angeles. *Journal of Family Strengths* 12(1):1-23. http://digitalcommons.library.tmc.edu/jfs/vol12/iss1/5 (accessed August 6, 2013).

Merkel-Holguin, L., C. Kaplan, and A. Kwak. 2006. *National study on differential response in child welfare.* Washington, DC: Child Welfare League of America.

Mor Barak, M. E., D. J. Travis, H. Pyun, and B. Xie. 2009. The impact of supervision on worker outcomes: A meta analysis. *Social Service Review* 83(1):3-32.

National Evaluation of the Court Improvement Program. 2007. *The national evaluation of the Court Improvement Program (CIP): Synthesis of 2005 Court Improvement Program reform and activities-final report.* Washington, DC: U.S. Department of Health and Human Services. https://docs.google.com/viewer?a=v&q=cache:2e88RgueWEQJ:www.pal-tech. com/cip/files/FirstSynthesis.pdf+national+CIP+evaluation+final+report&hl=en&gl=us& pid=bl&srcid=ADGEEShtnHYZqHLyzoRzJZFouKT0ZaE9BRPT_IrFnBfc5l2fLhshHU9-kxuy5N73plkZeVTIu9WFrPaJHZ4Wq7DZX04V-m13is08bEyHm9tbdFpo ZDxb7vhL_c-yAlKxdSUZG_r_PVGA&sig=AHIEtbQKNjVeY9esdv_MeGJZ-1f1AzIVTg (accessed June 13, 2013).

NCCD (National Council on Crime and Delinquency). 2013. *Structured Decision Making (SDM) system.* http://www.nccdglobal.org/assessment/structured-decision-making-sdm-system (accessed May 3, 2013).

NCSL (National Conference of State Legislatures). 2012. *Mandatory reporting of child abuse and neglect: 2012 introduced state legislation (review from).* http://www.ncsl.org/issues-research/human-services/2012-child-abuse-mandatory-reporting-bills.aspx (accessed December 3, 2013).

Needell, B., M. A. Brookhart, and S. Lee. 2003. Black children and foster care placement in California. *Children and Youth Services Review* 25(5-6):393-408.

Newton, R. R., A. J. Litrownik, and J. A. Landsverk. 2000. Children and youth in foster care: Disentangling the relationship between problem behaviors and number of placements. *Child Abuse & Neglect* 24(10):1363-1374.

NRC (National Research Council). 1993. *Understanding child abuse and neglect.* Washington, DC: National Academy Press.

OPRE (Office of Planning, Research, and Evaluation). 2013. *National Survey of Child and Adolescent Well-Being (NSCAW), 1997-2013: Project overview.* http://www.acf.hhs.gov/programs/opre/research/project/national-survey-of-child-and-adolescent-well-being-nscaw-1 (accessed February 15, 2013).

Osterling, K. L., A. D'Andrade, and M. J. Austin. 2008. Understanding and addressing racial/ethnic disproportionality in the front end of the child welfare system. *Journal of Evidence-Based Social Work* 5(1-2):9-30.

Palmer, S. E. (1996). Placement stability and inclusive practice in foster care: An empirical study. *Children and Youth Services Review* 18(7):589-601.

Pardeck, J. T. 1984. Multiple placement of children in foster family care: An empirical analysis. *Social Work* 29(6):506-509.

Pardeck, J. T. 1985. A profile of the child likely to experience unstable foster care. *Adolescence* 20(79):689-696.

Pardeck, J. T., J. W. Murphy, and L. Fitzwater. 1985. Profile of the foster child likely to experience unstable care: A re-examination. *Early Child Development and Care* 22(2-3):137-146.

Patel, D., P. Matyanga, T. Nyamundaya, D. Chimedza, K. Webb, and B. Engelsmann. 2012. Facilitating HIV testing, care and treatment for orphans and vulnerable children aged five years and younger through community-based early childhood development playcentres in rural Zimbabwe. *Journal of the International AIDS Society* 15(Suppl 2):17404.

Pennell, J., and G. Burford. 2000. Family group decision making: Protecting children and women. *Child Welfare* 79(2):131-158.

Poertner, J., M. Bussey, and J. Fluke. 1999. How safe are out-of-home placements? *Children and Youth Services Review* 21(7):549-563.

Polinsky, M. L., L. Pion-Berlin, S. Williams, T. Long, and A. M. Wolf. 2010. Preventing child abuse and neglect: A national evaluation of parents anonymous groups. *Child Welfare* 89(6):43-62.

Proch, K., and M. A. Taber. 1985. Placement disruption: A review of research. *Children and Youth Services Review* 7(4):309-320.

Provence, S. 1989. Infants in institutions revisited. *Zero to Three* 9(4):1-4.

QIC-DR (National Quality Improvement Center on Differential Response in Child Protective Services). 2011. *Differential response in Child Protective Services: A literature review.* Version 2. CRDA Number: 93:670. Washington, DC: U.S. Department of Health and Human Services, Children's Bureau.

QIC-DR. 2012. *Differential response approach in Child Protective Services: An analysis of state legislative provisions.* Denver, CO: QIC-DR.

Redding, R. E., C. Fried, and P. A. Britner. 2000. Predictors of placement outcomes in treatment foster care: Implications for foster parent selection and service delivery. *Journal of Child and Family Studies* 9(4):425-447.

Ringeisen, H., C. Casanueva, M. Urato, and T. Cross. 2008. Special health care needs among children in the child welfare system. *Pediatrics* 122(1):e232-e241.

Rivaux, S. L., J. James, K. Wittenstrom, D. Baumann, J. Sheets, J. Henry, and V. Jeffries. 2008. The intersection of race, poverty, and risk: Understanding the decision to provide services to clients and to remove children. *Child Welfare* 87(2):151-168.

Rosner, D., and G. Markowitz. 1997. Race, foster care, and the politics of abandonment in New York City. *American Journal of Public Health* 87(11):1844-1849.

Ruppel, J., Y. Huang, and G. Haulenbeek. 2011. Differential response in child protective services in New York state. New York: New York State Office of Children and Family Services.

Rzepnicki, T. L., P. R. Johnson, D. Kane, D. Moncher, L. Coconato, and B. Shulman. 2010. Transforming child protection agencies into high reliability organizations: A conceptual framework. *Protecting Children* 25(1):48-62.

Sanders, D. 2012. Presentation at the Child Maltreatment, Research, Policy, and Practice for the Next Decade Workshop, January 31, 2012, Washington, DC.

Schwalbe, C. S. 2008. Strengthening the integration of actuarial risk assessment with clinical judgment in an evidence based practice framework. *Children and Youth Services Review* 30(12):1458-1464.

Sedlak, A. J., K. McPeherson, and B. Dias. 2010. *Supplementary analyses of race differences in child child abuse and neglect rates in the NIS-4.* Rockville, MD: Westat, Inc.

Shlonsky, A., and D. Wagner. 2005. The next step: Integrating actuarial risk assessment and clinical judgment into an evidence-based practice framework in CPS case management. *Child and Youth Services Review* 27(4):409-427.

Siegel, G. L., and L. A. Loman. 2006. *Extended follow up study of Minnesota's Family Assessment Response: Final report.* St. Louis, MO: Institute of Applied Research.

Siegel, G. L., C. S. Filonow, and L. A. Loman. 2010. *Differential response in Nevada.* St. Louis, MO: Institute of Applied Research.

Smith, D. K., E. Stormshak, P. Chamberlain, and R. B. Whaley. 2001. Placement disruption in treatment foster care. *Journal of Emotional and Behavioral Disorders* 9(3):200-205.

Social Work Policy Institute. 2011. *Supervision: The safety net for front-line child welfare practice.* http://www.socialworkpolicy.org/wp-content/uploads/2011/03/SWPI-ChildWelfare-Supervision-Final-Report.pdf (accessed December 3, 2013).

Social Work Policy Institute. 2012a. *Children at risk: Optimizing health in an era of reform.* Washington, DC: National Association of Social Workers. http://www.socialworkpolicy. org/wp-content/uploads/2012/06/childrenatrisk-report1.pdf (accessed August 15, 2013).

Social Work Policy Institute. 2012b. *Educating social workers for child welfare practice: The status of using Title IV-E funding to support BSW & MSW education.* Washington, DC: National Association of Social Workers. http://www.socialworkpolicy.org/wp-content/uploads/2013/01/SWPI-IVE-Policy-Brief.pdf (accessed August 15, 2013).

Staff, I., and E. Fein. 1995. Stability and change: Initial findings in a study of treatment foster care placements. *Children and Youth Services Review* 17(3):379-389.

Stahmer, A. C., L. K. Leslie, M. Hurlburt, R. P. Barth, M. B. Webb, J. Landsverk, and J. Zhang. 2005. Developmental and behavioral needs and service use for young children in child welfare. *Pediatrics* 116(4):891-900.

Stovall, K., and M. Dozier. 1998. Infants in foster care: An attachment theory perspective. *Adoption Quarterly* 2(1):55-88.

Sullivan, D. J., and M. A. van Zyl. 2008. The well-being of children in foster care: Exploring physical and mental health needs. *Children and Youth Services Review* 30(7):774-786.

Summers, A., S. Wood, and J. Russell. 2012. *Disproportionality rates for children of color in foster care.* http://www.ncjfcj.org/sites/default/files/Disproportionality%20Rates%20for%20Children%20of%20Color%202010.pdf (accessed June 24, 2013).

Terling-Watt, T. 2001. Permanency in kinship care: An exploration of disruption rates and factors associated with placement disruption. *Children and Youth Services Review* 23(2):111-126.

Testa, M. F. 2010. Flexibility, innovation, and experimentation: The rise and fall of child welfare waiver demonstrations. In *Fostering accountablilty: Using evidence to guide and improve child welfare policy,* edited by M. F. Testa and J. Poertner. New York: Oxford University Press. Pp. 269-290.

Testa, M. F. 2012. Fostering innovation through Title IV-E waiver demonstrations. *Policy and Practice* 70(3):28-30, 48.

Tittle, G., J. Poertner, and P. Garnier. 2001. *Child maltreatment in foster care: A study of retrospective reporting.* Urbana, IL: Children and Family Research Center.

Tittle, G., J. Poertner, and P. Garnier. 2008. *Child maltreatment in out of home care: What do we know now?* Urbana: Children and Family Research Center, School of Social Work, University of Illinois at Urbana-Champaign.

Usher, C. L., K. A. Randolph, and H. C. Gogan. 1999. Placement patterns in foster care. *Social Service Review* 73(1):22-36.

Walsh, J. A., and R. A. Walsh. 1990. Studies of the maintenance of subsidized foster placements in the Casey Family Program. *Child Welfare* 69(2):99-114.

Webb, M. B., K. Dowd, B. Jones Harden, J. Landsverk, and M. Testa. 2010. *Child welfare and child well-being: New perspectives from the National Survey of Child and Adolescent Well-Being.* New York: Oxford University Press.

Widom, C. S. 1991. Avoidance of criminality in abused and neglected children. *Psychiatry: Journal for the Study of Interpersonal Processes* 54(2):162-174.

Winokur, M., A. Holten, and D. Valentine. July 2009. Kinship care for the safety, permanency, and well-being of children removed from the home for maltreatment. *Cochrane Database of Systematic Reviews* (1):CD006546.

Wulczyn, F. 1986. *Child welfare caseloads: A sociological interpretation.* Unpublished doctoral dissertation, University of Chicago.

Wulczyn, F. 2012. *Multistate foster care data archive.* Chicago: Center for State Child Welfare Data, Chapin Hall, University of Chicago.

Wulczyn, F., L. Chen, and K. B. Hislop. 2007. *Foster care dynamics, 2000-2005: A report from the multistate foster care data archive.* Chicago: Chapin Hall Center for Children, University of Chicago.

Wulczyn, F., L. Chen, L. Collins, and M. Ernst. 2011. The foster care baby boom revisited: What do the numbers tell us? *Zero to Three* 31(3):4-10.

Wulczyn, F., R. Gibbons, L. Snowden, and B. Lery. 2013. Poverty, social disadvantage and the black/white placement gap. *Child and Youth Services Review* 35(1):65-74.

Yampolskaya, S., R. I. Paulson, M. Armstrong, N. Jordan, and A. C. Vargo. 2004. Child welfare privatization: Quantitative indicators and policy issues. *Evaluation Review* 28(2): 87-103.

Yang, K. F., and G. van Landingham. 2012. How hollow can we go? A case study of the Florida's efforts to outsource oversight of privatized child welfare services. *American Review of Public Administration* 42(5):543-561.

Zayas, L. E., J. C. McMillen, M. Y. Lee, and S. J. Books. 2013. Challenges to quality assurance and improvement efforts in behavioral health organizations: A qualitative assessment. *Administration and Policy in Mental Health and Mental Health Services Research* 40(3):190-198.

Zlotnik, J. L. 2009. *Social work and child welfare: A national debate.* University of Michigan Fauri Lecture, October 27, Ann Arbor, MI.

Zlotnik, J. L. 2010. Fostering and sustaining university/agency partnerships. In *Fostering accountability: Using evidence to guide and improve child welfare policy,* edited by M. F. Testa and J. Poertner. New York: Oxford University Press. Pp. 328-356.

Zlotnik, J. L., D. DePanfilis, C. Daining, and M. M. Lane. 2005. *Factors influencing recruitment and retention of child welfare workers: A systematic review of research.* Washington, DC: Institute for the Advancement of Social Work Research. http://www.socialworkpolicy.org/wp-content/uploads/2007/06/4-CW-SRRFinalFullReport.pdf (accessed August 6, 2013).

Zuravin, S. J., M. Benedict, and M. Somerfield. 1993. Child maltreatment in family foster-care. *American Journal of Orthopsychiatry* 63(4):589-596.

6

Interventions and Service Delivery Systems

Since the 1993 National Research Council (NRC) report was issued (NRC, 1993), significant advances have occurred in the development and dissemination of model programs for treating and preventing various forms of child abuse and neglect (Daro and Benedetti, 2014). In addition to the public child protection and child welfare systems found in all communities, a variety of treatment programs targeting victims and perpetrators of child abuse and neglect are offered through various mental health and social service agencies. Many communities also have access to primary and secondary prevention services designed to reduce the risk for child abuse or neglect for families experiencing difficulties. Among this growing array of service options, an increasing number of interventions have strong evidence of efficacy with at least a portion of their target populations. Many others are aggressively building their evidence base and now operate with increased awareness of the need for and the value of robust evaluative data.

The current evidence base also suggests that the availability of these services is uneven across communities and populations, leaving many of the most vulnerable children and families without adequate services. Even when identified, children who are victims of child abuse or neglect may not receive the therapeutic services needed to address their serious developmental and behavioral problems. Families at significant risk of child abuse or neglect as a result of mental health issues, domestic violence, or substance abuse are among those least likely to be adequately served by the current array of preventive and family support services. And when services are offered, their quality and potential impacts vary greatly (Paxson and Haskins, 2009). On balance, however, much progress has been made in the ability to successfully identify, engage, and assist a growing proportion of children and families that have experienced or are at risk for child abuse and neglect.

The purpose of this chapter is to describe those program models and intervention strategies with the strongest evidence of success, identify approaches that have been found lacking, and highlight the importance of building an integrated system of care to enhance the capacity to successfully prevent child abuse and neglect and treat victims. In developing this conceptual framework, the committee intentionally considered the collective challenges facing all relevant interventions instead of segmenting the discussion into the traditional silos of treatment and prevention services. Also highlighted are the common challenges faced with all interventions in attempting to enhance their assessment, implementation, replication, and sustainability.

The child abuse and neglect interventions reviewed here are aimed in part at improving the capacity of parents and caretakers to cease certain harmful behaviors or to adopt behaviors commonly accepted as contributing to healthy child development. The behaviors targeted include those that are illegal and wrong, as well as those for which evidence demonstrates a link to negative or positive impacts on a child's development or safety. Parental capacity and behaviors can be altered either directly by providing services to individual caretakers to improve their knowledge and skills, or indirectly by creating a context in which doing the "right thing" is easier, such as by reducing stress and increasing support within the immediate family and local community.

The child welfare system, as described in Chapter 5, provides a necessary public policy and service response but is insufficient to address the immediate and long-term consequences of child abuse and neglect or give families the support they need to prevent these outcomes. This chapter focuses on why it is important to develop, implement, assess, and sustain an array of strong interventions that address the consequences of child abuse and neglect (treatment) and offer promising pathways to improve parental capacity to support optimal child development by reducing risks and strengthening protective factors (prevention). The committee recognizes the wider range of interventions that address myriad issues associated with an elevated risk for child abuse and neglect, such as substance abuse treatment programs, domestic violence interventions, depression treatments, income support programs, child care, and community violence prevention programs. The discussion here, however, is limited to strategies whose core objectives include reducing child abuse and neglect, improving parental capacity, and ameliorating the consequences of child abuse and neglect.

The first two sections of the chapter identify an array of service strategies and program models that have demonstrated success in achieving their targeted outcomes, as well as those efforts that have failed to fulfill expectations. Because of variations in legal authority, target population, and scope across the various elements of the child abuse and neglect service continuum, this evidence is presented in two broad groupings: treatment programs designed to reduce reincidence and ameliorate the consequences of child abuse or neglect, and prevention efforts designed to enhance parental capacity, improve child outcomes, and reduce a child's risk for experiencing abuse or neglect. The third section of the chapter examines a set of issues that have limited the replication and efficacy of interventions designed to address child abuse and neglect. Although the issues addressed are not exhaustive, they illustrate the challenges facing both public child welfare systems and the direct services provided to children and families. Improving outcomes for a greater proportion of victims and those at risk of child abuse and neglect will require new research on such issues as cultural relevance, replication fidelity, cost-effectiveness, service delivery reform, and service integration. In addition to offering guidance on how to structure and target specific interventions, such research can guide reforms in public child welfare and other public service delivery systems to improve overall service quality and create an institutional infrastructure capable of sustaining such reforms. The fourth section examines important aspects of building an integrated system of care, including organization culture and interagency networks. The final section presents conclusions.

Any intervention or reform strategy, regardless of its target population or primary outcomes, appears to benefit from a set of "core ingredients" (Barth et al., 2012). Although identifying the exact nature of these ingredients is a work in progress, they generally include building on a strong theoretical foundation that links intended outcomes to a clearly articulated theory of change, offering the program at a sufficient dosage and duration to make it possible to achieve the intended outcomes, staffing the program with individuals who have the knowledge and competencies to work with participants to achieve the desired outcomes, and operating within a system of quality assurance to ensure that the program is delivered properly and the desired outcomes are achieved (Chorpita et al., 2005; Duncan et al., 2010; Wulczyn et al., 2010). As noted in the following sections, these characteristics, among others, help distinguish successful efforts from those with less promise.

TREATMENT PROGRAMS

The greatest change in the development of treatment programs to address child abuse and neglect has been an emphasis on evidence-based practices rather than new theories that might suggest radically different treatment areas. Two primary advances have occurred. The first is the development of therapies that specifically target the impact of trauma or abuse on children. These approaches deal mainly with posttraumatic stress, depression, and anxiety—the primary emotional impacts of abuse. There is a robust literature on interventions addressing these outcomes, but it is not exclusive to child abuse. This research base acknowledges the importance of screening for trauma (including abuse) and validating its occurrence, but encompasses strategies that operate within the traditional framework of mental health interventions. Treatment clinically targets the outcomes or the mental health condition, not the event or cause per se. This focus is consistent with the evidence showing that not all children exposed to child abuse, various forms of trauma, or even terrible lives in general develop mental health disorders. The emphasis also is on modular approaches that address multiple clinical outcomes rather than a single presenting problem.

The second main advance in treatment interventions is in approaches to problematic parenting and behavior problems in children. Child abuse and neglect represent extreme forms of problematic parenting, and parenting interventions are the most common service recommendation in child welfare. It has long been known that parenting approaches, parental behaviors, and their interaction with child behaviors are primary determinants of behavioral problems in children. In child abuse and neglect situations, behavioral problems are both a consequence of abuse or neglect and a potential risk factor for triggering physical abuse. It is not only physical or sexual abuse that may produce behavioral problems in children; the inconsistent or coercive parenting that often characterizes neglect is also implicated (Gardner, 1989; Patterson et al., 1990; Stormshak et al., 2000). Neglecting parents may be inattentive, unresponsive, or inconsistent. Therefore, effective parenting interventions are the first-line treatments both for dealing with behavior problems in child victims and for reducing the risk for subsequent child abuse and neglect.

The empirical literature is unanimous that behavioral problems are addressed most effectively through interventions that target parents as the primary change agents. In many cases, especially those involving younger children, the interventions are fully parent mediated (Carlson et al., 1989); the children need not be the recipients of individual treatment. This targeting of parents is particularly apt in the context of child abuse and neglect as compared with the typical nonabusive scenario in which children have behavioral problems. Wolfe and others (Graziano and Diament, 1992; Wolf et al., 1987; Wolfe et al., 1988) demonstrated early on that a behavioral parent training program was effective with abusive parents. However, the idea of applying this well-established approach to child abuse and neglect situations did not fully take hold until Urquiza and McNeil (1996) published a paper in *Child Maltreatment* advancing the application of parent-child interaction therapy (PCIT) in these cases (Urquiza and McNeil, 1996) (PCIT is further discussed below). The emphasis on promoting positive parent-child relationships to address behavioral problems in abused or neglected children resonated with the child abuse and neglect community because behavioral problems in these cases are the result of abusive or neglectful parenting. In other words, applying a proven parent-mediated intervention would simultaneously address the child's behavior problems and the deficits in the parent-child relationship. Ideally, enhancing the parent-child relationship promotes more secure attachment and stronger bonding, which in turn not only improves child behavior but also lowers the risk for future abuse or neglect.

The focus on parenting interventions is not new; they have always been a primary service for child abuse and neglect cases. What changed was the recognition that parenting practices and child behavior problems are inextricably interrelated and are best addressed through a single parenting-focused intervention, as opposed to sending parents to parent education classes and children to individual therapy when abuse or neglect results in behavior problems. Moreover, the parenting interventions typically offered were didactic classes or peer support, neither of which involve learning and using new skills in difficult parenting interactions. While parenting classes are still common, it is increasingly appreciated that they are unlikely to produce behavior change in abusive or neglectful parents.

Evidence for Effectiveness

The standard, well-established parent management training or behavioral parent training programs have now been applied extensively to child abuse and neglect situations, and in some cases subjected to specific clinical trials. Findings on parent management training suggest robust effects across cultural groups (Lau, 2006; Martinez and Eddy, 2005). PCIT is effective with abusive or neglectful parents (Timmer et al., 2005), as well as with foster parents (Timmer et al., 2006), when children have behavioral problems. For example, the Incredible Years (Herman et al., 2011; Webster-Stratton et al., 2011a,b) has been tested extensively with low-income Head Start families, many of which are at high risk for abuse or neglect or have been involved in the child welfare system.

The Parent Management Training Oregon (PMTO) model is one of the earliest and most well-established interventions for behavior problems. It is the basis for two interventions that have been used in child welfare populations. The first, Multi-dimensional Treatment Foster Care (Chamberlain et al., 2008), is a treatment foster care model for severely behaviorally disturbed children that teaches foster parents to deliver the PMTO model with the active consultation and support of a consultant. Under the model, youth can be transitioned to regular foster care or their family home in less than 6 months. The second intervention is Keeping Foster and Kin Parents

Supported and Trained, a less intensive version of the model for foster parents and kinship caretakers that has been found to be effective in reducing behavior problems and promoting placement stability (Chamberlain et al., 2008). As discussed later in this chapter, another well-established parent management training program—the Positive Parenting Program, commonly known as Triple P (Sanders et al., 2002)—also is increasingly being used in child welfare cases.

A number of these parenting interventions have been shown to improve child welfare outcomes in addition to improving behavior problems in abused and neglected children. PCIT with a motivational enhancement component significantly reduces referrals to the child welfare system compared with services as usual (Chaffin, 2004; Chaffin et al., 2004). In fact, PCIT by itself outperforms PCIT combined with other services (Chaffin, 2004). Alternatives for Families-Cognitive-Behavioral Therapy (AF-CBT) entails parent-child cognitive-behavioral therapy for physically abusive families. It incorporates standard parent management training; coping skills for children and parents; and a process for parents to make amends for the abuse, which reduces behavior problems and violence in both children and parents. Parent-Child CBT (PC-CBT), a similar approach for physically abusing families in which the intervention is delivered in child and parent groups, also has been shown to improve behavior problems and reduce future aggression (Runyon et al., 2009). And Triple P delivered as a population-based intervention has been shown to offset increases in child abuse referrals and placement rates (Prinz et al., 2009).

Infant mental health interventions have been developed for the very youngest victims of abuse and neglect. These programs are fully parent mediated and focus on enhancing parents' sensitivity and responsiveness to their children, as well as basic protective parenting. Parents learn to recognize child cues, especially for distress, and to respond in ways that are consistently comforting. Several programs have been tested in clinical trials involving abusive or neglectful situations and been found to be effective in improving parent sensitivity and child adjustment (Bernard et al., 2012; Spieker et al., 2012).

SafeCare is a parenting-focused intervention for neglect situations involving young children. It is a brief structured home-based program, delivered by trained professionals or paraprofessionals, consisting of three components: safety proofing the home, teaching parents how to monitor and manage child health, and coaching in parenting. The parenting coaching component is not intended for cases in which the children have significant behavioral problems, but teaches basic positive parenting skills. In a recent statewide randomized trial taking the intervention to scale, families receiving SafeCare in addition to the usual array of home-based services had significantly lower rates of rereferral to child protective services (Chaffin et al., 2012a). Implemented in a trial with American Indian families, SafeCare not only was effective but also was highly acceptable to these families (Chaffin et al., 2012b).

Not infrequently, children show more than one internalizing impact of abuse and neglect, including posttraumatic stress, anxiety, and depression. The literature is robust for the effectiveness of Trauma-Focused CBT (TF-CBT) (Mannarino et al., 2012), a structured intervention for children and caregivers that directly targets the impact of traumatic experiences, including physical and sexual abuse. It reduces not only posttraumatic stress, but also depression and moderate behavior problems when present. The intervention consists of standard CBT elements such as psychoeducation, relaxation and emotion regulation skills, and positive parenting. The trauma-specific CBT component is the trauma narrative, which entails gradual exposure to trauma memories and cognitive processing to correct maladaptive trauma-related beliefs. TF-CBT has been tested extensively with children involved with the child welfare system, including those in foster care placement. It has also been widely disseminated in a variety of public mental health settings through the National Child Traumatic Stress Network. CBT is well established for children with depression or anxiety (Walkup et al., 2008), although research has not specifically addressed whether the proven interventions are equally effective with abused and neglected children.

Child and Family Posttraumatic Stress Intervention (Berkowitz, 2011), a brief trauma-focused intervention, has been shown to be effective in preventing chronic posttraumatic stress disorder when delivered shortly after a trauma. It consists of assessing trauma impact with feedback to families, providing psychoeducation and normalizing about traumatic stress, and teaching coping skills. Although not yet specifically tested in child abuse or neglect cases, this intervention has been shown to be effective in domestic violence cases and is potentially applicable as an early intervention in cases of child abuse and neglect.

There are also well-established interventions for anxiety and depression in children. CBT is the first-line treatment and may be combined with medication in some cases (Walkup et al., 2008). Children are given information about anxiety or depression; are taught relaxation and coping skills; undergo cognitive restructuring designed to change maladaptive and unhelpful thoughts; and in the case of depression, are taught exposure to unrealistic fears and behavioral activation. Parents may or may not be actively involved in this therapy. The literature has not established that these models work specifically with abused and neglected children, but there is no reason to believe that they would not.

TF-CBT and many parent management training programs have been found to be equally effective for minority youth and their families among the samples included in clinical trials. For example, equivalent outcomes for TF-CBT have been observed for African Americans (Scheeringa et al., 2010). A school-based group version of TF-CBT (Cognitive-Behavioral Intervention for Trauma in Schools [CBITS]) was initially tested and found effective in the highly diverse Los Angeles school district, where a majority of children are immigrants (Jaycox et al., 2002). Culturally adapted versions of CBITS for Latinos and American Indians have been developed (Chaffin et al., 2012b; Workgroup on Adapting Latino Services, 2008). Another trauma-focused intervention (Resilient Peer Treatment) has been identified as probably efficacious for abused African American youth. Several interventions for anxiety have shown some efficacy with ethnic minority youth (Huey and Polo, 2008). Group cognitive-behavioral therapy (GCBT) has been identified as possibly efficacious for African American and Latino youth (see Huey and Polo, 2008). In addition, anxiety management training and CBT have been identified as possibly efficacious for African American youth. For conduct problems, a variety of approaches show some degree of efficacy; specific approaches tend to differ for African American and Hispanic/Latino youth. Consistent efficacy has been found for Multisystemic Therapy (MST) and Coping Power with African American youth, and for Brief Strategic Family Therapy (BSFT) with Latino youth. In addition, MST has been effective with Native Hawaiian youth (Rowland et al., 2005), and in a small randomized controlled trial, The Incredible Years was found to be effective for maladjusted Chinese American youth (Lau et al., 2011). While these interventions have not been tested specifically with abused and neglected youth, there is no reason to believe they would not be effective with this population.

In 2013 a comparative effectiveness review of parenting interventions, trauma-focused treatments, and enhanced foster care approaches that address child abuse and neglect was conducted under the auspices of the Agency for Healthcare Research and Quality (Forman-Hoffman et al., 2013). While the authors note the support for a number of promising treatment strategies, the review found that methodological gaps in the evidence limit the ability to compare results across studies adequately.

The Bottom Line

There are two big success stories in interventions for children affected by abuse and neglect. The first is TF-CBT. Tested extensively, it has been found effective for children and families from diverse backgrounds and circumstances and has been adapted specifically for foster children and children in residential care (Mannarino et al., 2012). TF-CBT has been widely disseminated throughout the United States, and there are well-established training models for the program.

The second big success story is the application of well-established parent management training programs to child welfare populations. Many of these programs have been found not only to improve behavior problems caused by child abuse and neglect but also to impact child welfare outcomes such as reabuse and rereferral.

The most pressing remaining questions relate to how these interventions can be taken to scale in the mental health and service settings where abused and neglected children receive their care. These questions about implementation and sustainability are not specific to interventions in child abuse and neglect. Questions specific to child welfare relate more to service planning and to how many of what types of interventions should be readily available or ordered for families in the child welfare system. The current approach is to order a single, limited intervention for each problem, which often results in a long list of services that families must complete as part of their child welfare case plan (Society for Prevention Research, 2004). As demonstrated by Chaffin and colleagues (2004), a single evidence-based intervention may actually be more effective for both child and system outcomes than multiple services designed to address the many different problems families may have.

Finding: Significant advances have been achieved in the development of therapies that specifically target the impact of trauma or abuse on children. These advances include the extensive testing of TF-CBT models that have been shown to be effective.

Finding: The application of well-established parent management training programs with proven success to children and families involved in the child welfare system has been highly successful with regard to improved outcomes across behavioral problems caused by child abuse and neglect, as well as a reduced need for further involvement in the child welfare system across metrics such as reabuse and rereferral.

Finding: More research is needed to explore how better to deploy effective treatment intervention programs in the mental health and service settings where abused and neglected children receive care. Questions to be addressed relate to the types and breadth of services to provide for children and families, as well as how to sustain the impact of effective programs over the long term.

PREVENTION STRATEGIES

Over the past 50 years, child abuse and neglect prevention strategies evolved to draw on what was known about the scope of the problem at the time and beliefs about how best to prevent its initial occurrence. Responding to the diverse causes of child abuse and neglect suggested by ecological theory, prevention strategists emphasized the development of a continuum of separate but integrated interventions designed to provide the array of therapeutic and support services necessary to shore up failing or vulnerable families. Within this framework, each component was equally important to achieving positive outcomes regardless of its target population; its targeted outcomes; and, in some cases, evidence of its effects.

At the time of the 1993 NRC report, the concept of prevention had begun to shift from a horizontal to a more vertical structure in which particular emphasis was placed on initiating a strong relationship between parent and child at the moment a woman became pregnant or at the time a child was born (Daro, 2009; Daro and Cohn-Donnelly, 2002). The message changed from providing a plethora of prevention services to placing highest priority on building a network of services that would strengthen the supports available to new parents and link these services in a more intentional and effective manner than had previously been the case.

Support for new parents has taken many forms over the past 20 years, with leadership in these programs generally being shared by state health and human service administrators and community-based program advocates. A comprehensive review conducted in 1993 identified 37 major parent support initiatives operating in 25 states; 9 states (Delaware, Florida, Hawaii, Kentucky, Minnesota, Missouri, Rhode Island, Vermont, and West Virginia) offered statewide parent education and support programs, generally through their department of maternal and child health (Bryant, 1993). Key components of these state efforts included parent education, child health and developmental assessments, and health and social service referrals.

These state initiatives, coupled with the continued expansion of several national home visiting models, have increased public policy interest in the pivotal role of early home visiting in this emerging system of early intervention services. The seminal work of Olds and colleagues showing initial and long-term benefits from regular nurse visiting during pregnancy and a child's first 2 years of life provided the most robust evidence for the effectiveness of this intervention (Olds et al., 2007). Equally important, however, were the growing number of national home visiting programs being developed and successfully implemented by public agencies and community-based service organizations. Although initially not rigorous in their evaluation methodologies, programs such as Parents as Teachers, Healthy Families America, and the Parent-Child Home Program demonstrated respectable gains in parent-child attachment, access to preventive medical care, parental capacity and functioning, and early identification of developmental delays (Daro, 2011).

The call for a major federal investment in home visiting programs was first voiced by the U.S. Advisory Board on Child Abuse and Neglect (1990), which cited the statewide system operating in Hawaii and the early findings of Olds and colleagues. While the U.S. Advisory Board's recommendation was well received by child abuse and neglect advocates, substantial federal support for this strategy has only recently been provided. Authorized under the Patient Protection and Affordable Care Act (ACA) of 2010, the Maternal, Infant and Early Childhood Home Visiting Program will provide $1.5 billion to states, territories, and tribal entities to expand the availability of home visiting programs and create a system of support for families with children aged 0-8. As of the end of the 2012 federal fiscal year, the federal government had awarded $340 million in formula grants to 56 states and territories and an additional $182 million in competitive grants to selected states and territories that demonstrated the interest and capacity to expand and/or enhance their home visiting programs. A total of $21 million in funding also has been provided to multiple tribal entities for purposes of establishing home visiting programs targeting the unique needs of the Native American population. In terms of direct research support, the legislation provides funding for an interdisciplinary, multicenter research forum to support scientific collaboration and infrastructure building related to home visiting research.

Beyond the broad implementation of home visiting programs, those seeking to prevent child abuse and neglect continue to design, implement, and assess a range of initiatives. These initiatives include, among others, parent education services; crisis intervention programs that provide telephone numbers for families facing an immediate crisis or seeking parenting advice, as well as crisis nurseries; education for children and adolescents on assault prevention, antibullying behaviors, and nonviolence; efforts to assess new parental concerns and service needs; public education to raise awareness and alter parental behaviors; and initiatives designed to change how health care professionals and others working directly with children recognize and respond to potential child abuse and neglect. In addition to targeting change at the individual level, prevention efforts focus on altering community context and implementing a variety of strategies to create social service networks and social environments more conducive to positive parenting and healthy child development (Daro and Dodge, 2009). Compared with early home visiting, these efforts, in general, are more diffuse and less governed by national standards or expectations.

Evidence for Effectiveness

Today, prevention research is guided by a set of rigorous standards addressing research design and quality, such as the criteria for efficacy, effectiveness, and dissemination established by the Society for Prevention

Research (2004). The adoption of shared evidentiary standards in the field allows for the identification and testing of programs deemed effective and suitable for replication, adoption, or dissemination. Alternatively, these standards facilitate the identification of programs that lack a sound theoretical model or clinical base, show no effect, and should not be implemented further.

This section focuses primarily on those effective prevention interventions for which evidence shows a reduction in child abuse and neglect reports and other child safety outcomes, such as a lack of reported injuries and accidents. Also identified are programs with documented effects on risk and protective factors that are correlated with child abuse and neglect, including parent characteristics, child characteristics, and the parent-child relationship.

Home Visiting

As noted, the provision of home-based interventions at the time a woman becomes pregnant or gives birth is one of the most widely disseminated child abuse and neglect prevention strategies (Daro, 2010). Although findings remain inconsistent across program models, target populations, and outcome domains, the approach continues to demonstrate impacts on the frequency of child abuse and neglect and harsh punishment (Chaffin et al., 2012a; DuMont et al., 2010; Lowell et al., 2011; Olds et al., 2010; Silovsky et al., 2011), parental capacity and positive parenting practices (Connell et al., 2008; Dishion et al., 2008; DuMont et al., 2010; LeCroy and Krysik, 2011; Nievar et al., 2011; Roggman et al., 2009; Zigler et al., 2008), and healthy child development (DuMont et al., 2010; Lowell et al., 2011; Olds et al., 2007; Shaw et al., 2009). Likewise, home visiting programs that engage families with older children (aged 5-11) have demonstrated an ability to reduce depressive symptoms, parental stress, and life stress and enhance parental competence and social support (DePanfilis and Dubowitz, 2005).

Findings of a 15-year follow-up study of families enrolled in the Nurse Family Partnership's randomized clinical trials support that program's long-term positive impacts on both parents (Eckenrode et al., 2010) and children (Kitzman et al., 2010; Olds, 2010). In contrast to control families, mothers who received the program were involved in fewer substantiated reports for maltreatment, abuse, and neglect, and children were less likely to report running away or to have had contact with the juvenile justice system. These and similar gains were most concentrated among families with the fewest material and emotional resources at the time they enrolled in the program.

As noted earlier, confidence in home visiting as an effective way to address child abuse and neglect, as well as other poor child developmental and behavioral outcomes, contributed to the inclusion of the Maternal, Infant and Early Childhood Home Visitation Program in the ACA. As of this writing, 12 home visiting models that serve young children have met the criteria for identification as an evidence-based model appropriate for this initiative in that one or more rigorous evaluations have documented impacts in one of eight core outcome domains (child health; child development and school readiness; family economic self-sufficiency; linkages and referrals to other services; maternal health; positive parenting practices; reduction in child abuse and neglect; or reduction in juvenile delinquency, family violence, or crime) (Avellar et al., 2012). However, only 3 of the 12 approved models have had a measurable and significant impact in reducing either child abuse or neglect reports or the incidence of harsh parenting.

While home visiting programs continue to build an evidence base around a wide range of outcomes, preventing child abuse and neglect as measured by a reduction in initial or subsequent abuse and neglect reports remains an area in which consistent findings are lacking. Also, as promising models are taken to scale, sustaining their impacts is proving problematic. For example, a broad replication of the Nurse Family Partnership in Pennsylvania resulted in no significant differences in visits to hospital emergency departments for serious injuries between families enrolled in the program and a comparison group (Matone et al., 2012). Other studies also have raised concern about the extent to which home visiting services are able to prevent the recurrence of physical abuse or neglect (MacMillan et al., 2005) or alter the developmental consequences of abuse or neglect (Chaffin, 2004; Cicchetti and Toth, 2005).

For the past several years, a number of states and local communities have explored ways of extending support to a greater proportion of newborns and their parents. In contrast to targeted approaches that limit services to parents identified as high risk, these more universal initiatives are built on a public health model aimed at altering the context in which parents raise their children. Specifically, these initiatives offer comprehensive assessments and a limited number of service contacts to all parents or all first-time parents living within a specific geographic area (e.g., neighborhood, city, county) (Daro and Dodge, 2010). Assessments of the impacts of this approach have found that families are receptive to offers of such assistance and are able to access additional services in a more timely and appropriate manner (Dodge et al., 2013; Urban Institute, 2012).

At least one randomized study of this approach, conducted in Durham County, North Carolina, found that families with access to an initial nurse home visit at the time their child was born were less likely to use hospital emergency room services; less likely to present with anxiety; and more likely to exhibit positive parenting behaviors, to have strong community connections, and to participate in higher-quality out-of-home care (Dodge et al.,

2013). Additional research is required to fully understand the implementation challenges associated with such universal strategies and their ultimate impacts on parental behaviors and child outcomes.

Parenting Education

Improving parents' capacity to meet the developmental and emotional needs of their children has long been viewed as an effective strategy for preventing child abuse and neglect (Helfer, 1982; Kempe, 1976). Parenting education programs designed to increase knowledge of child development, enhance care, promote positive parent-child interaction and emotional sensitivity, and address child discipline and behavior management are considered a strong theoretical and practical approach to reducing risk and strengthening protective factors (Barth et al., 2005; Johnson et al., 2008). Since parenting education programs can occur in diverse settings, including both home-based and center-based models, and often include additional service components, such as child care services and family support groups, it is difficult to distinguish those impacts that may be attributable to specific parenting education activities (Barth, 2009; Reynolds et al., 2009). Further, the populations utilizing these programs are diverse. While unique challenges are faced by parents and families dealing with difficult circumstances, such as substance abuse, mental illness, poverty, domestic violence, or divorce, and those parenting a child with behavioral or developmental difficulties, these parents would not all be expected to engage in abusive or neglectful behavior in the absence of parenting education services.

An assessment of parenting education models by the California Evidence-Based Clearinghouse for Child Welfare identified several social learning-based educational efforts with robust results supported by repeated randomized controlled trials, including two that are often cited as demonstrating strong potential to reduce the risk for child abuse and neglect. Participants in Webster-Stratton's The Incredible Years, a multifaceted and developmentally based curriculum for parents, teachers, and children delivered in both primary school and early education settings, demonstrated more positive affective responses and a corresponding decrease in the use of harsh discipline, reduced parental depression, and improved self-confidence and better communication and problem solving within the family (Daro and McCurdy, 2007; Gardner et al., 2010; Reid et al., 2001, 2004; Webster-Stratton et al., 2011b). Significant aspects of the model include group-based training in parenting skills; classroom management training for teachers; and peer support groups for parents, children, and teachers.

Triple P, mentioned earlier, is another well-established and well-researched parent management training program. It consists of a series of integrated or scaled interventions "designed to provide a common set of information and parenting practices to parents who face varying degrees of difficulty or challenges in caring for their children. Based on social learning theory, research on child and family behavior therapy, and developmental research on parenting in everyday contexts, each intervention is designed to reduce child behavior problems by teaching healthy parenting practices and how to recognize negative or destructive practices. Parents are taught self-monitoring, self-determination of goals, self-evaluation of performance, and self-selection of change strategies (Daro and Dodge, 2009, p. 75). A geographically randomized study illustrated the effectiveness of Triple P at a population level (Prinz et al., 2009). Triple P was implemented in 18 randomized medium-sized southeastern U.S. counties over a 2-year period, demonstrating a decrease in child abuse and neglect. Additionally, multiple randomized controlled trials of the model in various cultural contexts have found it to have positive impacts on parent-reported child behavior problems, reducing dysfunctional parenting and improving parental competence (Bor et al., 2002; Leung et al., 2003; Martin and Sanders, 2003).

Most recently, those examining parenting education programs have focused on identifying those elements of the programs that appear to have the most consistent impact on participant outcomes (Barth et al., 2012). A meta-analysis conducted by the Centers for Disease Control and Prevention on training programs for parents of children aged 0-7 identified components of programs that have a positive impact on acquiring parenting skills as demonstrated by increased use of effective discipline and nurturing behaviors (CWIG, 2011). The 77 studies selected for the review all assessed parenting programs that incorporate active learning strategies such as completing homework assignments, modeling, or practicing skills. Among the 14 content and program delivery characteristics examined, the factors most frequently associated with positive outcomes were teaching parents emotional communication skills, helping them acquire positive parent-child interaction skills, and giving them opportunities to demonstrate and practice these skills while observed by a service provider (CWIG, 2011; Kaminski et al., 2008). The study also found small program effects on parent behaviors and skills outcomes with those programs having ancillary services. The researchers hypothesized that these ancillary services were a burden for the parents and program staff, and could impede skills development focused on parent-child interactions.

Universal Antiviolence Education Programs

In contrast to efforts designed to alter the behavior of adults who might commit child abuse or neglect, a category of prevention programs that emerged in the 1980s was designed to alter the behavior of potential victims (CWIG, 2011). Initially, such efforts focused exclusively on providing children information on physical and sexual assault; how to avoid risky situations; and if abused, how to respond. Meta-analyses and evaluations of these programs found they were effective in conveying safety information to children and imparting skills to avoid or lower the risk of assault (Berrick and Barth, 1992; Daro, 1994; MacMillan et al., 1994; Rispens et al., 1997). It remains unclear, however, to what extent these programs can alter adult behavior and responsiveness or change institutional culture in ways that reduce the likelihood of children being victimized and if they are, having their case addressed in an appropriate and transparent manner (Daro, 2010).

More recently, the focus of these universal education programs has expanded to encompass issues of bullying and aggressive behavior, particularly among elementary and middle school students. While the immediate goal of these interventions is to reduce levels of bullying and aggressive behavior among children and youth, accomplishing this goal might potentially contribute to a reduction in these behaviors in adulthood, thereby reducing levels of child abuse. A 2006 Cochrane review of school-based violence prevention programs targeting children identified as being or at risk of being aggressive found that aggressive behavior was significantly reduced in the intervention groups compared with the control groups in 34 trials with data on this outcome, and that positive impacts were maintained in the seven studies reporting 12-month follow-up data (Mytton et al., 2006).

These programs also may impact the response of bystanders to bullying behavior. A randomized controlled trial of a whole-school intervention provided universally to students by teachers found that the program moderated the developmental trend of increasing peer-reported victimization, self-reported aggression, and aggressive bystanding compared with schools randomly assigned to the control group. The program also moderated a decline in empathy and an increase in the percentage of children victimized compared with the other intervention conditions (Fonagy et al., 2009). Likewise, an observational study of playground interactions in schools randomly assigned to a bullying prevention program found declines in bullying and argumentative behavior, increases in agreeable interactions, and a trend toward reduced destructive bystander behaviors (Frey et al., 2005). Children in the intervention group reported enhanced bystander responsibility, greater perceived adult responsiveness, and less acceptance of bullying/aggression (Frey et al., 2005). While not well researched, the observed impacts on children's response to acts of peer aggression and their increased willingness to speak up and support the victim may have implications for subsequent reductions in various forms of child abuse and neglect. Adolescents and young adults who become increasingly comfortable with the concept of actively resisting aggression toward their peers may be more likely to support normative standards by which such behavior toward children is less tolerated and individuals feel more empowered to seek ways to stop it.

Public Education and Awareness

A consistent feature of child abuse and neglect prevention programming has been the development of public awareness campaigns. Initially, these efforts focused on raising awareness of the problem and enhancing the public's understanding of behaviors that constitute abuse and neglect and their impact on child well-being (Daro and Cohn-Donnelly, 2002). In recent years, broadly targeted prevention campaigns have been used to alter specific parental behaviors. For example, the U.S. Public Health Service, in partnership with the American Academy of Pediatrics (AAP) and the Association of SIDS and Infant Mortality Programs, launched its "Back to Sleep" campaign in 1994 to educate parents and caretakers about the importance of placing infants on their back to sleep so as to reduce the rate of sudden infant death syndrome (SIDS). Campaign strategies included media coverage; the availability of a nationwide toll-free information and referral hotline; the production of television, radio, and print ads; and the distribution of informational brochures to new parents. As of 2002, the National Center for Health Statistics reported a 50 percent drop in SIDS deaths and a decrease in stomach sleeping from 70 percent to 15 percent. Although the evidence linking the campaign to changes in these population-level indicators is exploratory, the data are suggestive of how public education might be used to change normative practices (Mitchell et al., 2007).

One of the most thoroughly examined public education and awareness campaigns addressing child abuse has been the effort to prevent shaken baby syndrome, now termed abusive head trauma. In an evaluation of a 1992 federal campaign to educate the public about the dangers of this practice ("Never Shake a Baby"), one-third of those providing feedback on the campaign indicated that they had no prior knowledge of the potential danger of shaking an infant (Showers, 2001).

Moving beyond basic awareness, Dias and colleagues (2005) developed a universal education program on shaken baby syndrome, which they implemented in an eight-county region in western New York. The program provided information on shaking to parents of all newborns prior to the infants' discharge from the hospital. During the 6 years before the program, 40 cases of substantiated abusive head injuries were identified in the targeted New York counties—an average of 8.2 cases per year, or 41.5 cases per 100,000 live births. During the 5.5-year period of the intervention, 21 cases of substantiated abusive head injury were identified—3.8 cases per year (a 53 percent reduction), or 22.2 cases per 100,000 live births (a 47 percent reduction). In the Pennsylvania comparison communities, there was no change in the number of such cases observed during the same two time periods (Dias et al., 2005).

Another promising public education and awareness program, The Period of PURPLE Crying, focuses on helping parents understand and cope with the stresses of normal infant crying. The program was tested through four different types of delivery systems: maternity services, pediatric offices, prenatal classes, and nurse home visitor programs. More than 4,200 parents participated in the program. A randomized controlled trial of the program found that it succeeded in enhancing mothers' knowledge about infant crying. Women who participated in the program were more likely to differentiate "inconsolable crying" from other types of crying that signaled hunger, discomfort, or pain in an infant (Barr et al., 2009).

While these findings are encouraging, others implementing these types of broadly targeted efforts have not achieved comparable results. The extent to which these programs can result in sustained population-level change in parenting behaviors remains unclear.

Professional Practice Reforms

In addition to the provision of direct services to new parents, increased consideration is being given to how best to use existing service delivery systems that regularly interact with families to address the potential for abuse and neglect. For example, the medical field has long sought ways to better address healthy child development and child abuse and neglect within clinical settings. Historically, health professionals have faced barriers to using the traditional checkup appointment to carry out this responsibility. Doctors are often uncomfortable discussing sensitive issues, and they frequently lack the training to instigate such conversations and the ability to recognize key warning signs (Benedetti, 2012). Additionally, adequate and comprehensive screening tools have not been made available to all primary care providers (Benedetti, 2012; Dubowitz et al., 2009). The Healthy Steps program, an evidence-based model that places child development specialists within selected pediatric practices, was initially created in 1994 to address this issue. Today, Healthy Steps is available in 17 states and has demonstrated consistent impacts on child health, child development and school readiness, and positive parenting practices (Benedetti, 2012; Caughy et al., 2003; Minkovitz et al., 2003, 2007).

More recently, the Safe Environment for Every Kid (SEEK) program was created to help health professionals address risk factors for child abuse and neglect through a training course, the introduction of a Parent Screening Questionnaire, and the addition of an in-house social worker team to work with families. Two studies were recently conducted to test existing SEEK programs: one to determine outcomes for children and families and one to measure effects on the health professionals participating in the intervention (Benedetti, 2012; Dubowitz et al., 2009). The first was a randomized trial conducted between 2002 and 2005 in resident clinics in Baltimore, Maryland. Families enrolled in the SEEK treatment group showed significantly lower rates of abuse and neglect across all measures compared with controls (Dubowitz et al., 2009). The second study, conducted 2 years later, investigated whether the program changed doctors' attitudes, behaviors, and competence in addressing child abuse and neglect among their patients (Dubowitz et al., 2011). Eighteen private practice primary care clinics participated in a cluster randomized controlled trial. The pediatricians in the SEEK group showed significant improvement in their abilities to address substance use, intimate partner violence, depression, and stress, and they reported higher levels of comfort and perceived competence in doing so (Dubowitz et al., 2011).

Community Prevention

A focus on the community as an appropriate prevention target is supported by findings of public health surveillance efforts and research on the effects of neighborhood contexts (Coulton et al., 1997; Pinderhughes et al., 2001; Zimmerman and Mercy, 2010). Research using population- and community-level data underscores the pressing need to design, target, and promote preventive service programs in jurisdictions exhibiting the greatest need (Putnam-Hornstein et al., 2011; Wulczyn, 2009). Accordingly, a number of strategies have emerged that focus on ways to better coordinate and integrate services provided through multiple domains and to alter the context in which parents rear their children (Daro and Dodge, 2009). The goal of such efforts is to move from simply assessing the prevention impacts on program participants to achieving population-level change by creating safe and nurturing environments for all children, as well as communities in which parents are supported through both formal services and normative values that foster mutual reciprocity. Although such initiatives are not fully operational in any community, the goal of altering both individuals and the context in which they live potentially provides a potent programmatic and policy response (Daro et al., 2009).

In a recent review of five multicomponent community initiatives, Daro and Dodge (2009) conclude that the implementation of multifaceted interventions that combine direct service reforms with attempts to alter residents' access to and use of both formal and informal supports are promising but largely unproven. Based on comparisons of administrative data, at least some of the models they reviewed had successfully reduced reported rates of child abuse and injury to young children at the county or community level (Dodge et al., 2004, Prinz et al., 2009), and repeated population-based surveys revealed that the models had altered adverse parent-child interactions, reduced parental stress, and improved parental efficacy (Daro et al., 2008). When focusing on community building, several models demonstrated a capacity to mobilize volunteers and engage diverse sectors within the community, such as first responders, the faith community, local businesses, and civic groups, in preventing child abuse (Daro et al., 2008; Melton et al., 2008). At present, however, little information is available on how these attitudes and willingness to support one's neighbors will translate into a measurable or sustained reduction in child abuse and neglect and enhanced parental support (CDC Essentials for Children, available at http://www.cdc. gov/ViolencePrevention/childmaltreatment/essentials/index.html [accessed March 7, 2014].

Designing and implementing a high-quality multifaceted community prevention initiative is costly. The models examined by Daro and Dodge (2009), each of which focused on only a single county or community within a county, cost approximately $1-$1.5 million annually to implement and evaluate. Moving forward, policy makers need to consider the trade-offs of investing in diffuse strategies designed to alter community context versus expanding the availability of services for known high-risk individuals. For the research community, a potential area of inquiry may lie in examining key mediators of either individual- or population-level outcomes and identifying less costly ways to create these mediators within prevention efforts.

The Bottom Line

Investments in preventing child abuse and neglect increasingly are being directed to evidence-based interventions that target pregnant women, new parents, and young children. Since the 1993 NRC report was issued, the prevention field has become stronger and more rigorous both in how it defines its services and in its commitment to evaluative research. And although greater attention is being paid to the development of home visiting interventions, the field embraces a plethora of prevention strategies. Communities and public agencies continue to demand and support broadly targeted primary prevention strategies such as school-based violence-prevention education, public awareness campaigns, and professional practice reforms, as well as a variety of parenting education strategies and support services for families facing particular challenges.

None of these program approaches are perfect, and they often fail to reach, engage, and retain their full target population successfully. Notable gaps exist in service capacity, particularly in communities at high risk and among populations facing the greatest challenges. And a substantial proportion of those families that do engage in intensive, long-term early intervention programs will exit the services before achieving their targeted program goals. That said, the committee finds the progress in prevention programming to be impressive, but the strategies employed to be underdeveloped and inadequately researched.

> *Finding:* A broad range of evidence-based child abuse and neglect prevention programs increasingly are being supported at the community level to address the needs of different populations. Strategies such as early home visiting, targeting pregnant women and parents with newborns, are well researched and have demonstrated meaningful improvements in mitigating the factors commonly associated with an elevated risk for poor parenting, including abuse and neglect. Promising prevention models also have been identified in other areas, including school-based violence prevention education, public awareness campaigns, parenting education, and professional practice reforms.

> *Finding:* Despite substantial progress in the development of effective prevention models, many of these models require more rigorous evaluation. Research is needed to devise strategies for better reaching, engaging, and retaining target populations, as well as to develop the capacity to deliver services to communities at high risk and among populations facing the greatest challenges.

COMMON ISSUES IN IMPROVING PROGRAM IMPACTS

Developing a pool of high-quality interventions is essential to address the problem of child abuse and neglect. Equally important is understanding how best to replicate, sustain, and integrate these programs into an effective system of care. Unfortunately, in child abuse and neglect as in other areas of health, mental health, and social services, a wide gap exists between available evidence-based interventions and practices and effective methods for their dissemination, implementation, and sustainment. This is a critical concern because the potential public health benefit of these interventions will be severely limited or unrealized if they are not implemented and sustained effectively in usual-care practice, be it in child welfare, mental health, substance abuse, or primary health care settings (Balas and Boren, 2000). Indeed, the success of efforts to improve services designed to support the well-being of children and families is influenced as much by the process used to implement innovative practices as by the practices selected for implementation (Aarons and Palinkas, 2007; Fixsen et al., 2009; Greenhalgh et al., 2004; Palinkas and Aarons, 2009; Palinkas et al., 2008). It is increasingly recognized that investment in the development of interventions without attention to how they align with service systems, organizations, providers, and consumers results in poor application of evidence-based practices.

Indeed, once evidence-based practices are taken to scale, the outcomes and effect sizes documented in their initial clinical trials often are not replicated. One reason for this is that complex interventions frequently are simplified over time in ways that impact key program objectives and strategies (Mildon and Shlonsky, 2011). Poor implementation has been cited as the reason for weakened effects in programs addressing conduct problems (Lee et al., 2008), learning delays (Hagermoser Sanetti and Kratochwill, 2009), crime prevention (Welsh et al., 2010), home visiting (Matone et al., 2012), and various child welfare reforms (Daro and Dodge, 2009). If replicating an evidence-based intervention does not produce a corresponding replication of impact, the intervention cannot be expected to reduce the incidence of the problem it was designed to address. Unless incidence is significantly reduced, the dramatic cost savings purported to follow major investments in high-quality treatment and prevention services may not materialize.

As evidence-based practices move from controlled settings to a real-world context, tension arises between remaining rigidly faithful to the original model and adapting it to local circumstances and needs (Backer, 2001; Bauman et al., 1991). Although adaptation may or may not be a deliberate choice, some form of adaptation is likely to be the rule rather than the exception in community care (Aarons et al., 2012). Ideally, such adaptation does not change the core elements of evidence-based practices, that is, those required elements that fundamentally define the nature of the practices and produce their main effects (Backer, 2001; Bauman et al., 1991; Cardona et al., 2009; Gandelman and Rietmeijer, 2004; Harshbarger et al., 2006; McKleroy et al., 2006; Veniegas et al., 2009).

Understanding when and how to alter a program in ways that enhance rather than diminish its effects represents a major social service challenge. Since the 1993 NRC report was issued, significant research has been conducted on how to define the concept of program fidelity, understand the role of race and culture in determining when and how to adapt evidence-based practices, identify those factors that facilitate or compromise the replication of evidence-based practices with fidelity, and clarify how research can be incorporated into the overall programming planning process. In addition, increased attention is being paid to the costs of interventions relative to their overall impact, resulting in an increased demand for more consistent and comparable methods of quantifying and tracking program expenditures and their long-term impacts on public budgets. This section summarizes this body of research and identifies those areas in need of additional study.

Fidelity as a Strategy for Enhancing Impact

At the most basic level, faithfully replicating programs that have been found effective in rigorous experimental studies is believed to result in a higher likelihood of achieving desired outcomes than replicating programs that lack a strong evidentiary base (Fixsen et al., 2005). Investing in direct service programs with a proven track record offers policy makers a hedge on their investment and provides increased confidence that outcomes also can be replicated. Central to this hypothesis, however, is ensuring that sites replicating a model maintain fidelity to its original design and intent.

As replication of evidence-based programs becomes more commonplace, it is increasingly important to design and implement frameworks for defining program fidelity, as well as data management systems that can track the implementation process at the level of specificity needed to ensure consistent replication. Researchers use several theoretical frameworks to define fidelity and address issues of appropriate modification. In summarizing work in this area, Carroll and colleagues (2007) identify five elements of implementation fidelity: (1) adherence to the service model as specified by the developer, (2) service exposure or dosage, (3) the quality or manner in which services are delivered, (4) participants' response or engagement, and (5) understanding of essential program elements not subject to adaptation or variation.

The rise of implementation science and the need to replicate and scale up evidence-based programs with fidelity across a range of disciplines has led to the development of a number of frameworks identifying an array of factors that should be considered to ensure that replication is faithful to both the structure and intent of the original model (Bagnato et al., 2011; Berkel et al., 2011; Damschroder and Hagedorn, 2011; Dane and Schneider, 1998; Gearing et al., 2011; Hagermoser et al., 2011). These factors include an appropriate target population, staff skills and training, supervision, caseloads, curriculum, and service dosage and duration, as well as the manner in which services are provided and participants are engaged in the service delivery process. Maintaining fidelity is especially important in practice-based research networks and learning collaboratives because it allows networks to gauge outcomes that can be used to make necessary practice and science improvements. Attention to these factors is necessary both in the initial planning process and throughout implementation.

Evidence-Based Treatments and Culturally Diverse Populations

The importance of cultural processes in shaping human functioning is increasingly being recognized. It is therefore critical to understand whether child abuse and neglect interventions are effective with ethnic minority youth who are at risk for or experience child abuse or neglect. A number of scholars have argued that culture matters in the development and testing of prevention and intervention strategies, as well as in the replication and adaptation of evidence-based practices for distinct populations or groups (e.g., Barrera et al., 2011; Bernal et al., 2009; Lau, 2006). According to this perspective, the culturally related processes underlying parenting and sociocultural risks that can lead to or exacerbate abuse and neglect must be considered to ensure the social validity and practical application of an intervention (Lau, 2006).

Another body of literature comprises evaluation of evidence-based interventions with ethnic minority youth and families, focusing on such questions as (1) Are evidence-based interventions effective for ethnic minority youth?, (2) Do minority youth benefit more when interventions are responsive to their cultural context?, and (3) Is there evidence for either culturally specific or culturally adapted youth interventions? (Huey and Polo, 2008, 2010). This literature is still in its infancy. As discussed earlier in this chapter, the extant literature shows that evidence-based interventions delivered to African American and Latino youth can be effective (for additional discussion of this issue, see Huey and Polo, 2008, 2010). These interventions target a range of concerns, including anxiety-related problems, attention-deficit hyperactivity disorder (ADHD), conduct problems, depression, substance use problems, trauma-related problems, and mixed/comorbid problems. Of note, only four interventions have shown effectiveness with ethnic minority youth across multiple trials: CBT, MST, interpersonal therapy (IPT), and brief solution-focused therapy (BSFT). In addition to these interventions targeting mental health and adjustment problems, a child welfare intervention targeting American Indian parents (Chaffin et al., 2012b) has shown effectiveness. Evidence-based interventions appear to work equally well for African American and Latino youth and European American youth, indicating no consistent effects of moderation (Huey and Polo, 2008).

Although most of the interventions investigated in these studies did not explicitly target ethnic minority youth who were abused and neglected, those interventions that did explicitly include this population yielded similar findings regarding effectiveness, moderation, and the impact of cultural adaptation. However, the discussion of cultural elements in reports on evidence-based interventions varies considerably (Huey and Polo, 2008), which may impede understanding of the impact of cultural adaptation; in particular, reporting of the development and evaluation of many culturally adapted interventions is characterized by a relative lack of theory and conceptual framing. Thus, more research is needed to test key assumptions and hypotheses regarding minority youth and the effectiveness of interventions.

A critical gap in this literature is that evidence-based interventions have been tested primarily with African American and Latino youth; with few exceptions, little is known about the effectiveness of evidence-based interventions with Asian American and American Indian youth. For example, there have been few studies on the effectiveness of home visiting models that involve structured, protocol-driven approaches with families in tribal communities (Del Grosso et al., 2012). One noteworthy effort is the randomized controlled trial of Family Spirit, modeled on Healthy Families America, which found that a family-strengthening home visiting program delivered by paraprofessionals significantly increased mothers' child care knowledge and involvement (Walkup et al., 2009).

To illustrate these issues, interventions targeting American Indian and Alaska Native families and communities need to take account of their history, culture, and tribal diversity (DeBruyn et al., 2001; Weaver, 2003). Thus, addressing child abuse and neglect and trauma among these populations presents unique opportunities to develop culturally sensitive interventions that align with traditional circular and contextual world views and to adapt or enhance evidence-based practices that are based in authentic practitioner-researcher partnerships (Poupart et al., 2009; Spicer et al., 2012). One prominent example, Project Making Medicine, provides training in the clinical treatment of child physical and sexual abuse based on the cultural adaptation of TF-CBT. Entitled Honoring Children, Mending the Circle, the curriculum features an indigenous orientation to well-being and the use of traditional healing practices. Cultural adaptations to family preservation approaches involve using genograms, wraparounds, talking circles, kinship care, healing ceremonies, and traditional adoptions with Native families. This intervention also incorporates tribal elders and extended family in the use of specific cultural approaches, such as storytelling, sweat lodges, feasts, and use of Native languages (Bigfoot and Funderburk, 2011). The effectiveness of these adaptations of clinical tools and interventions merits further research.

In sum, the field of evidence-based interventions for cultural minority populations is still developing. Research is needed on understudied populations, as well as on key assumptions, hypotheses, and implementation issues of culturally adapted evidence-based interventions. Guidelines on when to consider making a cultural adaptation and how specifically to do so would provide important support for the field. Lau (2006) offers an evidence-based approach to making such decisions. Her framework calls for the selective identification of target problems and/or communities for which adaptations are appropriate. More specifically, populations that face unique sociocultural contexts of risk or resilience that differ from those targeted by the original evidence-based intervention may be appropriate candidates for cultural adaptation. When it is determined that cultural adaptation is warranted, Lau further suggests a data-based approach to decisions on the adaptations to implement. Surface-structure adaptations (Resnicow et al., 2000) (e.g., language translation, use of videos or books that depict a cultural group, interventionists who share the same cultural background as target families) are designed to make interventions more accessible, whereas deep-structure changes are designed to make interventions more effective and target underlying cultural values.

One example of this data-based approach is the cultural adaption of the evidence-based program Guiando a Niños Activos (Guiding Active Children, or GANA), a version of PCIT for Mexican American families (McCabe et al., 2005). A multistep process was used, including a review of the clinical literature on Mexican American families; identification of known barriers to treatment access and effectiveness; use of focus groups; and interviews with Mexican American mothers, fathers, and therapists to learn how PCIT could be modified to be more culturally effective. The process culminated in an expert panel review of the intervention (Lau, 2006). Another example, The Children and Families (as part of the National Child Traumatic Stress Network), addressed the treatment and service needs of traumatized Latino children and families through the creation of adaptation guidelines for practitioners and researchers. These guidelines address micro- and macro-level domains related to child abuse and neglect, including assessment, provision of therapy, communication and linguistic competence, cultural values, immigration/documentation, child welfare/resource families, service utilization and case management, diversity among Latinos, research, therapist training and support, organizational competence, system challenges, and policy (Workgroup on Adapting Latino Services, 2008). Child welfare staff were trained to implement a systems of care approach— an existing evidence-based framework—to improve practice and service delivery for immigrant Latino children at the system level (Dettlaff and Rycraft, 2010).

In such efforts, it is important to attend to the theoretical, implementation, and evaluation issues involved. Perhaps the data-based framework articulated by Lau (2006) can help inform a more rigorous articulation of the circumstances in which evidence-based interventions should be culturally adapted and of the methods that should be used to evaluate the adapted interventions.

The Implementation Process

Since the 1993 NRC report was issued, significant work has been done on how to define and monitor the program implementation process itself and on the critical factors related to higher-quality implementation and sustainability. Consensus exists on important key factors, such as availability of funding; leadership in implementation efforts; ongoing consultation and training, especially in the early implementation phases; and the need to address the impact of staff turnover. In many cases, however, research on these factors is lacking (Aarons et al., 2009a). Consensus also exists that multicomponent implementation strategies are needed, as many different factors need to be addressed in sequence or in tandem for effective implementation that sustains public health impact (Ferlie and Shortell, 2001; Fixsen et al., 2009; Glisson and Schoenwald, 2005; Grimshaw et al., 2001; Grol and Grimshaw, 1999).

Implementation frameworks have been developed to expand and distill theories, structures, and processes into manageable approaches for understanding and identifying key facilitators of and barriers to effective implementation. Most theories provide guidance regarding implementation research and practice, while particular tenets and assumptions of frameworks require further empirical testing to determine whether they actually lead to more effective implementation (Aarons et al., 2011). Implementation researchers typically test components of models (e.g., technology-assisted coaching, organizational improvement) rather than more comprehensive implementation and scale-up strategies. Notable exceptions include studies of system-level implementation in the context of child welfare, such as the use of community development teams to scale up multidimensional treatment foster care in multiple counties (Chamberlain et al., 2012) and the use of interagency collaborative teams to scale up SafeCare across an entire large county.

To support program fidelity, effective and efficient measurement methods that can be readily utilized in usual care settings are needed (Schoenwald et al., 2011). In addition, there must be a feedback system coupled with supportive quality improvement or coaching to help providers maintain fidelity (Aarons et al., 2012). In many cases, however, little ongoing attention is paid to fidelity once an intervention has been implemented. Delivery of an intervention without attention to its fidelity fails to ensure that services are effective.

Efforts have been made to integrate fidelity assessment for psychosocial interventions in systems that involve child abuse and neglect; however, these efforts may or may not be part of implementation studies. One effectiveness trial found that incorporating ongoing coaching to direct service providers in the delivery of a child neglect intervention supported service efficacy (Chaffin et al., 2012a). This statewide trial was also examined in an implementation study that found benefits for organizations and service teams in reduced provider burnout and turnover. There is also increasing interest in the use of technology to support real-time fidelity assessment.

It is important to recognize that many program implementation efforts have occurred in the context of funded research studies. Outside research funding often covers the costs associated with initial monitoring and documentation of the implementation process, including the collection and analysis of participant-level data to document service dosage, duration, and content. In some cases, study subjects have been paid for their participation in the program and may have received reimbursement for child care or transportation expenses related to their participation. As evidence-based practices move from the research venue to standard practice, some entity must pay these costs.

Increasingly, evidence-based practice models are factoring into their per-participant cost projections those expenses associated with initial and ongoing training for direct service staff, supervisory standards, and data reporting requirements. State agencies or community-based service providers seeking to implement these models are required to cover these costs as part of purchasing the program. It remains unclear whether these program-driven standards will be sufficient to sustain program fidelity and quality over time and achieve the level of participant engagement required to both sustain program fidelity and replicate outcomes.

Integration of Research into Practice

Most implementation plans for evidence-based practices include methods for transferring research evidence from the program developers to potential users. Some of these models focus explicitly on the use of research evidence (Honig and Coburn, 2008; Kennedy, 1984; Nutley et al., 2007); in other cases, the use of research evidence is embedded in broader processes of innovation, including the dissemination and implementation of evidence-based practices (Fixsen et al., 2005; Greenhalgh et al., 2004).

Many of these models represent typologies of research use. For instance, several researchers have distinguished between an *instrumental model*, in which "use" consists of making a decision, and research evidence is assumed to be instructive to that decision, and a *conceptual model*, in which "use" consists of thinking about the evidence. Whereas the central feature of the instrumental model is the decision, the central feature of the conceptual model is the human information processor. Hence, the instrumental model focuses on the outcome of using evidence, while the conceptual model focuses on the process of using evidence (Kennedy, 1984).

Conceptual models of evidence acknowledge that the use of research evidence to make or support decisions is often a collective endeavor rather than an activity performed by any individual decision maker (Spillane et al., 2001). This collective endeavor involves the utilization of social capital (Honig and Coburn, 2008; Spillane et al., 2001), social networks (Valente, 1995; Valente et al., 2003), and the exchange of knowledge or information between researchers and practitioners and within networks of practitioners (Lomas, 2000; Mitton et al., 2007; Nutley et al., 2007).

Preliminary research (Palinkas et al., 2012) conducted on leaders in child welfare, mental health, and juvenile justice systems implementing multidimensional treatment foster care (Chamberlain et al., 2007) found that published information (journal articles, treatment manuals, Internet searches) was the most frequently accessed source of information on evidence-based practices, followed by local experts and knowledgeable personal contacts. Feasibility of implementation was the primary criterion used to evaluate this evidence. However, further research is needed to identify components of feasibility that may drive implementation decisions.

Capacity to Identify Costs and Cost-Effectiveness Across Approaches

Policy makers, program administrators, and researchers increasingly acknowledge the importance of understanding the costs, cost-effectiveness, and returns on investment of child abuse and neglect programs.

> Policy makers want information on costs and how they compare with outcomes of interest for determining how to allocate scarce resources; program administrators want to identify which programs to implement; and researchers are interested in economic evaluation because it makes their program evaluations more comprehensive (Corso and Lutzker, 2006; Courtney, 1999). The demand for economic analysis is evident in strategic planning being developed at the federal level. In the Centers for Disease Control and Prevention's research plan for injury and violence prevention, for example, a top priority is to describe the use and impact of service delivery as well as the costs of interventions for child abuse and neglect. (Corso and Filene, 2009, p. 78)

Assessment of the economic costs of implementing an intervention is called programmatic cost analysis. The process involves the systematic collection, categorization, and analysis of intervention delivery costs, including those entailed during the preimplementation (developing the program delivery infrastructure) and implementation (delivering the program) phases (Corso and Filene, 2009). A standardized methodology for determining costs for child abuse and neglect interventions does not currently exist, although guidelines available in other fields could be applied (Foster et al., 2003, 2007; Haddix et al., 2003; Yates, 2009). To address this need, efforts are under way at the Children's Bureau within the Administration for Children and Families to develop a manual on how to conduct programmatic cost analyses specifically within the child welfare community.

Once the costs of a program have been determined, they can be compared with a program's expected and realized short- and long-term outcomes. This comparison of costs with outcomes is referred to as economic evaluation and includes a number of analyses, such as benefit-cost analysis and return on investment, whereby outcomes are valued in monetary terms, and cost-effectiveness analysis, whereby outcomes are valued in natural units, such as cases of child abuse and neglect prevented or improvements in quality of life. Although some guidelines for conducting economic evaluations do exist for community-level interventions in general (Haddix et al., 2003; Shiell et al., 2008), the literature is sparse on how specifically to conduct economic evaluations of family and child development interventions.

Despite the need for information on the economic cost and impact of implementing child and family development or child abuse and neglect prevention programs, few cost analyses (Corso and Filene, 2009) or economic evaluations have been conducted in this area since the 1993 NRC report was issued (Barlow et al., 2007; Dalziel and Segal, 2012; DePanfilis et al., 2008; Karoly et al., 1998; McIntosh et al., 2009; Olds, 1993). More studies have focused specifically on economic evaluation of interventions designed to improve outcomes for children at risk for or currently involved in the child welfare system (these studies are systematically reviewed and summarized by Goldhaber-Fiebert and colleagues [2011]).

Remaining challenges to conducting programmatic cost analysis and economic evaluation in the fields of child abuse and neglect intervention and child welfare include the need for (1) the development and consistent use of standardized methodology for assessing program costs; (2) multisite assessment of programs in which program-, provider-, and community-level variables may impact program-level costs and outcomes; (3) better tools for assessing the impact of child abuse and neglect on health-related quality of life, which is an important outcome measure in economic evaluations within other health fields; (4) assessment of the long-term costs of child abuse and neglect to determine the potential benefits of prevention and successful child welfare services; and (5) the development and use of model-based economic evaluations to support decision making within the child welfare system (Goldhaber-Fiebert et al., 2011).

The Bottom Line

As policy makers place greater emphasis on evidence-based decision making and the implementation of programs that have been proven effective through rigorous evaluation, research will be needed to understand how these high-quality interventions are replicated, adapted to diverse populations, and incorporated into the overall service delivery system. At present, little is known about the most effective strategies for ensuring that evidence-based practices are replicated with fidelity to their intent and structural elements. Central here is determining which service attributes are most essential to achieving the desired impacts and therefore should not be altered and which can or should be modified to address the needs of specific subpopulations. Equally important is understanding the costs associated with the emphasis on replicating with fidelity in terms of (1) monitoring the service delivery process; (2) providing the required levels of supervision and infrastructure support, including the development of data collection systems; and (3) determining how the data will be integrated into subsequent practice and policy decisions.

Finding: Despite a growing body of theoretical and applied research in the area, a wide gap exists between available evidence-based interventions and practices for treating and preventing child abuse and neglect and methods of effective dissemination, implementation, and sustainment of those interventions. It is increasingly recognized that investment in developing interventions alone, without attention to how they align with service systems, organizations, providers, and consumers, results in poor application of evidence-based practices. Therefore, more research is needed to support the translation of model programs for effective use in real-world settings.

Finding: Little is known about the most effective strategies for ensuring that evidence-based interventions are replicated with fidelity to their intent and structural elements. Further research is needed to determine which service attributes are most essential to achieving the desired impacts and therefore should not be altered and which can or should be modified to address the needs of specific subpopulations.

Finding: More research is needed on the development of evidence-based interventions for cultural minority populations, with a particular focus on understudied populations. Also needed is research that carefully examines key assumption, hypotheses, and implementation issues of culturally adapted evidence-based interventions. Guidelines on when to consider making a cultural adaptation and what the specific adaptation should be would provide important support to the field.

Finding: Significant advances have been achieved in how the program implementation process itself is defined and monitored and in the identification of critical factors related to higher-quality implementation and sustainability. Consensus exists on key factors, but in many cases, research on these factors is lacking. Consensus also exists that multicomponent implementation strategies are needed to address the challenges of effective implementation.

Finding: Despite the need for information on the economic cost and impact of implementing child and family development or child abuse and neglect prevention programs, few studies have conducted programmatic cost analyses or economic evaluations in this area. This type of research is needed to guide policy makers and program administrators.

BUILDING AN INTEGRATED SYSTEM OF CARE

As the discussion in this chapter has made clear, several of the challenges faced in replicating promising programs and their outcomes lie in the process by which programs are designed and implemented. Equally important, however, is considering the programs' institutional, organizational, and political context. Elements of this broader infrastructure can support or complicate the implementation and sustainability of a promising approach (Tibbits et al., 2010; Wandersman et al., 2008).

Social service programs benefit from an array of elements that strengthen their capacity to deliver high-quality services consistently. These elements have been organized conceptually into three groups: (1) foundational infrastructure (planning and collaboration); (2) implementation infrastructure (operations and workforce development); and (3) sustaining infrastructure (fiscal capacity, community and political support, communications, and evaluation) (Paulsell et al., 2012).

Child abuse and neglect is a complex issue with diverse causal pathways, manifestations, and affected populations. Therefore, multiple high-quality interventions are needed to address it. An effective response to the problem would be facilitated by a more explicit focus on building an infrastructure that can support the most promising interventions as they emerge and link them in ways that maximize their collective impact.

Unfortunately, limited research has been conducted on the potential impact of infrastructure reforms on program implementation and participant outcomes. Although efforts aimed at enhancing the knowledge and skills of the workforce in order to strengthen organizational capacity to support evidence-based practices or at reducing barriers to service access through better interagency coordination make sense, relatively little is known about how to accomplish these improvements. This section briefly reviews the literature on the impact of organizational culture and interagency networks on the implementation and sustainability of evidence-based programs.

Organizational Culture

The quality of services provided to families and children is influenced not only by the rigor of a program's design and its implementation but also by the organizations in which services are embedded. Studies of organizational context have found associations between an organizational culture and climate and participant outcomes (Glisson and Hemmelgarn, 1998). Organizational culture also can result in improved service engagement, reduced staff turnover, and improved child outcomes, independent of the implementation of evidence-based practices (Glisson et al., 2010).

This relationship between organizational culture and program implementation is reciprocal. The implementation of evidence-based practices can adversely impact organizations by adding to the workload of an already overworked labor force or by leading to increased employee turnover as staff are asked to change their practices and adopt new strategies that may restrict their sense of control over the therapeutic process (Glisson et al., 2008; Sheidow et al., 2007; Woltmann et al., 2008). On the other hand, organizations also can benefit from the implementation of evidence-based practices. These benefits include enhanced professional identity, improved client outcomes, and the gratification of contributing to a process of knowledge generation (Aarons and Palinkas, 2007; Palinkas and Aarons, 2009). One statewide study of implementing evidence-based practices found that ongoing fidelity coaching predicted decreased staff burnout and reduced staff turnover (Aarons et al., 2009b).

These benefits aside, the culture of evidence-based practices that stems from an empirically based research perspective and the culture of child abuse and neglect practice may be at odds, engendering a gap that must be bridged if effective implementation is to be achieved (Palinkas et al., 2009). Even something as basic as the reporting of child abuse and neglect may be impacted by organizational context (Ashton, 2007). Thus, for example, an examination of child sexual abuse in the Catholic Church implicates a strong organizational culture as a major factor limiting the institution's appropriate response to the problem (Keenan, 2011).

While some of the above-mentioned studies assess or deliberately alter organizational context, others examine or cite organizational context as important in the implementation of evidence-based practices (Kolko et al., 2012). Yet while there have been calls for increased attention to organizational context in the dissemination and implementation of evidence-based practices (Chaffin, 2006; Kessler et al., 2005), much research remains to be done on how organizational context in child abuse and neglect settings impacts the implementation process.

Interagency Networks

Although many factors influence the diffusion of evidence-based practices in general, "researchers have consistently found that interpersonal contacts within and between organizations and communities are important influences on the adoption of new behaviors" (Brekke et al., 2007; Palinkas et al., 2005, 2011, p. 8; Rogers, 2003). Based on diffusion of innovations theory (Rogers, 2003) and social learning theory (Bandura, 1986), Valente's (1995) social network thresholds model calls for identification and matching of champions within peer networks that manage organizational agenda setting, change, and evaluation of change (e.g., data collection, evaluation, and feedback) and use information technology processes consistent with continuous quality improvement strategies (Palinkas et al., 2011).

Studies and meta-analyses have shown that both the influence of trusted others in one's personal network and access and exposure to external information are important influences on rates of adoption of innovative practices (Palinkas et al., 2011). Across a series of studies, Valente and colleagues found that individuals who were most innovative almost always had the highest exposure to external influences (Valente and Davis, 1999; Valente et al., 2003, 2007). Although external influence played a crucial role in bringing an innovation to an individual's attention, it was usually the persuasion of trusted others that finally convinced the individual to adopt the innovation (Valente, 1995). Other empirical studies have confirmed the importance and influence of opinion leaders (e.g., Jung et al., 2003). It has also been hypothesized that leaders in dense or centralized groups may have more power than leaders not in such groups (Valente, 2006), although this has not been found in all influence networks (Valente et al., 2007).

Applying this theoretical framework to child abuse and neglect, Palinkas and colleagues (2011) found that the social networks of county-level child welfare, mental health, and juvenile justice system leaders and staff play a significant role in the implementation of evidence-based practices for abused and neglected youth. System leaders develop and maintain networks of information and advice based on roles, responsibilities, geography, and friendship ties. Networks expose leaders to information about evidence-based practices and opportunities to adopt them, and also influence decisions to adopt. In that study, individuals in counties at the same stage of implementation of multidimensional treatment foster care accounted for 83 percent of all network ties. Networks in counties that decided not to implement a specific evidence-based practice had no extracounty ties. Implementation of multidimensional treatment foster care at the 2-year follow-up of a randomized controlled trial funded by the National Institute of Mental Health was associated with the size of the county, urban versus rural counties, and in-degree centrality (i.e., the extent to which others interacted with specific network members).

Successful, large-scale incorporation of evidence-based practices in existing child-serving systems is likely to involve multiple levels of constituents, in part because the new practices affect multiple stakeholders in the funding, planning, coordination, delivery, and receipt of services. Further, the successful implementation of many evidence-based practice models requires substantial interagency linkages.

In their report from the Blueprints programs, Mihalic and colleagues (2004) found these linkages to be a crucial factor in whether the programs had stable funding, a stable referral base, and coordinated case planning activities, especially for youth involved in multiple systems. In addition to interagency coordination, these linkages often include system-level factors that impact the implementing organization's operation; that relate to federal and state laws and regulations; and that impact larger human resource decisions (e.g., collocation of staff from multiple agencies), access to funding streams, and contracting issues.

Most evidence-based practice implementation studies that focus on interorganizational collaboration fail to consider the wider context within which collaboration occurs, including such factors as the involvement of external stakeholders, sociopolitical processes, and the roles of relationships and leadership (Horwath and Morrison, 2007). Increasingly, this context is characterized by government mandates and fiscal realities that require collaboration in the form of integrative multidisciplinary practice in the delivery of children's services (Ehrle et al., 2004; Hogan and Murphey, 2002). In a sociopolitical climate in which organizations face increasing budget restrictions and are challenged to do more with less, collaboration across agencies and organizations appears to be critical for successful implementation of evidence-based practices. In turn, an understanding of effective collaboration appears to be at the core of many evidence-based practices developed to improve outcomes in child-serving systems (Prince and Austin, 2005).

An extensive literature exists on the nature of interagency collaboration for the delivery of health and human services in general and child welfare services in particular. Although many consider such collaboration to be essential to the delivery of a complex array of services (Jones et al., 2004; Lippitt and van Til, 1981; Stroul and Friedman, 1986), others have questioned its usefulness on both theoretical (Scott, 1985) and empirical (Glisson and Hemmelgarn, 1998; Longoria, 2005) grounds. Several studies have pointed to improved access to services and improved outcomes associated with interagency collaboration (Bai et al., 2009; Cottrell et al., 2000; Hurlburt et al., 2004). However, Glisson and Hemmelgarn (1998) found that efforts to coordinate the services of public child-serving agencies in Tennessee were negatively associated with the quality of services provided. And Chuang and Wells (2010) found that while interagency sharing of administrative data increased the odds of youth receiving inpatient behavioral health services, having a single agency accountable for youth care increased the odds of receiving both inpatient and outpatient services.

In part, this inconsistency in findings may be attributable to differences in the definition and operationalization of key terms. For instance, some researchers have distinguished among collaboration, cooperation, coordination, and networking, whereas others have used these terms interchangeably (Grace et al., 2012; Hodges et al., 1999). Others view interagency collaboration as an aspect of organizational culture, defined as "the way things are done in an organization" (Glisson, 2007, p. 739).

Specific factors that have been found to contribute to successful inter-agency collaboration for child welfare and other agencies include shared goals, a high level of trust, mutual responsibility, open lines of communication, and strong leadership (Johnson et al., 2003; Weinberg et al., 2009). Barriers to effective collaboration include deeply ingrained mistrust and continued lack of other agencies' values, goals, and perspectives; different organizational priorities; confusion over how services should be funded and who has jurisdiction over participants; and difficulty in tracking cases across organizations (Conger and Ross, 2006; Green et al., 2008; Sedlak et al., 2006).

The Bottom Line

Treatment and prevention programs generally are delivered by public agencies or community-based organizations. The operating culture within these entities has an impact on the quality of services and the extent to which evidence-based practices will be implemented and sustained over time. Research suggests that a degree of reciprocity exists between service models and their host agencies. In some instances, the rigor and quality of these innovations may alter the standards of practice throughout an agency, thereby improving the overall service delivery process and enhancing participant outcomes. In other cases, organizations that provide little incentive for staff to adopt new ideas or reduce the dosage or duration of evidence-based models to accommodate an agency's limited resources contribute to poor implementation and reduced impacts. Maximizing the impact of evidence-based models and proven approaches will require more explicit attention to the organizational strengths and weaknesses of the agencies in which such models and approaches are embedded and how these factors impact service implementation.

Equally important is developing a research base that can inform the process of building a collaborative culture and a set of working relationships across the institutions and community-based agencies that constitute the child maltreatment response system. Because child abuse and neglect is a complex, multifaceted problem with myriad causes, promising treatment and prevention strategies lie within a variety of disciplines and multiple institutions. Additional research is needed to understand how these multiple institutional resources can be integrated in ways that reinforce the impact of these individual strategies in the most efficient and cost-effective manner.

Finding: Maximizing the impact of evidence-based models and proven approaches will require more explicit attention to the organizational strengths and weaknesses of the agencies in which such models and approaches are embedded and how these factors impact service implementation.

Finding: Multiple high-quality interventions and strategies must be sustained to address child abuse and neglect—a complex problem with diverse causal pathways, manifestations, and affected populations. An effective response to the problem would be facilitated by a more explicit focus on building an infrastructure that can support the most promising interventions as they emerge and link them in ways that maximize their collective impact.

Finding: Because child abuse and neglect are complex, multifaceted problems with myriad causes, a variety of disciplines and multiple institutions support treatment and prevention programs. Additional research is needed to understand how these multiple institutional resources can be integrated in ways that reinforce the impact of individual strategies in the most efficient and cost-effective manner.

Finding: Limited research has been conducted on the impact of infrastructure reforms on program implementation and participant outcomes. More research is needed to determine how best to direct efforts aimed at enhancing the knowledge and skills of the workforce, strengthening organizational capacity to support evidence-based practices, and reducing barriers to service access through better interagency coordination.

CONCLUSIONS

Significant advances in the development of child abuse and neglect treatment and prevention strategies have been realized since the 1993 NRC report was issued. This work has been informed by the growing body of research on the causes and consequences of abuse and neglect, as well as research assessing the efficacy and effectiveness of interventions. In the treatment domain, TF-CBT, a brief structured program based on well-established theory and treatment elements, has been tested extensively and found to be effective with children affected by abuse and other traumatic experiences. Equally important has been the successful application of a number of well-established parent management training programs to children and families involved in the child welfare system. Again, these are programs with well-established theory and large bodies of knowledge. As this chapter has reported, outcomes include not only improvements in behavior problems caused by child abuse and neglect but also reduced need for subsequent child welfare involvement.

With respect to prevention, strategies such as early home visiting targeting pregnant women and parents with newborns are well researched and have demonstrated meaningful improvements in factors commonly associated with an elevated risk for poor parenting, including abuse and neglect. Promising prevention models also have been identified in other areas, including school-based education in violence prevention, public awareness campaigns, parenting education programs, and professional practice reforms. As in the past, communities continue to invest in and support a broad continuum of prevention services that address the needs of different populations and utilize different institutional resources. In contrast to the reality in 1993, policy makers and practitioners have a much stronger pool of candidate programs on which to draw in both remediating the impacts of abuse and neglect and reducing its incidence.

Also important is tracking the long-term, second-generation effects of current interventions. Few program evaluations have tracked participants longitudinally, and even fewer have examined the potential effects of high-quality treatment and prevention services on the parenting practices and abuse or neglect potential of children whose parents receive these interventions. Such research is needed to determine the most promising investments.

Improving the performance of evidence-based programs is the subject of considerable ongoing theoretical and applied research designed to increase understanding of how interventions are implemented, replicated, and sustained. The most pressing questions relate to how to take interventions to scale in the public mental health, child welfare, and community-based service settings where children who have experienced child abuse or neglect and families in need of preventive services receive their care. As policy makers place greater emphasis on evidence-based decision making and the implementation of programs that have been proven effective through rigorous evaluation, research will be needed to understand how these high-quality interventions can best be replicated, adapted to diverse populations, and incorporated into the overall service delivery system.

At present, little is known about the most effective strategies for ensuring that evidence-based practices are replicated with fidelity to their intent and structural elements. Central to this discussion is determining which service attributes are most essential to achieving the desired impacts and therefore should not be altered and which can or should be modified to address the needs of specific subpopulations. Equally important is understanding the costs associated with an emphasis on replicating with fidelity in terms of (1) monitoring the service delivery process; (2) providing the required levels of supervision and infrastructure support, including the development of time-sensitive data collection systems; and (3) determining how the data will be integrated into subsequent practice and policy decisions.

Research suggests that a degree of reciprocity exists between service models and their host agencies. In some instances, the rigor and quality of innovations may alter the standards of practice throughout an agency, thereby improving the overall service delivery process and enhancing participant outcomes. In other cases, organizations that provide little incentive for staff to adopt new ideas or reduce the dosage or duration of evidence-based models to accommodate an agency's limited resources contribute to poor implementation and reduced impacts. Maximizing the impact of evidence-based models and proven approaches will require more explicit attention to the organizational strengths and weaknesses of the agencies in which such efforts are embedded and how these factors impact service implementation.

Finally, this chapter's review underscores the absence of research on the question of system reform and the infrastructure required to institutionalize and support it. Little research exists on how best to improve interventions and agency performance in the areas of workforce development, data management, and system integration. Although some preliminary research has been conducted in the area of system integration, clarity is lacking on which strategies are most effective in building a collaborative culture and set of working relationships across public institutions and between these institutions and the community-based agencies that constitute the child abuse and neglect response system. Because child abuse and neglect is a complex, multifaceted problem with myriad causes, a variety of disciplines and multiple institutions support treatment and prevention programs. Additional research is needed to understand how these multiple institutional resources can be integrated in ways that reinforce the impact of individual strategies in the most efficient and cost-effective manner.

REFERENCES

Aarons, G. A., and L. A. Palinkas. 2007. Implementation of evidence-based practice in child welfare: Service provider perspectives. *Administration and Policy in Mental Health and Mental Health Services Research* 34(4):411-419.

Aarons, G. A., D. L. Fettes, L. E. Flores, and D. H. Sommerfeld. 2009a. Evidence-based practice implementation and staff emotional exhaustion in children's services. *Behaviour Research and Therapy* 47(11):954-960.

Aarons, G. A., D. H. Sommerfeld, D. B. Hecht, J. F. Silovsky, and M. J. Chaffin. 2009b. The impact of evidence-based practice implementation and fidelity monitoring on staff turnover: Evidence for a protective effect. *Journal of Consulting and Clinical Psychology* 77(2):270-280.

Aarons, G. A., M. Hurlburt, and S. M. Horwitz. 2011. Advancing a conceptual model of evidence-based practice implementation in child welfare. *Administration and Policy in Mental Health and Mental Health Services Research* 38(1):4-23.

Aarons, G. A., A. E. Green, L. A. Palinkas, S. Self-Brown, D. J. Whitaker, J. R. Lutzker, and M. J. Chaffin. 2012. Dynamic adaptation process to implement an evidence-based child maltreatment intervention. *Implementation Science* 7:32.

Ashton, V. 2007. The impact of organizational environment on the likelihood that social workers will report child maltreatment. *Journal of Aggression, Maltreatment and Trauma* 15(1):1-18.

Avellar, S., D. Paulsell, E. Sama-Miller, and P. Del Grosso. 2012. *Home visiting evidence of effectiveness review: Executive summary.* Washington, DC: Office of Planning, Research and Evaluation, Administration for Children and Families, U.S. Department of Health and Human Services.

Backer, T. E. 2001. *Finding the balance: Program fidelity and adaptation in substance abuse prevention: A state-of-the-art review.* Rockville, MD: Center for Substance Abuse Prevention.

Bagnato, S. J., H. K. Suen, and A. V. Fevola. 2011. Dosage effects on developmental progress during early childhood intervention: Accessible metrics for real-life research and advocacy. *Infancy and Young Children* 24(2):117-132.

Bai, Y., R. Wells, and M. Hillemeier. 2009. Coordination between child welfare agencies and mental health services providers, children's service use, and outcomes. *Child Abuse & Neglect* 33(6):372-381.

Balas, E. A., and S. A. Boren. 2000. Managing clinical knowledge for healthcare improvements. *Yearbook of medical informatics 2000: Patient-centered systems,* edited by J. Bemmel and A. T. McCray. Stuttgart, Germany: Schattauer Verlagsgesellschaft mbH. Pp. 65-70.

Bandura, A. 1986. *Social foundations of thought and action: A social cognitive theory.* Upper Saddle River, NJ: Prentice-Hall.

Barlow, J., H. Davis, E. McIntosh, P. Jarrett, C. Mockford, and S. Stewart-Brown. 2007. Role of home visiting in improving parenting and health in families at risk of abuse and neglect: Results of a multicentre randomised controlled trial and economic evaluation. *Archives of Disease in Childhood* 92(3):229-233.

Barr, R. G., M. Barr, T. Fujiwara, J. Conway, N. Catherine, and R. Brant. 2009. Do educational materials change knowledge and behavior about crying and shaken baby syndrome?: A randomized controlled trial. *Canadian Medical Association Journal* 180(7):727-733.

Barrera, M., Jr., F. G. Castro, and L. K. Steiker. 2011. A critical analysis of approaches to the development of preventive interventions for subcultural groups. *American Journal of Community Psychology* 48(3-4):439-454.

Barth, R. 2009. Preventing child abuse and neglect with parent training: Evidence and opportunities. *The Future of Children* 19(2):95-118.

Barth, R. P., J. Landsverk, P. Chamberlain, J. B. Reid, J. A. Rolls, M. S. Hurlburt, E. M. Z. Farmer, S. James, K. M. McCabe, and P. L. Kohl. 2005. Parent-training programs in child welfare services: Planning for a more evidence-based approach to serving biological parents. *Research on Social Work Practice* 15(5):353-371.

Barth, R. P., B. R. Lee, M. A. Lindsey, K. S. Collins, F. Strieder, B. F. Chorpita, K. D. Becker, and J. A. Sparks. 2012. Evidence-based practice at a crossroads the timely emergence of common elements and common factors. *Research on Social Work Practice* 22(1): 108-119.

Bauman, L. J., R. E. Stein, and H. T. Ireys. 1991. Reinventing fidelity: The transfer of social technology among settings. *American Journal of Community Psychology* 19(4):619-639.

Benedetti, G. 2012. *Innovations in the field of child abuse and neglect prevention: A review of the literature.* Chicago: Chapin Hall at the University of Chicago. http://www.chapinhall. org/research/report/innovations-field-child-abuse-and-neglect-prevention-review-literature (accessed December 6, 2013).

Berkel, C., A. M. Mauricio, E. Schoenfelder, and I. N. Sandler. 2011. Putting the pieces together: An integrated model of program implementation. *Prevention Science* 12(1):23-33.

Berkowitz, S. J., C. S. Stover, and S. R. Marans. 2011. The Child and Family Traumatic Stress Intervention: Secondary prevention for youth at risk of developing PTSD. *Journal of Child Psychology and Psychiatry* 52(61):676-685.

Bernal, G., E. Saez-Santiago, and A. Galloza-Carrero. 2009. Evidence-based approaches to working with Latino youth and families. In *Handbook of U.S. Latino psychology. Development and community-based perspectives*, edited by F. A. Villarruel, G. Carlo, J. M. Grau, M. Azmitia, N. J. Cabrera, and T. J. Chahin. Los Angeles, CA: Sage. Pp. 309-332.

Bernard, K., M. Dozier, J. Bick, E. Lewis-Morrarty, O. Lindhiem, and E. Carlson. 2012. Enhancing attachment organization among maltreated children: Results of a randomized clinical trial. *Child Development* 83(2):623-636.

Berrick, J., and R. Barth. 1992. Child sexual abuse prevention: Research review and recommendations. *Social Work Research and Abstracts* 28(4):6-15.

Bigfoot, D. S., and B. W. Funderburk. 2011. Honoring children, making relatives: The cultural translation of parent-child interaction therapy for American Indian and Alaska native families. *Journal of Psychoactive Drugs* 43(4):309-318.

Bor, W., M. R. Sanders, and C. Markie-Dadds. 2002. The effects of Triple P—Positive Parenting Program on preschool children with co-occurring disruptive behavior and attentional/hyperactive difficulties. *Journal of Abnormal Child Psychology* 30(6):571-587.

Brekke, J. S., K. Ell, and L. A. Palinkas. 2007. Translational science at the National Institutes of Mental Health: Can social work take its rightful place? *Research on Social Work Practice* 17(1):123-133.

Bryant, P. 1993. *Availability of existing statewide parent education and support programs.* Working Paper 861. Chicago: National Committee to Prevent Child Abuse.

Cardona, J. P., K. Holtrop, D. Cordova, A. R. Escobar-Chew, S. Horsford, L. Tams, and H. E. Fitzgerald. 2009. Queremos aprender: Latino immigrants' call to integrate cultural adaptation with best practice knowledge in a parenting intervention. *Family Process* 48(2):211-231.

Carlson, V., D. Cicchetti, D. Barnett, and K. Braunwald. 1989. Disorganized/disoriented attachment relationships in maltreated infants. *Developmental Psychology* 25(4):525.

Carroll, C., M. Patterson, S. Wood, A. Booth, J. Rick, and S. Balain. 2007. A conceptual framework for implementation fidelity. *Implementation Science* 2:40.

Caughy, M. O., T. Miller, J. L. Genevro, K. Huang, and C. Nautiyal. 2003. The effects of Healthy Steps on discipline strategies of parents of young children. *Journal of Applied Developmental Psychology* 24(5):517-534.

Chaffin, M. 2004. Is it time to rethink healthy start/healthy families? *Child Abuse & Neglect* 28(6):589-595.

Chaffin, M. 2006. Organizational culture and practice epistemologies. *Clinical Psychology: Science and Practice* 13(1):90-93.

Chaffin, M., J. F. Silovsky, B. Funderburk, L. A. Valle, E. V. Brestan, T. Balachova, S. Jackson, J. Lensgraf, and B. L. Bonner. 2004. Parent-child interaction therapy with physically abusive parents: Efficacy for reducing future abuse reports. *Journal of Consulting and Clinical Psychology* 72(3):500.

Chaffin, M., D. Hecht, D. Bard, J. F. Silovsky, and W. Beasley. 2012a. A statewide trial of SafeCare home-based services model with parents in child protective services. *Pediatrics* 129(3):509-515.

Chaffin, M., D. Bard, D. S. Bigfoot, and E. J. Maher. 2012b. Is a structured, manualized, evidence-based treatment protocol culturally competent and equivalently effective among American Indian parents in child welfare? *Child Maltreatment* 17(3):242-252.

Chamberlain, P., L. D. Leve, and D. S. DeGarmo. 2007. Multidimensional treatment foster care for girls in the juvenile justice system: 2-year follow-up of a randomized clinical trial. *Journal of Consulting and Clinical Psychology* 75(1):187-193.

Chamberlain, P., J. Price, L. D. Leve, H. Laurent, J. A. Landsverk, and J. B. Reid. 2008. Prevention of behavior problems for children in foster care: Outcomes and mediation effects. *Prevention Science* 9(1):17-27.

Chamberlain, P., R. Roberts, H. Jones, L. Marsenich, T., Sosna, and J. M. Price. 2012. Three collaborative models for scaling up evidence-based practices. *Administration and Policy in Mental Health* 39(4):278-290.

Chorpita, B. F., E. L. Daleiden, and J. R. Weisz. 2005. Identifying and selecting the common elements of evidence based interventions: A distillation and matching model. *Mental Health Services Research* 7(1):5-20.

Chuang, E., and R. Wells. 2010. The role of inter-agency collaboration in facilitating receipt of behavioral health services for youth involved with child welfare and juvenile justice. *Children and Youth Services Review* 32(12):1814-1822.

Cicchetti, D., and S. L. Toth. 2005. Child maltreatment. *Annual Review of Clinical Psychology* 1:409-438.

Conger, D., and T. Ross. 2006. Project Confirm: An outcome evaluation of a program for children in the child welfare and juvenile justice systems. *Youth Violence and Juvenile Justice* 4(1):97-115.

Connell, A., B. M. Bullock, T. J. Dishion, D. Shaw, M. Wilson, and F. Gardner. 2008. Family intervention effects on co-occurring early childhood behavioral and emotional problems: A latent transition analysis approach. *Journal of Abnormal Child Psychology* 36(8):1211-1225.

Corso, P., and J. H. Filene. 2009. Programmatic cost analysis of the family connections program. *Protecting Children* 24(3):77-87.

Corso, P. S., and J. R. Lutzker. 2006. The need for economic analysis in research on child maltreatment. *Child Abuse & Neglect* 30(7):727-738.

Cottrell, D., D. Lucey, I. Porter, and D. Walker. 2000. Joint working between child and adolescent mental health services and the Department of Social Services: The Leeds Model. *Clinical Child Psychology and Psychiatry* 5(4):481-489.

Coulton, C., J. Korbin, and M. Sue. 1997. Neighborhoods and child maltreatment: A multilevel analysis. *Child Abuse & Neglect* 23(11):1019-1040.

Courtney, M. E. 1999. National call to action: Working toward the elimination of child maltreatment. The economics. *Child Abuse & Neglect* 23(10):975-986.

CWIG (Child Welfare Information Gateway). 2011. *Child maltreatment prevention: Past, present, and future.* https://www.childwelfare.gov/pubs/issue_briefs/cm_prevention.cfm (accessed December 6, 2013).

Dalziel, K., and L. Segal. 2012. Home visiting programmes for the prevention of child maltreatment: Cost-effectiveness of 33 programmes. *Archives of Disease in Childhood* 97(9):787-798.

Damschroder, L. J., and H. J. Hagedorn. 2011. A guiding framework and approach for implementation research in substance use disorders treatment. *Psychology of Addictive Behaviors* 25(2):194-205.

Dane, A. V., and F. H. Schneider. 1998. Program integrity in primary and early secondary prevention: Are implementation effects out of control? *Clinical Psychology Review* 18(1):23-45.

Daro, D. 1994. Prevention of childhood sexual abuse. *The Future of Children* 4(2):198-223.

Daro, D. 2009. Science and child abuse prevention: A reciprocal relationship. In *Community prevention of child maltreatment,* edited by K. Dodge and D. Coleman. New York: Guilford Press. Pp. 9-28.

Daro, D. 2010. Preventing child abuse and neglect. In *APSAC handbook on child maltreatment,* 3rd ed., edited by J. Myers. Beverly Hills, CA: Sage Publications. Pp. 17-38.

Daro, D. 2011. Home visitation. In *The preschool education debates*, edited by E. Zigler, W. Gilliam, and S. Barnett. Baltimore, MD: Paul H. Brookes Publishing Co. Pp. 169-173.

Daro, D., and G. Benedetti. 2014. Sustaining progress in preventing child maltreatment: A transformative challenge. In *Handbook of child maltreatment*. Springer. Pp. 281-300.

Daro, D., and A. Cohn-Donnelly. 2002. Charting the waves of prevention: Two steps forward, one step back. *Child Abuse & Neglect* 26(6/7):731-742.

Daro, D., and K. Dodge. 2009. Creating community responsibility for child protection: Expanding partnerships, changing context. *The Future of Children* 19(2):67-94.

Daro, D., and K. Dodge. 2010. Strengthening home-visiting intervention policy: Expanding reach, building knowledge. In *Investing in young children: New directions for America's preschool policies*, edited by R. Haskins and W. S. Barnett. Washington, DC: National Institution for Early Education Research and Brookings Institution. Pp. 79-86.

Daro, D. A., and K. P. McCurdy. 2007. Interventions to prevent child maltreatment. *Handbook of injury and violence prevention*. Pp. 137-155. http://link.springer.com/chapter/1 0.1007%2F978-0-387-29457-5_8 (accessed December 6, 2013).

Daro, D., L. A. Huang, and B. English. 2008. *The Duke endowment child abuse prevention: Mid point assessment*. Chicago: Chapin Hall at the University of Chicago.

Daro, D., E. Barringer, and B. English. 2009. *Key trends in prevention: Report for the National Quality Improvement Center on Early Childhood Education (QIC-EC)*. Chicago: Chapin Hall at the University of Chicago.

DeBruyn, L., M. Chino, P. Serna, and L. Fullerton-Gleason. 2001. Child maltreatment in American Indian and Alaska native communities: Integrating culture, history, and public health for intervention and prevention. *Child Maltreatment* 6(2):89-102.

Del Grosso, P., R. Kleinman, A. M. Esposito, E. Sama-Miller, and D. Paulsell. 2012. Assessing the evidence of effectiveness of home visiting program models implemented in tribal communities. Washington, DC: Office of Planning, Research and Evaluation, Administration for Children and Families, U.S. Department of Health and Human Services. http://homvee.acf.hhs.gov/Tribal_Report_2012.pdf (accessed November, 26, 2013).

DePanfilis, D., and H. Dubowitz. 2005. Family connections: A program for preventing child neglect. *Child Maltreatment* 10(2):108-123.

DePanfilis, D., H. Dubowitz, and J. Kunz. 2008. Assessing the cost-effectiveness of family connections. *Child Abuse and Neglect* 32(3):335-351.

Dettlaff, A. J., and J. R. Rycraft. 2010. Adapting systems of care for child welfare practice with immigrant Latino children and families. *Evaluation and Program Planning* 33(3):303-310.

Dias, M. S., K. Smith, K. DeGuehery, P. Mazur, V. Li, and M. L. S. Shaffer. 2005. Preventing abusive head trauma among infants and young children: A hospital-based, parent education program. *Pediatrics* 115(4):e470-e477.

Dishion, T. J., D. Shaw, A. Connell, F. Gardner, C. Weaver, and M. Wilson. 2008. The family check-up with high-risk indigent families: Preventing problem behavior by increasing parents' positive behavior support in early childhood. *Child Development* 79(5):1395-1414.

Dodge, K. A., L. J. Berlin, M. Epstein, A. Spitz Roth, K. O'Donnell, M. Kaufman, L. Amaya-Jackson, J. Rosch, and C. Christopoulos. 2004. The Durham Family Initiative: A preventive system of care. *Child Welfare* 83(2):109-128.

Dodge, K. A., W. B. Goodman, R. A. Murphy, K. O'Donnell, and J. Sato. 2013. Toward population impact from home visiting. *Zero to Three* 33(3):17-23.

Dubowitz, H., S. Feigelman, W. Lane, and J. Kim. 2009. Pediatric primary care to help prevent child maltreatment: The Safe Environment for Every Kid (SEEK) model. *Pediatrics* 123(3):858-864.

Dubowitz, H., W. G. Lane, J. N. Semiatin, L. S. Magder, M. Venepally, and M. Jans. 2011. The Safe Environment for Every Kid Model: Impact on pediatric primary care professionals. *Pediatrics* 127(4):e962-e970.

DuMont, K., K. Kirkland, S. Mitchell-Herzfeld, S. Ehrhard-Dietzel, M. L. Rodriguez, E. Lee, C. Layne, and R. Greene. 2010. *A randomized trial of Healthy Families New York (HFNY): Does home visiting prevent child maltreatment?* New York: University at Albany, State University of New York.

Duncan, B. L., S. D. Miller, B. E. Wampold, and M. A. Hubble. 2010. *The heart and soul of change: Delivering what works in therapy,* 2nd ed. Washington, DC: American Psychological Association.

Eckenrode, J., M. Campa, D. W. Luckey, C. R. Henderson, Jr., R. Cole, H. Kitzman, and D. Olds. 2010. Long-term effects of prenatal and infancy nurse home visitation on the life course of youths: 19-year follow-up of a randomized trial. *Archives of Pediatrics and Adolescent Medicine* 164(1):9-15.

Ehrle, J., C. Andrews Scarcella, and R. Geen. 2004. Teaming up: Collaboration between welfare and child welfare agencies since welfare reform. *Children and Youth Services Review* 26(3):265-285.

Ferlie, E. B., and S. M. Shortell. 2001. Improving the quality of health care in the United Kingdom and the United States: A framework for change. *Milbank Quarterly* 79(2):281-315.

Fixsen, D. L., S. F. Naoom, K. A. Blase, R. M. Friedman, and F. Wallace. 2005. *Implementation research: A synthesis of the literature.* Tampa: University of South Florida, Louis de la Parte Florida Mental Health Institute, the National Implementation Research Network.

Fixsen, D., K. Blase, S. Naoom, and F. Wallace. 2009. Core implementation components. *Research on Social Work Practice* 19(5):531-540.

Fonagy, P., S. W. Twemlow, E. M. Vernberg, J. M. Nelson, E. J. Dill, T. D. Little, and J. A. Sargent. 2009. A cluster randomized controlled trial of child-focused psychiatric consultation and a school systems-focused intervention to reduce aggression. *Journal of Child Psychology and Psychiatry and Allied Disciplines* 50(5):607-616.

Forman-Hoffman, V., S. Knauer, J. McKeeman, A. Zolotor, R. Blanco, S. Lloyd, E. Tant, and M. Viswanathan. 2013. *Child and adolescent exposure to trauma: Comparative effectiveness of interventions addressing trauma other than maltreatment or family violence. Comparative effectiveness review no. 107 (AHRQ publication no. 13-ehc054-ef).* Rockville, MD: Agency for Healthcare Research and Quality. http://effectivehealthcare.ahrq.gov/index.cfm/search-for-guides-reviews-and-reports/?productid=1396&pageaction=displayproduct (accessed November 26, 2013).

Foster, E. M., K. A. Dodge, and D. Jones. 2003. Issues in the economic evaluation of prevention programs. *Applied Developmental Science* 7(2):76-86.

Foster, E. M., M. M. Porter, T. S. Ayers, D. L. Kaplan, and I. Sandler. 2007. Estimating the costs of preventive interventions. *Evaluation Review* 31(3):261-286.

Frey, K. S., M. K. Hirschstein, J. L. Snell, L. V. Edstrom, E. P. MacKenzie, and C. J. Broderick. 2005. Reducing playground bullying and supporting beliefs: An experimental trial of the steps to respect program. *Developmental Psychology* 41(3):479-490.

Gandelman, A., and C. Rietmeijer. 2004. Translation, adaptation, and synthesis of interventions for persons living with HIV: Lessons from previous HIV prevention interventions. *Acquired Immune Deficiency Syndrome* 37(2):S126-S129.

Gardner, F. M. 1989. Inconsistent parenting: Is there evidence for a link with children's conduct problems? *Journal of Abnormal Child Psychology* 17(2):223-233.

Gardner, R., J. Hutchings, T. Bywater, and C. Whitaker. 2010. Who benefits and how does it work? Moderators and mediators of outcomes in an effectiveness trail of a parenting intervention. *Journal of Clinical Child and Adolescent Psychology* 39(4):568-580.

Gearing, R. E., N. El-Bassel, A. Ghesquiere, S. Baldwin, J. Gillies, and E. Ngeow. 2011. Major ingredients of fidelity: A review and scientific guide to improving quality of intervention research implementation. *Clinical Psychology Review* 31(1):71-98.

Glisson, C. 2007. Assessing and changing organizational culture and climate for effective services. *Research on Social Work Practice* 17(6):736-747.

Glisson, C., and A. Hemmelgarn. 1998. The effects of organizational climate and interorganizational coordination on the quality and outcomes of children's service systems. *Child Abuse & Neglect* 22(5):401-421.

Glisson, C., and S. Schoenwald. 2005. The ARC organizational and community intervention strategy for implementing evidence-based children's mental health treatments. *Mental Health Services Research* 7(4):243-259.

Glisson, C., J. Landsverk, S. Schoenwald, K. Kelleher, K. Hoagwood, S. Mayberg, and P. Green. 2008. Assessing the Organizational Social Context (OSC) of mental health services: Implications for research and practice. *Administration and Policy in Mental Health and Mental Health Services Research. Special Issue: Improving Mental Health Services* 35(1-2):98-113.

Glisson, C., S. K. Schoenwald, A. Hemmelgarn, P. Green, D. Dukes, K. S. Armstrong, and J. E. Chapman. 2010. Randomized trial of MST and ARC in a two-level evidence-based treatment implementation strategy. *Journal of Consulting and Clinical Psychology* 78(4):537-550.

Goldhaber-Fiebert, J. D., L. R. Snowden, F. Wulczyn, J. Landsverk, and S. M. Horwitz. 2011. Economic evaluation research in the context of child welfare policy: A structured literature review and recommendations. *Child Abuse & Neglect* 35(9):722-740.

Grace, M., L. Coventry, and D. Batterham. 2012. The role of interagency collaboration in "joined-up" case management. *Journal of Interprofessional Care* 26(2):141-149.

Graziano, A. M., and D. M. Diament. 1992. Parent behavioral training: An examination of the paradigm. *Behavior Modification* 16(1):3-38.

Green, B. L., A. Rockhill, and S. Burrus. 2008. The role of interagency collaboration for substance-abusing families involved with child welfare. *Child Welfare* 87(1):29-61.

Greenhalgh, T., G. Robert, F. Macfarlane, P. Bate, and O. Kyriakidou. 2004. Diffusion of innovations in service organizations: Systematic review and recommendations. *Milbank Quarterly* 82(4):581-629.

Grimshaw, J., L. Shirran, R. Thomas, G. Mowatt, C. Fraser, L. Bero, and M. O'Brien. 2001. Changing provider behavior: An overview of systematic reviews of interventions. *Medical Care* 39(8):II2-II45.

Grol, R., and J. Grimshaw. 1999. Evidence-based implementation of evidence-based medicine. *Joint Commission Journal on Quality Improvement* 25(10):503-513.

Haddix, A. C., S. M. Teutsch, and P. S. Corso. 2003. *Prevention effectiveness: A guide to decision analysis and economic evaluation.* New York: Oxford University Press.

Hagermoser Sanetti, L. M., and L. M. Fallon. 2011. Treatment integrity assessment: How estimates of adherence, quality, and exposure influence interpretation of implementation. *Journal of Educational and Psychological Consultation* 21(3):209-232.

Hagermoser Sanetti, L. M., and T. R. Kratochwill. 2009. Toward developing a science of treatment integrity: Introduction to the special issue. *School Psychology Review* 38(4):445-459.

Harshbarger, C., G. Simmons, H. Coelho, K. Sloop, and C. Collins. 2006. An empirical assessment of implementation, adaptation, and tailoring: The evaluation of CDC's national diffusion of VOICES/VOCES. *AIDS Education and Prevention. Special Issue: Moving Science into Practice: The Role of Technology Exchange for HIV/STD Prevention* 18(Suppl. A):184-197.

Helfer, R. 1982. A review of the literature on the prevention of child abuse and neglect. *Child Abuse & Neglect* 6:251-261.

Herman, K. C., L. A. Borden, W. M. Reinke, and C. Webster-Stratton. 2011. The impact of the incredible years parent, child, and teacher training programs on children's co-occurring internalizing symptoms. *School Psychology Quarterly* 26(3):189-201.

Hodges, S., T. Nesman, and M. Hernandez. 1999. *Promising practices: Building collaboration in systems of care*, Vol. 6. Washington, DC: Center for Effective Collaboration and Practice, American Institutes for Research.

Hogan, C., and D. Murphey. 2002. *Outcomes: Reframing responsibility for well-being*. Baltimore, MD: Annie E. Casey Foundation.

Honig, M. I., and C. Coburn. 2008. Evidence-based decision making in school district central offices: Toward a policy and research agenda. *Educational Policy* 22(4):578-608.

Horwath, J., and T. Morrison. 2007. Collaboration, integration and change in children's services: Critical issues and key ingredients. *Child Abuse & Neglect* 31(1):55-69.

Huey, S. J., and A. J. Polo. 2008. Evidence-based psychosocial treatments for ethnic minority youth. *Journal of Clinical Child and Adolescent Psychology* 37(1):262-301.

Huey, S. J., and A. J. Polo. 2010. Assessing the effects of evidence-based psychotherapies with ethnic minority youths. In *Evidence-based psychotherapies for children and adolescents*, edited by J. R. Weisz and A. E. Kazdin. New York: Guilford Press. Pp. 451-469.

Hurlburt, M. S., L. K. Leslie, J. Landsverk, R. P. Barth, B. J. Burns, R. D. Gibbons, D. J. Slymen, and J. Zhang. 2004. Contextual predictors of mental health service use among children open to child welfare. *Archives of General Psychiatry* 61(12):1217-1224.

Jaycox, L. H., B. D. Stein, S. H. Kataoka, M. Wong, A. Fink, P. I. A. Escudero, and C. Zaragoza. 2002. Violence exposure, posttraumatic stress disorder, and depressive symptoms among recent immigrant schoolchildren. *Journal of the American Academy of Child & Adolescent Psychiatry* 41(9):1104-1110.

Johnson, M. A., S. Stone, C. Lou, J. Ling, J. Claassen, and M. J. Austin. 2008. Assessing parent education programs for families involved with child welfare services: Evidence and implications. *Journal of Evidence-Based Social Work* 5(1/2):191-236.

Johnson, P., G. Wistow, R. Schulz, and B. Hardy. 2003. Interagency and interprofessional collaboration in community care: The interdependence of structures and values. *Journal of Interprofessional Care* 17(1):69-83.

Jones, N., P. Thomas, and L. Rudd. 2004. Collaborating for mental health services in Wales: A process evaluation. *Public Administration* 82(1):109-121.

Jung, D. I., C. Chow, and A. Wu. 2003. The role of transformational leadership in enhancing organizational innovation: Hypotheses and some preliminary findings. *The Leadership Quarterly* 14(4-5):525-544.

Kaminski, J. W., L. A. Valle, J. H. Filene, and C. L. Boyle. 2008. A meta-analytic review of components associated with parent training program effectiveness. *Journal of Abnormal Child Psychology* 36(4):567-589.

Karoly, L. A., P. W. Greenwood, S. S. Everingham, J. Houbé, and M. R. Kilburn. 1998. Investing in our children: What we know and don't know about the costs and benefits of early childhood interventions. Santa Monica, CA: RAND Corporation.

Keenan, M. 2011. *Child sexual abuse and the Catholic church: Gender, power, and organizational culture*. New York: Oxford University Press.

Kempe, C. H. 1976. Approaches to preventing child abuse: The health visitors concept. *American Journal of Diseases of Children* 130(9):941-947.

Kennedy, M. M. 1984. How evidence alters understanding and decisions. *Educational Evaluation and Policy Analysis* 6(3):207-226.

Kessler, M. L., E. Gira, and J. Poertner. 2005. Moving best practice to evidence-based practice in child welfare. *Families in Society* 86(2):244-250.

Kitzman, H. J., D. L. Olds, R. E. Cole, C. A. Hanks, E. A. Anson, K. J. Arcoleo, and J. R. Holmberg. 2010. Enduring effects of prenatal and infancy home visiting by nurses on children: Follow-up of a randomized trial among children at age 12 years. *Archives of Pediatrics and Adolescent Medicine* 164(5):412-418.

Kolko, D. J., B. L. Baumann, A. D. Herschell, J. A. Hart, E. A. Holden, and S. R. Wisniewski. 2012. Implementation of AF-CBT by community practitioners serving child welfare and mental health: A randomized trial. *Child Maltreatment* 17(1):32-46.

Lau, A. S. 2006. Making the case for selective and directed cultural adaptations of evidence-based treatments: Examples from parent training. *Clinical Psychology: Science and Practice* 13(4):295-310.

Lau, A. S., J. J. Fung, L. Y. Ho, L. L. Liu, and O. G. Gudiño. 2011. Parent training with high-risk immigrant Chinese families: A pilot group randomized trial yielding practice-based evidence. *Behavior Therapy* 42(3):413-426.

LeCroy, C. W., and J. Krysik. 2011. Randomized trial of the healthy families Arizona home visiting program. *Children and Youth Services Review* 33(10):1761-1766.

Lee, C.-Y., G. August, G. Realmuto, J. Horowitz, M. Bloomquist, and B. Klimes-Dougan. 2008. Fidelity at a distance: Assessing implementation fidelity of the Early Risers prevention program in a going to scale intervention trial. *Prevention Science* 9:215-229.

Leung, C., M. R. Sanders, S. Leung, R. Mak, and J. Lau. 2003. An outcome evaluation of the implementation of the Triple P-Positive Parenting Program in Hong Kong. *Family Process* 42(4):531-544.

Lippitt, R., and J. van Til. 1981. Can we achieve a collaborative community? Issues, imperatives, potentials. *Nonprofit and Voluntary Sector Quarterly* 10(3-4):7-17.

Lomas, J. 2000. Using "linkage and exchange" to move research into policy at a Canadian foundation. *Health Affairs* 19(3):236-240.

Longoria, R. A. 2005. Is inter-organizational collaboration always a good thing? *Journal of Sociology and Social Welfare* 32:123-138.

Lowell, D. I., A. S. Carter, L. Godoy, B. Paulicin, and M. J. Briggs-Gowan. 2011. A randomized controlled trial of child first: A comprehensive home-based intervention translating research into early childhood practice. *Child Development* 82(1):193-208.

MacMillan, H., J. MacMillan, D. Offord, L. Griffith, and A. MacMillan. 1994. Primary prevention of child sexual abuse: A critical review. Part II. *Journal of Child Psychology and Psychiatry* 35(5):857-876.

MacMillan, H. L., B. H. Thomas, E. Jamieson, C. A. Walsh, M. H. Boyle, H. Shannon, and A. Gafni. 2005. Effectiveness of public health nurse home visitation in preventing the recurrence of child physical abuse and neglect: A randomized, controlled trial. *Lancet* 365(9473):1786-1793.

Mannarino, A. P., J. A. Cohen, E. Deblinger, M. K. Runyon, and R. A. Steer. 2012. Trauma-focused cognitive-behavioral therapy for children: Sustained impact of treatment 6 and 12 months later. *Child Maltreatment* 17(3):231-241.

Martin, A. J., and M. R. Sanders. 2003. Balancing work and family: A controlled evaluation of the Triple P—Positive Parenting Program as a work-site intervention. *Child and Adolescent Mental Health* 8(4):161-169.

Martinez, C. R., and M. Eddy. 2005. Effects of culturally adapted parent management training on Latino youth behavioral health outcomes. *Journal of Consulting and Clincal Psychology* 73(4):841-851.

Matone, M., A. O-Reilly, X. Luan, A. R. Localio, and D. Rubin. 2012. Emergency department visits and hospitalizations for injuries among infants and children following statewide implementation of a home visitation model. *Maternal and Child Health Journal* 16(9):1754-1761.

McIntosh, E., J. Barlow, H. Davis, and S. Stewart-Brown. 2009. Economic evaluation of an intensive home visiting programme for vulnerable families: A cost-effectiveness analysis of a public health intervention. *Journal of Public Health* 31(3):423-433.

McKleroy, V. S., J. S. Galbraith, B. Cummings, P. Jones, C. Harshbarger, C. Collins, and J. W. Carey. 2006. Adapting evidence-based behavioral interventions for new settings and target populations. *AIDS Education and Prevention* 18(4 Suppl. A):59-73.

Melton, G., B. Holaday, and R. Kimbrough-Melton. 2008. Community life, public health, and children's safety. *Family and Community Health* 31(2):84-99.

Mihalic, S. F., A. Fagan, K. Irwin, D. Ballard, and D. M. Elliott. 2004. *Blueprints for violence prevention.* Washington, DC: U.S. Department of Justice, Office of Juvenile Justice and Delinquency Prevention.

Mildon, R., and A. Shlonsky. 2011. Bridge over troubled water: Using implementation science to facilitate effective services in child welfare. *Child Abuse & Neglect* 35(9):753-756.

Minkovitz, C. S., N. Hughart, B. A. Strobino, D. Scharfstein, H. Grason, W. Hou, T. Miller, D. Bishai, M. Augustyn, K. T. McLearn, and B. Guyer. 2003. A practice-based intervention to enhance quality of care in the first 3 years of life: The Healthy Steps for Young Children Program. *Journal of the American Medical Association* 290(23):3081-3091.

Minkovitz, C. S., D. Strobino, K. B. Mistry, D. O. Scharfstein, H. Grason, W. Hou, and B. Guyer. 2007. Healthy steps for young children: Sustained results at 5.5 years. *Pediatrics* 120(3):658-668.

Mitchell, E., L. Hutchison, and A. Stewart. 2007. The continuing decline in SIDS mortality. *Archives of Disease in Childhood* 92(7):625-626.

Mitton, C., C. E. Adair, E. McKenzie, S. B. Patten, and B. Waye Perry. 2007. Knowledge transfer and exchange: Review and synthesis of the literature. *Milbank Quarterly* 85(4):729-768.

Mytton, J., C. DiGuiseppi, D. Gough, R. Taylor, and S. Logan. 2006. School-based secondary prevention programmes for preventing violence. *Cochrane Database of Systematic Reviews* 3:CD004606.

Nievar, M. A., J. Arminta, C. Qi, J. Ursula, and D. Shannon. 2011. Impact of HIPPY on home learning environments of Latino families. *Early Childhood Research Quarterly* 26:268-277.

NRC (National Research Council). 1993. *Understanding child abuse and neglect.* Washington, DC: National Academy Press.

Nutley, S. M., I. Walter, and H. T. O. Davies. 2007. *Using evidence: How research can inform public services.* Bristol, UK: The Policy Press.

Olds, D. 2010. The Nurse Family Partnership. In *New directions for America's preschool policies,* edited by R. Haskins and W. Barnett. Washington, DC: National Institution for Early Education Research and Brookings Institution. Pp. 69-78.

Olds, D. L., L. Sadler, and H. Kitzman. 2007. Programs for parents of infants and toddlers: Recent evidence from randomized trials. *Journal of Child Psychology and Psychiatry* 48(3-4):355-391.

Olds, D. L., H. J. Kitzman, R. E. Cole, C. A. Hanks, K. J. Arcoleo, E. A. Anson, D. W. Luckey, M. D. Knudtson, C. R. Henderson, J. Bondy, and A. Stevenson. 2010. Enduring effects of prenatal and infancy home visiting by nurses on maternal life course and government spending. *Archives of Pediatrics and Adolescent Medicine* 164(5):419-424.

Palinkas, L. A., and G. A. Aarons. 2009. A view from the top: Executive and management challenges in a statewide implementation of an evidence-based practice to reduce child neglect. *International Journal of Child Health and Human Development* 2(1):47-55.

Palinkas, L. A., C. A. Allred, and J. A. Landsverk. 2005. Models of research-operational collaboration for behavioral health in space. *Aviation, Space, and Environments Medicine* 76(Suppl. 6):B52-B60.

Palinkas, L. A., S. K. Schoenwald, K. Hoagwood, J. Landsverk, B. F. Chorpita, and J. R. Weisz. 2008. An ethnographic study of implementation of evidence-based treatments in child mental health: First steps. *Psychiatric Services* 59(7):738-746.

Palinkas, L. A., G. A. Aarons, B. F. Chorpita, K. Hoagwood, J. Landsverk, and J. R. Weisz. 2009. Cultural exchange and implementation of evidence-based practices. *Research on Social Work Practice* 19(5):602-612.

Palinkas, L. A., I. W. Holloway, E. Rice, D. Fuentes, Q. Wu, and P. Chamberlain. 2011. Social networks and implementation of evidence-based practices in public youth-serving systems: A mixed-methods study. *Implementation Science* 6(1):1-11.

Palinkas, L. A., A. R. Garcia, G. A. Aarons, I. Holloway, M. Finno, D. Fuentes, and P. Chamberlain. 2012. *Measurement of implementation process: The Structured Interview of Evidence Use (SIEU) and Cultural Exchange Inventory (CEI).* Paper presented at the 5th Annual NIH Conference on the Science of Dissemination and Implementation, Washington, DC.

Patterson, G. R., B. DeBarhyshe, and E. Ramsey. 1990. A developmental perspective on antisocial behavior. *American Psychologist* 44(2):329-335.

Paulsell, D., M. Hargreaves, B. Coffee-Borden, and K. Boller. 2012. *Evidence-based home visiting systems evaluation update: 2011 draft report.* Princeton, NJ: Mathematica Policy Research.

Paxson, C., and R. Haskins. 2009. Introducing the issue. *The Future of Children* 19(2):3-17.

Pinderhughes, E., R. Nix, E. M. Foster, D. Jones, and the Conduct Problems Prevention Research Group. 2001. Parenting in context: Impact of neighborhood poverty, residential stability, public services, social networks, and danger on parental behaviors. *Journal of Marriage and the Family* 63(4):941-953.

Poupart, J., L. Baker, and J. R. Horse. 2009. Research with American Indian communities: The value of authentic partnerships. *Children and Youth Services Review* 31(11):1180-1186.

Prince, J., and M. J. Austin. 2005. Inter-agency collaboration in child welfare and child mental health systems. *Social Work in Mental Health* 4(1):1-16.

Prinz, R. J., M. R. Sanders, C. J. Shapiro, D. J. Whitaker, and J. R. Lutzker. 2009. Population-based prevention of child maltreatment: The U.S. Triple P System Population Trial. *Prevention Science* 10(1):1-12.

Putnam-Hornstein, E., D. Webster, B. Needell, and J. Magruder. 2011. A public health approach to child maltreatment surveillance: Evidence from a data linkage project in the United States. *Child Abuse Review* 20(4):356-373.

Reid, M. J., C. Webster-Stratton, and R. P. Beauchaine. 2001. Parent training in Head Start: A comparison of program response among African American, Asian America, Caucasian, and Hispanic mothers. *Prevention Science* 2(4):209-227.

Reid, M. J., C. Webster-Stratton, and N. Baydar. 2004. Halting the development of conduct problems in Head Start children: The effect of parent training. *Journal of Clinical Child and Adolescent Psychology* 33(2):279-291.

Reynolds, A., L. Mathieson, and J. Topitzes. 2009. Do early childhood interventions prevent child maltreatment? A review of research. *Child Maltreatment* 14(2):182-206.

Rispens, J., A. Aleman, and P. P. Goudena. 1997. Prevention of child sexual abuse victimization: A meta-analysis of school programs. *Child Abuse & Neglect* 21(10):975-987.

Rogers, E. M. 2003. *Diffusion of innovations,* 5th ed. New York: Free Press.

Roggman, L. A., L. K. Boyce, and G. A. Cook. 2009. Keeping kids on track: Impacts of a parenting-focused Early Head Start program on attachment security and cognitive development. *Early Education and Development* 20(6):920-941.

Rowland, M. D., C. A. Halliday-Boykins, S. W. Henggeler, P. B. Cunningham, T. G. Lee, M. J. P. Kruesi, and S. B. Shapiro. 2005. A randomized trial of multisystemic therapy with Hawaii's felix class youths. *Journal of Emotional & Behavioral Disorders* 13(1):13-23.

Runyon, M. K., E. Deblinger, and C. M. Schroeder. 2009. Pilot evaluation of outcomes of combined parent-child cognitive-behavioral group therapy for families at risk for child physical abuse. *Cognitive and Behavioral Practice* 16(1):101-118.

Sanders, M. R., K. M. Turner, and C. Markie-Dadds. 2002. The development and dissemination of the Triple P—Positive Parenting Program: A multilevel, evidence-based system of parenting and family support. *Prevention Science* 3(3):173-189.

Scheeringa, M. S., C. F. Weems, J. A. Cohen, L. Amaya-Jackson, and D. Guthrie. 2011. Trauma-focused cognitive-behavioral therapy for posttraumatic stress disorder in three-through six year-old children: A randomized clinical trial. *Journal of Child Psychology and Psychiatry* 52(8):853-860.

Schoenwald, S. K., A. F. Garland, J. E. Chapman, S. L. Frazier, A. J. Sheidow, and M. A. Southam-Gerow. 2011. Toward the effective and efficient measurement of implementation fidelity. *Administration and Policy in Mental Health and Mental Health Services Research* 38(1):32-43.

Scott, W. R. 1985. Systems within systems. *American Behavioral Scientist* 28:601-618.

Sedlak, A. J., D. Schultz, S. J. Wells, P. Lyons, H. J. Doueck, and F. Gragg. 2006. Child protection and justice systems processing of serious child abuse and neglect cases. *Child Abuse & Neglect* 30(6):657-677.

Shaw, D. S., A. Connell, T. J. Dishion, M. N. Wilson, and F. Gardner. 2009. Improvements in maternal depression as a mediator of intervention effects on early childhood problem behavior. *Development and Psychopathology* 21(2):417-439.

Sheidow, A. J., S. K. Schoenwald, H. R. Wagner, C. A. Allred, and B. J. Burns. 2007. Predictors of workforce turnover in a transported treatment program. *Administration and Policy in Mental Health* 34(1):45-56.

Shiell, A., P. Hawe, and L. Gold. 2008. Complex interventions or complex systems? Implications for health economic evaluation. *British Medical Journal* 336(7656):1281.

Showers, J. 2001. Preventing shaken baby syndrome. *Journal of Aggression, Maltreatment and Trauma* 5(1):349-365.

Silovsky, J. F., D. Bard, M. Chaffin, D. Hecht, L. Burris, A. Owora, L. Beasley, and J. Lutzker. 2011. Prevention of child maltreatment in high-risk rural families: A randomized clinical trial with child welfare outcomes. *Children and Youth Services Review* 33(8):1435-1444.

Society for Prevention Research. 2004. *Standards of evidence: Criteria for efficacy, effectiveness, and dissemination.* Falls Church, VA. http://www.preventionresearch.org/StandardsofEvidencebook.pdf (accessed November 11, 2013).

Spieker, S. J., M. L. Oxford, J. F. Kelly, E. M. Nelson, and C. B. Fleming. 2012. Promoting first relationships: Randomized trial of a relationship-based intervention for toddlers in child welfare. *Child Maltreatment* 17(4):271-286.

Spillane, J. P., J. B. Diamond, L. J. Walker, R. Halverson, and L. Jita. 2001. Urban school leadership for elementary science instruction: Identifying and activating resources in an undervalued school subject. *Journal of Research in Science Teaching* 38(8):918-940.

Stormshak, E. A., K. L. Bierman, R. J. McMahon, and L. J. Lengua. 2000. Parenting practices and child disruptive behavior problems in early elementary school. *Journal of Clinical Child Psychology* 29(1):17-29.

Stroul, B. A., and R. M. Friedman. 1986. *A system of care for children and adolescents with severe emotional disturbance.* Washington, DC: Georgetown University, Child development Center, National Technical Assistance Center for Child Mental Health.

Tibbits, M., B. Bumbarger, S. Kyler, and D. Perkins. 2010. Sustaining evidence-based interventions under real-world conditions: Results from a large-scale diffusion project. *Prevention Science* 11(3):252-262.

Timmer, S. G., A. J. Urquiza, N. M. Zebell, and J. M. McGrath. 2005. Parent-child interaction therapy: Application to maltreating parent-child dyads. *Child Abuse & Neglect* 29(7):825-842.

Timmer, S. G., A. J. Urquiza, and N. M. Zebell. 2006. Challenging foster caregiver-maltreated child relationships: The effectiveness of parent-child interaction therapy. *Child and Youth Services Review* 28(1):1-19.

Urban Institute. 2012. *Best Start LA Pilot community evaluation; annual outcomes report, year 3*. Washington, DC: Urban Institute.

Urquiza, A. J., and C. B. McNeil. 1996. Parent-child interaction therapy: An intensive dyadic intervention for physically abusive families. *Child Maltreatment* 1(2):134-144.

U.S. Advisory Board on Child Abuse and Neglect. 1990. *Child abuse and neglect: Critical first steps in response to a national emergency (No. 017-092-001045)*. Washington, DC: U.S. Department of Health and Human Services.

Valente, T. W. 1995. *Network models in the diffusion of innovations*. Creskill, NJ: Hampton Press.

Valente, T. W. 2006. Opinion leader interventions in social networks. *British Medical Journal* 333(7578):1082.

Valente, T. W., and R. L. Davis. 1999. Accelerating the diffusion of innovations using opinion leaders. *The ANNALS of the American Academy of Political and Social Science* 566(1):55-67.

Valente, T. W., B. R. Hoffman, A. Ritt-Olson, K. Lichtman, and C. A. Johnson. 2003. Effects of a social-network method for group assignment strategies on peer-led tobacco prevention programs in schools. *American Journal of Public Health* 93(11):1837-1843.

Valente, T. W., C. P. Chou, and M. A. Pentz. 2007. Community coalitions as a system: Effects of network change on adoption of evidence-based substance abuse prevention. *American Journal of Public Health* 97(5):880-886.

Veniegas, R. C., U. H. Kao, and R. Rosales. 2009. Adapting HIV prevention evidence-based interventions in practice settings: An interview study. *Implementation Science* 4:9.

Walkup, J. T., A. M. Albano, J. Piacentini, B. Birmaher, S. N. Compton, J. T. Sherrill, G. S. Ginsburg, M. A. Rynn, J. McCracken, and B. Waslick. 2008. Cognitive behavioral therapy, sertraline, or a combination in childhood anxiety. *New England Journal of Medicine* 359(26):2753-2766.

Walkup, J. T., A. Barlow, B. C. Mullany, W. Pan, N. Goklish, R. Hasting, B. Cowboy, P. Fields, E. V. Baker, K. Speakman, G. Ginsburg, and R. Reid. 2009. Randomized controlled trial of a paraprofessional-delivered in-home intervention for young reservation-based American Indian mothers. *Journal of the American Academy of Child & Adolescent Psychiatry* 48(6):591-601.

Wandersman, A., J. Duffy, P. Flaspohler, R. Noonan, K. Lubell, L. Stillman, M. Blachman, and J. Saul. 2008. Bridging the gap between prevention research and practice: The interactive systems framework for dissemination and implementation. *American Journal of Community Psychology* 41(3-4):171-181.

Weaver, H. N. 2004. The elements of cultural competence: Applications with native American clients. *Journal of Ethnic and Cultural Diversity in Social Work* 13(1):19-35.

Webster-Stratton, C., J. Rinaldi, and J. M. Reid. 2011a. Long-term outcomes of incredible years parenting program: Predictors of adolescent adjustment. *Child and Adolescent Mental Health* 16(1):38-46.

Webster-Stratton, C., W. M. Reinke, K. C. Herman, and L. L. Newcomer. 2011b. The incredible years teacher classroom management training: The methods and principles that support fidelity of training delivery. *School Psychology Review* 40(4):509-529.

Weinberg, L. A., A. Zetlin, and N. M. Shea. 2009. Removing barriers to educating children in foster care through interagency collaboration: A seven county multiple-case study. *Child Welfare* 88(4):77-111.

Welsh, B., C. Sullivan, and D. Olds. 2010. When early crime prevention goes to scale: A new look at the evidence. *Prevention Science* 11(2):115-125.

Wolf, M. M., C. J. Braukmann, and K. A. Ramp. 1987. Serious delinquent behavior as part of a significantly handicapping condition: Cures and supportive environments. *Journal of Applied Behavior Analysis* 20(4):347-359.

Wolfe, D. A., B. Edwards, I. Manion, and C. Koverola. 1988. Early intervention for parents at risk of child abuse and neglect: A preliminary investigation. *Journal of Consulting and Clinical Psychology* 56(1):40-47.

Woltmann, E., R. Whitley, G. McHugo, M. Brunette, W. Torrey, L. Coots, D. Lynde, and R. Drake. 2008. The role of staff turnover in the implementation of evidence-based practices in mental health care. *Psychiatric Services* 59(7):732-737.

Workgroup on Adapting Latino Services. 2008. *Adaptation guidelines for serving Latino children and families affected by trauma (1st ed.).* San Diego, CA: Chadwick Center for Children and Families. http://www.chadwickcenter.org/WALS/wals.htm (accessed November 26, 2013).

Wulczyn, F. 2009. Epidemiological perspectives on maltreatment prevention. *The Future of Children* 19(2):39-66.

Wulczyn, F., D. Daro, J. Fluke, S. Feldman, C. Glodek, and K. Lifanda. 2010. *Adapting a systems approach to child protection: Key concepts and considerations.* New York: United Nations Children's Fund.

Yates, B. T. 2009. Cost-inclusive evaluation: A banquet of approaches for including costs, benefits, and cost-effectiveness and cost–benefit analyses in your next evaluation. *Evaluation and Program Planning* 32(1):52-54.

Zigler, E., J. Pfannenstiel, and V. Seitz. 2008. The Parents as Teachers Program and school success: A replication and extension. *Journal of Primary Prevention* 29(2):103-120.

Zimmerman, F., and J. A. Mercy. 2010. *A better start: Child maltreatment prevention as a public health priority.* Washington, DC: Zero To Three: National Center for Infants, Toddlers, and Families.

7

Research Challenges and Infrastructure

To be productive, high-quality scientific research requires a sophisticated infrastructure. This is especially true for research in which multiple fields, disciplines, methodologies, and levels of analysis are required to fully address key questions. Research on child abuse and neglect is especially complex, involving diverse independent service systems, multiple professions, ethical issues that are particularly complicated, and levels of outcome analysis ranging from the individual child to national statistics. Coordinating these multiple layers and systems requires a cohesive response from the federal government, private foundations, and academic institutions. All of these entities work together to build a research enterprise that can address the preventable problems of child abuse and neglect, making it possible to better understand, intervene in, and evaluate the pathways from causes to consequences and improve children's lives. This chapter describes the current landscape of research on child abuse and neglect, highlights the multiple challenges encountered in conducting such research, and considers opportunities for increasing and improving this research as a coordinated field. The final section presents conclusions.

COMPONENTS OF THE CHILD ABUSE AND NEGLECT RESEARCH INFRASTRUCTURE

Several components must be in place if a research infrastructure that is both effective in the short term and sustainable over time is to be built. Box 7-1 lists the human and physical capital components of a scientific research infrastructure. Building the research infrastructure needed to sup-

---

BOX 7-1
Basic Infrastructure Requirements for
Research on Child Abuse and Neglect

Human Capital
- Workforce
  - Professionals
  - Support staff
- Training and mentoring
  - Funded researchers
  - Training funds
  - Competent mentors
- Access to specialty consultation
- Larger research community
  - Colleagues
  - Robust partnerships with agency-based and community collaborators
  - Representation in study sections and journal reviews
  - General consensus on methodology, priorities, and key problems
  - Results valued by policy makers and funders

Physical Capital
- Space
  - Clinical
  - Office
  - Administrative and support staff
  - Research
- Basic instrumentation
- Information technology

Management and Capacity
- Data management
- Access to specialized instruments and services
- Patient/participant recruitment and flow
- Grant management and regulatory compliance
- Capacity in service sectors working with children and families who experience child abuse and neglect to engage in and use research

---

port and sustain a field of child abuse and neglect that can inform practices, programs, and policies requires a coordinated, comprehensive approach. The infrastructure should be designed to (1) incorporate multidisciplinary and multimethod perspectives in research design; (2) initiate research focused on determining the role of cultural factors; (3) incorporate additional longitudinal data, improved surveillance mechanisms, and registries; (4) coordinate the allocation of sufficient research funding; and (5) develop a robust workforce through training and mentorship. Each of these elements is examined in turn in this section.

Multidisciplinary and Multimethod Perspectives

Child abuse and neglect research encompasses a wide range of disciplines and research problems. Figure 7-1 depicts 11 of the most salient domains identified by the committee: mental health, physical health, implementation science, child development, policy research, neurobiology, court interventions, child welfare, public health, forensic sciences, and ethical issues. Under each domain are examples of the types of problems, missions, and tasks addressed by investigators, as well as key disciplines that may be engaged in this research. Each of these domains has unique research infrastructure needs, methodologies, and agendas. This list is not comprehensive, but provides a general overview of the breadth of disciplinary involvement in child abuse and neglect research. Selected domains are discussed below.

These domains, as well as many others that relate to the study of child abuse and neglect, have specific focuses with respect to the causes and consequences of child abuse and neglect, as well as the delivery of services to prevent or treat its effects. However, the topics of interest specific to each research domain do not exist in isolation from the others. Integrating multidisciplinary perspectives into research across these domains can allow researchers to examine the many contextual factors surrounding incidents of abuse and neglect, to disentangle its consequences from the many co-occurring risk factors, to examine the many outcomes of interest from the implementation of programs and services, and to understand the interactions among services from the many providers that encounter abused and neglected children.

Physical Health

Published medical research on child abuse and neglect has addressed its epidemiology; its clinical manifestations and presentation, diagnosis, treatment, and outcomes; issues related to the medical care needs of foster children; and prevention. The clinical manifestations and nature of the histories presented have been published for many forms of child abuse according to discrete sets of conditions (e.g., abusive head trauma, physical abuse, sexual abuse). Attention has been paid to improving diagnoses and avoiding false-positive diagnoses, as well as improving assessments of both future risk and safety. Epidemiological data have been accumulating. One area of great interest is screening in medical practice, given that this is the first line of defense in many cases.

Screening in medical practice is the process of looking for occult condi-

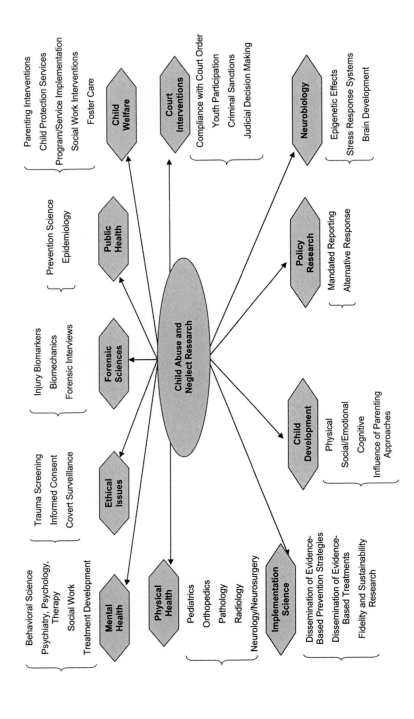

FIGURE 7-1 Child abuse and neglect research domains.

tions before they become manifest (Fletcher et al., 2005). The principles of screening include having a screening test that is acceptable with appropriate sensitivity and specificity, seeking an important condition, having effective interventions available, and seeing a better outcome if the condition is identified early rather than late (Fletcher et al., 2005). In 2004, the U.S. Preventive Services Task Force (USPSTF) considered whether the evidence supported recommending that physicians screen for child abuse and neglect in medical practice. The task force concluded: "We identified no studies meeting eligibility criteria that directly addressed the effectiveness of screening in a health care setting in reducing harm and premature death and disability, or the adverse effects of screening and interventions" (Nelson et al., 2004, p. 29). In January 2013, the USPSTF released a new systematic review addressing the same question (Selph et al., 2013). Although this review still does not offer strong support for screening, it is somewhat more supportive based on the impact of multiple home visiting trials (Duggan et al., 2004; Kitzman et al., 1997; Olds et al., 1986, 2007) and a single study of screening in pediatric primary care (Dubowitz et al., 2009). The task force states: "In conclusion, trials of risk assessment and behavioral interventions and counseling in pediatric clinics and early childhood home visitation programs indicated reduced abuse and neglect outcomes for children, although all trials had limitations and trials of home visitation reported inconsistent results.... More research is needed in key areas to provide clinicians with effective methods of [identifying children at risk for abuse and neglect]" (Selph et al., 2013, p. 188). Thus the USPSTF has called for more research on screening for child abuse and neglect in medical practices. New work is needed to document the process of screening (including asking parents or children directly), the proportion of children that receive the intervention and the proportion of refusals to participate, the beneficial impact for children or parents, and any adverse impacts.

Research on using the medical examination to detect abuse or neglect shows mixed results. For example, complete skeletal surveys have been recommended as an adjunct for assessing young injured children for physical abuse; however, there are gaps in knowledge about when, with whom, and how often X-rays should be obtained, aside from issues of the accuracy of readings or the appropriate technology for imaging. Rib fractures and multiple fractures are known to be associated with abuse more commonly than other fractures in young children (Kemp et al., 2008), but questions remain about when a diagnosis of abuse should be considered and X-rays ordered in potentially related conditions such as acute life-threatening events, seizures, burns, and abusive head injury. Unanswered questions include: What are the clinical indications for performing a radiographic skeletal survey?, What are the yields of X-rays in different populations of children?, and What is the utility of follow-up X-rays where data suggest improved sensitivity and specificity at the expense of increased radiation and monetary costs? Research is needed to ascertain the most sensitive, specific, and cost-effective methods for identifying skeletal injuries, with consideration of the hazards of increased radiation exposure. Comparative studies of findings across clinical centers using standardized reporting could improve understanding of fracture mechanics and identification of abusive versus accidental injuries.

With respect to sexual abuse, prior research has led the American Academy of Pediatrics (AAP) to publish interpretations of the relationship between some sexually transmitted infections and the likelihood of such abuse (Kellogg, 2005). However, many questions remain, such as: What is the specificity of ano-genital warts for a sexual abuse diagnosis in children?, How is this altered by the age and gender of the child, site of the lesions, or human papillomavirus type?, What is the natural history of this infection with vertical transmission or increasing age of the child?, What sensitivity and specificity do nucleic acid amplification tests have in detecting infection for the range of potential sexually transmitted infections?, Which diagnostic tests for sexually transmitted infections should be used for which parts of the body and at what time?, and What are the appropriate clinical indications for these tests?

Abusive head trauma was first described as shaken baby syndrome more than 40 years ago, yet intense public and legal controversy over this diagnosis persists. Several challenges are associated with the diagnosis. First, perhaps, is terminology and what is or is not included in this diagnosis category. As absolute certainty is rare with abusive head trauma cases, and a probabilistic or Bayesian approach to the diagnosis is consistent with this uncertainty. Another controversy in studies of abusive head trauma has to do with the relationship between hypoxia in isolation and subdural hemorrhage in infants. A clear characterization of the sensitivity and specificity of subdural hemorrhage, subarachnoid hemorrhage, and cervical epidural hemorrhage as markers for both neurotrauma and hypoxia/ischemia is lacking. The phenomena of scar retraction and spontaneous rebleed have been suggested as a challenge to determining the time of injury. Systematic study of subdural membranes and neuropathology related to rebleeds is needed to settle this controversy. Another area of controversy needing explication is the significance and location of beta amyloid precursor protein (APP) in the brain as a marker of trauma, hypoxia-ischemia, or infarction. Eye injuries, specifically retinal hemorrhages, have been interpreted as evidence of abusive head trauma by some and disputed by others.

Policy Research

As discussed in Chapter 8, there have been numerous changes to federal and state laws and policies designed to impact the incidence, reporting, and negative health and economic consequences of child abuse and neglect since the 1993 National Research Council (NRC) report was issued. In addition, states vary widely in policies regarding mandated reporters; definitions of abuse and neglect; inclusion of witnessing intimate partner violence; and expansions of what is included in the laws, the range of penalties, and stipulations of such things as shaken baby prevention in the nursery. However, research examining the impact of policy changes and variations across state laws on outcomes for children and families, as well the systems responsible for implementing the policies, has been scant. Despite an increased federal focus on implementing evidence-based policies, support has been lacking for research efforts to evaluate policies related to child abuse and neglect.

Child Welfare

A number of new research opportunities are emerging in the child welfare field. Large administrative datasets now available can be analyzed to inform practice, as well as case-linked to other electronic records to permit multidimensional and longitudinal evaluations of outcomes. Child welfare providers and funders increasingly are required to employ evidence-based practices and thus are active consumers of research, as described in Chapter 6. Areas of research, including in many instances testing of interventions, include addressing child neglect, parent engagement, infant mental health, community-based prevention and parenting education, addressing trauma and meeting the mental health needs of children who experience abuse and neglect, risk and safety assessment, decision making, the impact of substance abuse on child abuse and neglect, links between child abuse and neglect prevention and economic well-being, achieving permanency through guardianship, reducing long-term foster care, and accountability and performance-based contracting. The social work profession provides a large part of this research community, and successful collaborations between child welfare agencies and universities offer a range of examples of how to create productive research partnerships.

Funding for research evaluating child welfare programs is potentially available through many discretionary programs advanced through the multiple initiatives and priorities of the Children's Bureau and its Office on Child Abuse and Neglect. Other potential funding sources are the Centers for Disease Control and Prevention (CDC); the National Institutes of Health (NIH); the Department of Justice; and several foundations, including the Doris Duke Charitable Foundation and the William T. Grant

Foundation. Since the 1993 NRC report was issued, the Children's Bureau has strengthened the rigor of the required evaluations. In addition, federal legislation—for example, Title IV-E waivers for demonstration projects—has required rigorous evaluation, and many demonstrations have included randomized designs. As noted in Chapter 5, however, the 2011 waiver authority stipulates that the review of applications for Title IV-E waivers for fiscal years (FYs) 2012-2014 cannot consider whether the applicants will use an experimental design, reducing the impetus for the use of random assignment in Title IV-E waiver demonstrations (Testa, 2012).

Moreover, although there have been recent federal investments such as funding for training under Titles IV-E and IV-B, there have been no commensurate investments in child welfare research capacity. In fact, the small discretionary research program of the Children's Bureau, which also included some funding for doctoral students, was terminated in 1996, when the funds were used to launch the National Study of Child and Adolescent Well-Being as part of the Personal Responsibility and Workforce Investment Act. Unless potential investigators seeking support for field-initiated research approach NIH or CDC, there will be no national funding source for such research or for training for child welfare researchers. Given the few child welfare researchers being supported by these latter organizations, the number of mentors or reviewers for such research is limited, and there is little experience in the field with these funding sources.

Public Health

Child abuse and neglect is now recognized as a major public health problem by the World Health Organization and CDC (CDC, 2010, 2012a; Fang et al., 2012; Putnam-Hornstein et al., 2011; WHO, 2013). Research such as the seminal Adverse Childhood Experiences studies of Felitti and colleagues demonstrates the significant associations between childhood adversities and chronic medical conditions such as heart disease, diabetes, cancer, and obesity, as well as HIV risk (Anda et al., 1999, 2007; Chapman et al., 2004; Dong et al., 2003; Dube et al., 2001, 2003a,b; Felitti et al., 1998).

The classic public health approach is often conceptualized as a four-step process (Putnam-Hornstein et al., 2011). The first step is the implementation of a good surveillance system to collect and analyze data with which to detect and describe the condition, thereby informing the planning and implementation of public health interventions. The second step is the identification of risk and protective factors. The third is the development and testing of interventions focused on the identified risk and protective factors. The fourth and final step is the implementation of effective prevention and control strategies. Steps three and four require an ongoing surveillance infrastructure to evaluate the effectiveness of interventions and prevention strategies.

Suggestions for improving surveillance of child abuse and neglect include using data from multiple independent sources, linking cases across different databases, and enforcing the standard case definitions (Medina et al., 2012).[1] Pilot efforts entailing each of these strategies have yielded improvements in surveillance (Medina et al., 2012; Putnam-Hornstein et al., 2011; Schnitzer et al., 2004). Because abused and neglected children come in contact with multiple systems (e.g., health care, social services, education, law enforcement, and child death reviews), aggregating data across multiple independent sources can improve the identification of cases not referred to child welfare agencies. Linking case-based data from two or more datasets has proven especially informative about risk factors. In California, linking birth certificate data with child protection records for more than 2 million children aged 5 and younger enabled the identification of variables associated with high rates of child abuse and neglect (Putnam-Hornstein et al., 2011). The study found, for example, that 1 of every 3 children born without established paternity were reported to child protective services for abuse and neglect; about 1 in 10 children born to teenage mothers were victims of abuse and neglect.

Case-linkage studies are proving important for the early identification of groups that are at highest risk and therefore most likely to benefit from public health interventions. Case-linkage methodology requires quality datasets and sophisticated data management expertise to merge information reliably. Open-source software (e.g., Link Plus, developed by CDC) is increasingly available, as are standards for evaluating the probability of case matching. For research purposes, there are methodological and practical advantages to linking administrative data across systems. As noted by Jonson-Reid and Drake (2008), such linkage mitigates the underreporting biases found when single-agency data sources are used to understand immediate and longer-term outcomes. Analysis of administrative data in conjunction with survey data offsets the limitations of retrospective accounts of victimization based on respondent recall (Brown et al., 1998; Widom et al., 2004) and the use of resource-intensive, prospective in-person sampling methods (Dubowitz et al., 2006). For the field of child maltreatment, such analysis allows for greater research, practice, and policy synthesis (Drake and Jonson-Reid, 1999) and the examination of risk factors, recurrence or

---

[1]The term surveillance is used here in the public health sense to refer to a systematic assessment of the extent and nature of the child abuse and neglect problem by counting children or cases in a way that makes it possible to know the rates of occurrence; assess trends in types of abuse or neglect; and understand relationships to other important variables, such as single parenthood, special populations, and child gender and age.

recidivism, and prevention and intervention outcomes (Jonson-Reid and Drake, 2008; Medina et al., 2012). Children and families presenting with comorbid problems are involved with multiple systems, including the medical, child welfare, early childhood, juvenile justice, legal and judicial, and public health systems, as well as community-based services. While emphasis has increased on coordination across child protection and local service delivery environments (e.g., one-stop approaches, systems of care, interoperability[2]) and on the use of data-driven decision making, the case record of a child's or family's contact, referral, and service receipt over time is often distributed across administrative datasets housed in different institutional settings (Jonson-Reid and Drake, 2008).

Although most child abuse and neglect agencies lack the in-house expertise to benefit from using multiple data sources or case linking across datasets, efforts are being made to build this capacity. In response to this need, for example, Chapin Hall at the University of Chicago instituted Administrative Data Institutes for child welfare managers in the early 1990s. To foster the integration of research with policy and practice, Chapin Hall has since 2007 offered annual sessions in Advanced Analytics for Child Welfare Administration, which focus on using longitudinal administrative data in child welfare decision making, program planning, and outcome monitoring (Chapin Hall, 2012). A timely, sensitive, and reliable surveillance system also is necessary to determine the effectiveness of child abuse and neglect prevention programs. A coordinated national public health approach to child abuse and neglect will not be possible without a modern, general population-based, epidemiological surveillance system. The enormous costs and lifelong consequences of child abuse and neglect call for investment in a surveillance infrastructure commensurate with the magnitude of the problem.

Ethical Issues

Abused and neglected children and adolescents are a vulnerable population (MacMillan et al., 2007). As a result, ethical issues raised by proposed research in the field receive intensive scrutiny from study sections and institutional review boards. Questions often raised include: (1) Who is authorized to provide informed consent when children are wards of child protection?; (2) Under what circumstances can adolescents provide

---

[2]Findings from the pilot Information Portability Project indicate that the use of mobile technologies and the sharing of information across child- and family-serving systems facilitates access to information in real time, making it possible to monitor safety and well-being, coordinate service delivery, promote data-informed decision making, and reduce service duplication (Schilling-Wolfe, 2010).

informed consent?; (3) Is it harmful to ask subjects about possible abuse and neglect experiences, and at what age is this permissible?; (4) How does mandated reporting affect research confidentiality?; (5) Are researchers required to provide treatment or services when they uncover abuse and neglect?; (6) What inducements to participate in research are appropriate and not coercive for children or families involved in child protection investigations?; and (7) What are ethical approaches to tracking subjects involved in longitudinal studies? (MacMillan et al., 2007). Box 7-2 presents an example of difficulties faced by child abuse and neglect researchers as a result of ethical concerns of institutional review boards.

The Role of Cultural Factors

There is a continuing need to understand the complex role of culture and context in the causes, consequences, prevention, and treatment of child abuse and neglect (Feiring and Zielinski, 2011), particularly in light of the increasing heterogeneity of U.S. families (IOM and NRC, 2011). Viewing culture as shared and dynamic (Korbin, 2002), focused on the learning and transmission of behavior and activity and the expression of internalized norms and models (Rogoff, 2003; Weisner, 2002), provides a lens for the examination of risk and protective factors for child abuse and neglect within families, neighborhoods, and communities. Examples of cultural factors relevant to child abuse and neglect and child well-being that have been examined across research disciplines include child-rearing practices (Earle and Cross, 2001; Ferrari, 2002; Waters and Sykes, 2009), fathers' parenting behaviors (Ferrari, 2002), adultification of young children (Burton, 2007), child care burdens (Roditti, 2005), perceptions of neglect (Evans-Campbell, 2008), sibling caretaking and self-care among children of immigrants (Greene et al., 2011; Hafford, 2010), expressions of familism[3] and the role of extended families in systems of parental authority and disciplinary practices (Fontes, 2002; Fuhua and Qin, 2009), and family cohesion and mutual aid (Fuhua and Qin, 2009). Context, place, and structural factors, including poverty and historical trauma, also interact with culture and family dynamics (Coulton et al., 2007; DeBruyn et al., 2001).

Understanding cultural factors related to risk and protective factors for child abuse and neglect or the effectiveness of interventions requires the complementary use of qualitative and quantitative research methodologies (Korbin and Spilsbury, 1999). Understanding the interplay of micro- and macro-level processes and establishing the evidence base also entails the use of methods and approaches that are culturally sensitive and responsive to

---

[3]Attitudes, behaviors, and family structures operating within an extended family system (Germán et al., 2009).

BOX 7-2
Challenges of Institutional Review Board Review
for Research on Child Abuse and Neglect

The Yale Department of Psychiatry's Child and Adolescent Research and Education (CARE) program had a long-standing research collaboration with the State of Connecticut's Department of Child and Families (DCF), which included evaluating the DCF SAFE Homes intervention for children temporarily placed in state-run facilities (DeSena et al., 2005) and examining genetic and environmental factors associated with risk and resiliency (e.g., Kaufman et al., 2004, 2006). The CARE program also has been at the forefront of research on the epigenetic effects of child abuse and neglect (Yang et al., 2013). Both the Yale University Human Investigations Committee and the DCF Institutional Review Board (IRB) approved all research involving DCF children. The children's legal guardians provided written consent for participation in the study, and all children provided written assent; when available (96 percent of the time), birth parents also provided written assent. Children were assessed and saliva was collected for DNA extraction during the week the children participated in a free day camp. Demographically matched comparison subjects were recruited through targeted mailings and newspaper advertisements.

In 2006, Yale received a National Institute of Mental Health (NIMH) grant (R01 MH077087) to study genetic and environmental modifiers of child depression. In August 2006, leadership of the DCF IRB changed, and further recruitment of DCF youth for the pending R01-funded study was denied. In addition, previously collected DNA could no longer be analyzed. Multiple efforts were made to resolve the DCF IRB's concerns, which focused on the possibility that because of the high percentage of minority children in DCF custody, any genetic findings could be interpreted as stigmatizing.

---

diverse populations that are vulnerable, hidden, and underresearched and whose experience of maltreatment is not well understood or adequately addressed. Examples of these populations include American Indian and Alaska Native children and families (Cross, 2012); Latino children and families; children with disabilities; children of immigrants; lesbian, gay, bisexual, and transgender (LGBT) youth (D'Augelli, 2012); and military families (Heyman and Slep, 2012). Such methods and approaches are illustrated by the use of ethnography in studies seeking to understand social capital and neighbors' supports for parenting (Korbin et al., 1998); how parental undocumented status affects the developmental contexts and early learning of children of immigrants (Yoshikawa, 2011); and the dynamics of complex, minority families (Burton, 2007). Illustrative as well are the use of participatory, inclusive research to study sensitive issues related to at-risk

Despite letters from the director of NIMH and others, the DCF IRB continued to deny permission to recruit new subjects or to allow previously collected DNA to be analyzed. An effort to relocate the study to New York State failed after passing the first four of five levels of review. As was the case in Connecticut, the New York State Office of Children and Family Services ultimately denied approval of the study, citing, in part, "the lack of racial diversity in the sample of foster children ... as it appears to single out a group of children who will in all probability be made up almost exclusively of children of color."

In February 2011, NIMH requested that Yale return the R01 funds as the proposed study could not be conducted. In June 2011, just days before the grant was to be revoked, the DCF IRB, under new leadership, gave permission for the stored DNA samples to be analyzed. Among the results was a finding of significant differences between abused and neglected and comparison children in methylation of CpG sites ($p < 5.0 \times 10^{-7}$) in genes that have been implicated in neuropsychiatric diseases, cardiovascular disease, obesity, and cancer (Yang et al., 2013). Although further replication is required, these findings suggest that the increased risk for lung, colorectal, prostatic, breast, colon, and ovarian neoplasms in individuals with a child abuse and neglect history may reflect preventable or reversible epigenetic effects in addition to the known contributions of the high rates of health risk behaviors, such as smoking and drug and alcohol abuse, highly associated with childhood abuse and adversity.

Investigators working with children who are in state custody generally must satisfy multiple levels of human subjects and policy review beyond that of their IRB. In some instances, even when the risk of harm is minimal, political and social concerns may block scientific investigations, denying these high-risk children the benefits that routinely accrue for children with other conditions and disorders as a result of their participation in state-of-the-art medical and psychiatric research.

American Indian and Alaska Native populations (The National Congress of American Indians, 2009; Sahota, 2010); the use of community-based participatory research to develop intervention strategies (Baum et al., 2013) and examine the effectiveness of culturally validated practices (Cross et al., 2011); and the translation of research findings into culturally competent strategies for prevention, intervention, and service delivery (Sahota, 2010).

The importance of a focus on culture goes beyond understanding the causes and consequences of child abuse and neglect and involvement with child protective services or other social service systems. Culture matters in developing and testing the effectiveness of prevention and intervention strategies and replicating and adapting evidence-based practices for distinct populations or groups to ensure cultural fit, reach, efficacy, and adoption (Barrera et al., 2011), as well as the social validity and practical application of an intervention (Lau, 2006). Examples of areas in which more work is needed on the development of interventions for vulnerable populations include the following topics, which were raised at a public workshop held by this committee in December 2012: suicide prevention among LGBT youth, stress and adaptation among families with LGBT youth (D'Augelli, 2005), and stressors within military families due to multiple deployments (IOM and NRC, 2012).

Illustrative of a cultural focus in the development of interventions are recent adaptations of evidence-based psychosocial treatments targeting Latino children and adolescents (Silverman et al., 2008). Culturally modified trauma-focused treatment, for example, is a cultural adaptation of trauma-focused cognitive-behavioral therapy (see Chapter 6) (Rivera and Arellano, 2008), used with Latino children aged 4-18 who have experienced sexual or physical abuse. Incorporated throughout are treatment modules that integrate cultural concepts such as familismo, personalismo, respeto, sympatia, and fatalismo, as well as spirituality and folk beliefs.

One understudied population is children with disabilities (see Chapter 3). Knowledge is lacking about the prevalence of these children in the child welfare system, as well as the prevalence of children who have parents with disabilities, including how they are served and what prevention strategies are effective for their families (Lightfoot and LaLiberte, 2006; National Council on Disability, 2012). There are barriers to research on this population. As identified by AAP, they include the lack of a universal definition of what constitutes a disability; the lack of correspondence between legal definitions and clinical data; and inconsistent identification, assessment, and documentation of children who enter the child protection system (Bonner et al., 1997; Hibbard et al., 2007).

More research has been conducted on the victimization and abuse and neglect of the heterogenous LGBT population (IOM, 2011), including American Indian youth who may self-identify as LGBT or two-spirit (Anguksuar et al., 1997; Balsam et al., 2004; Saewyc et al., 2006; Walters et al., 2001). Greater demographic diversity of study samples, including youth who are under age 18 and sampling in urban and rural settings, is needed to detect subgroup differences (Elze, 2009). LGBT youth need to be recruited to participate in small-scale, qualitative research studies so that more can be learned about their abuse and neglect experiences, the consequences of their victimization, and their service needs and outcomes (Elze, 2009).[4] Incorporating questions about sexual identity and same-

---

[4]Topics to address include (1) demographic characteristics (race/ethnicity, sexual orientation, gender identity, socioeconomic status, education, geographic location); (2) family and interpersonal relations (including acceptance or rejection); (3) social supports (family, friends, peers); (4) needs and unmet needs; (5) the coming-out process; (6) experiences of stigma and

gender attraction and sexual behaviors in population-based surveys would increase the representation of LGBT youth (Elze, 2009; IOM, 2011) and limit reliance on convenience samples. Information on transgender youth (Grossman and D'Augelli, 2006, 2007) is particularly limited. Further guidance is needed on the incorporation of at-risk protocols into research studies and human subject protections (e.g., waivers of parental consent for minors who may be subject to exposure or risk of harm) (Grossman and D'Augelli, 2007).

Longitudinal Studies, Surveillance, and Registries

In addition to a compilation of state child abuse and neglect reports issued annually by the federal government (the Child Welfare Information Gateway), four National Incidence Studies (NISs) (Sedlak, 1988; Sedlak et al., 1997, 2010) have been conducted at about 10-year intervals, as well as surveys of parents or children (e.g., Straus et al., 1998), studies of trends in admission of children to hospitals and to intensive care units (e.g., Leventhal et al., 1997), and a population-based comparison of clinical and outcome characteristics of young children with serious inflicted and non-inflicted traumatic brain injury. As a result of this work, the demographics and trends of child abuse and neglect have become clearer. Nonetheless, as highlighted in the preceding chapters, more comprehensive and accurate data are needed to enable a better understanding of the incidence of and circumstances surrounding child abuse and neglect. The following sections examine longitudinal studies, more comprehensive surveillance systems, and registries as possible means to fill this data gap.

Longitudinal Studies

Longitudinal studies are essential for identifying causal pathways between abuse- and neglect-related biological changes and later adult outcomes (Trickett et al., 2011). Such studies are complicated and expensive in terms of both time and money, and require the dedication of stable research teams over long periods. Subjects must be tracked between measurement time points—often years apart—and periodically reengaged or reconsented to enhance sample retention. Longitudinal studies of developmental psychopathology also must grapple with validly issues in the

---

discrimination (including economic discrimination); (7) violence (sexual abuse, child abuse, intimate partner violence) and anti-LGBT victimization; (8) risk behaviors; (9) help-seeking behaviors and professional support; (10) barriers to access to human services; (11) interactions with service providers (cultural competency); (12) identification of services needed; and (13) ways to be better served.

measurement of central constructs such as depression, anxiety, and post-traumatic stress disorder across multiple developmental epochs associated with enormous cognitive and behavioral change. The few longitudinal studies that have been conducted—Longitudinal Studies of Child Abuse and Neglect (LONGSCAN) (Runyan et al., 1998), the Christchurch Health and Development Study (Trickett et al., 2011; Widom et al., 2004), and the Dunedin Multidisciplinary Health and Development Study—have yielded an extraordinarily rich perspective on the developmental progression of negative long-term outcomes associated with childhood abuse and neglect (MacMillan et al., 2007). Much of the accumulating knowledge base on the psychosocial consequences of child abuse and neglect (discussed in Chapter 4) derives from such longitudinal studies, along with continued hypothesis testing and secondary analyses of an increasing number of archived research studies in child abuse and case-level National Child Abuse and Neglect Data System (NCANDS) data.

The National Study of Child and Adolescent Well-Being (NSCAW) was conducted under a provision of the Personal Responsibility and Work Opportunity Act of 1996 that directed the Secretary of the Department of Health and Human Services (HHS) to conduct a national study of children at risk of abuse or neglect or in the child welfare system. The study was to include a longitudinal component that followed cases over the course of several years, and gather data on the types of abuse or neglect involved and the contacts and services provided by the child welfare agency, including out-of-home placement. The intent was to provide reliable state-level data for as many states as feasible regarding the characteristics of children and families served by the child welfare system, as well as system-level factors. The two rounds of the study over the past 15 years have yielded data whose analysis is making important contributions to enhancement of the delivery of child welfare services and their outcomes (see, for example, Casanueva, 2012a,b). It should be noted that the second round of the NSCAW has been truncated to 3 years without additional funding to follow this cohort further.

Surveillance Systems

Numerous limitations characterize the current child abuse and ne-glect surveillance system, which relies primarily on NCANDS data, supple-mented sporadically by the NIS. Critics note that NCANDS captures only children reported to child welfare agencies (Medina et al., 2012), who are believed to represent a minority of total abuse and neglect cases. Moreover, states submit data voluntarily to NCANDS, and their standards and case definitions vary greatly, preventing meaningful comparison across jurisdic-tions (GAO, 2008). The lack of definitional uniformity, compounded by local changes in case coding, makes it difficult to investigate geographic and chronological trends. NCANDS reports also have traditionally lagged about 2 years behind real time, preventing their use in public health responses to acute changes in rates. Furthermore, NCANDS does not collect data on many relevant risk factors, a primary function of a modern public health surveillance system. A recent study by the General Accounting Office estimates that about 50 percent of child abuse and neglect fatalities are missed by NCANDS (GAO, 2011).

Registries

Evidence-based classification schemes have brought conceptual and practical coherence to the maturing and interdisciplinary field of prevention research and the implementation of sound prevention strategies (Puddy and Wilkins, 2011). In the past decade, federal agencies have established a number of registries and clearinghouses with a focus on prevention of child abuse and neglect. Examples include the National Crime Victims Research and Treatment Center (Saunders et al., 2004) and the National Registry of Evidence-Based Programs and Practices (SAMHSA, 2013). University-based and other institutional efforts include the Chadwick Center for Children and Families; the California Evidence-Based Clearinghouse; and the Promising Practices Network for Children, Families, and Communities.

These registries serve to generate knowledge and advance the field; they are an important development in the infrastructure for prevention research and a valuable resource for the implementation of evidence-based models and strategies. Yet their varied institutional homes underscore the fragmentation of prevention research across federal agencies and the lack of a unified federal policy and research agenda. Universities and social science research organizations have attempted to unify the evidence base in child abuse and neglect and prevention research.

Research Funding

A wide array of federal agencies have provided funding for child abuse and neglect research through various legislative initiatives. Major funding sources include but are not limited to the Child Abuse Prevention and Treatment Act (CAPTA); CDC; NIH; the Administration on Children, Youth and Families (ACYF) within HHS; the Agency for Healthcare Research and Quality (AHRQ); and the Title IV-E waiver demonstration program. As noted earlier, several private foundations also provide support for child abuse and neglect research.

Child Abuse Prevention and Treatment Act

CAPTA was originally enacted in 1974 and was most recently amended and authorized on December 20, 2010 (P.L. 111-320). The act provides funding to states to support prevention, assessment, investigation, prosecution, and treatment for child abuse. It also supports grants for demonstration programs and projects to public agencies, tribal organizations, and nonprofits.

CAPTA requires that every 2 years, the Children's Bureau within ACYF issue for public comment a set of priorities for research topics to be covered in grants and contracts. On February 3, 2006, the Children's Bureau published in the *Federal Register* "Children's Bureau Proposed Research Priorities for Fiscal Year 2006-2008."[5] Despite this extensive published research agenda, limited funding—no more than $27 million for the entire CAPTA discretionary grant program in 2008—has precluded a full examination of most of these topics through CAPTA or other Children's Bureau research funding streams (IASWR, 2008). Some field-initiated research is funded through CAPTA; however, the funding announcements are often prescriptive as to the use of these funds. In 2003, for example, the Children's Bureau requested applications for replication of an evidence-based program, Family Connections (developed by DePanfilis and colleagues at the University of Maryland); the funding was used to support dissertation and other research through quality improvement centers and implementation grants.

Centers for Disease Control and Prevention

CDC established the National Center for Injury Prevention and Control (NCIPC) 20 years ago. This center is the nation's authority for prevention of violence and injury. It provides funding and technical assistance to 20 state health departments to strengthen capacity in injury prevention. Child abuse and neglect is one of NCIPC's priority areas, although funding for child abuse and neglect activities has been limited—a total of 25 grant awards or cooperative agreements for research projects in child abuse prevention since 2002. In FY 2011, the latest year shown on the NCIPC website, no new awards were made in the area of child abuse. In addition, several CDC-funded injury prevention centers, such as the Center for Violence and Injury Prevention at Washington University's Brown School of Social Work, target child abuse and neglect.

In 2001, CDC convened 15 abuse and neglect experts to establish

---

[5]71 FR 11427 Children's Bureau Proposed Research Priorities for Fiscal Years 2006-2008 (http://www.gpo.gov/fdsys/granule/FR-2006-03-07/06-2154/content-detail.html [accessed January 27, 2014]).

priorities related to surveillance (data collection, uniform definitions), etiological and risk factors, intervention and evaluation, and implementation and dissemination. The NCIPC research agenda was updated in 2009, with a plan to extend it through 2018. According to the updated agenda: "The mission of CDC's child maltreatment prevention program is to prevent maltreatment and its consequences through surveillance, research and development, capacity building, communication, and leadership. In pursuit of this mission, CDC's public health approach complements such other approaches as those of the criminal justice and mental health systems. In particular, CDC's approach emphasizes primary prevention of perpetration of child maltreatment or efforts that focus on preventing maltreatment before it occurs" (CDC, 2009, p. 75).

The foundation of CDC's child abuse and neglect prevention work is the promotion of safe, stable nurturing relationships (CDC, 2010). The agenda highlights the synergistic effects such relationships can have on health problems across the life span. These relationships also contribute to the development of skills that enhance the acquisition of healthy habits and lifestyles. CDC recognizes that to promote such relationships and reduce abuse and neglect, additional research is needed across the different social contexts in which children develop and interact, including the individual, the family, peers, the community, and society. The agenda draws on the Institute of Medicine (IOM) report *Reducing the Burden of Injury*, noting that "rigorous research is needed to assess the effectiveness of prevention programs and to determine which among them merit widespread use. To ensure the feasibility of widespread use of child abuse and neglect prevention programs, research is also needed to assess program cost-effectiveness and the cost of initiating or expanding effective programs" (CDC, 2009, p. 76).

CDC also has examined the economic costs of child abuse and neglect, finding that the costs for both victims and society are substantial (CDC, 2012a). According to Fang and colleagues (2012), the total lifetime estimated financial costs associated with just 1 year of confirmed cases of child physical abuse, sexual abuse, psychological abuse, and neglect is approximately $124 billion (see also the discussion of costs in Chapter 4).

National Institutes of Health

NIH pursues fundamental knowledge about the nature and behavior of living systems and the application of knowledge to enhance health, lengthen life, and reduce the burdens of illness and disability. It invests more than $30 billion annually in medical research; research in the area of child abuse and neglect generally accounts for about $30 million per year. Yet of the funding for child abuse and neglect research in FY 2011, just over one-half, or about $16 million, was awarded for grants whose abstract or title indicated that child abuse and neglect was either the major independent or dependent variable; the remainder of the grants were on a variety of other topics, such as treatment of suicide, delinquency, or drug treatment of mental disorders. Of the total NIH expenditures in the area of child abuse and neglect research in FY 2011, just over $4 million was spent on new, first-time R01 grants.

In 1997, the House of Representatives' Committee on Appropriations (House Report 104-659) directed that NIH "convene a working group of its component organizations currently supporting research on child abuse and neglect." The NIH Child Abuse and Neglect Working Group was established in response to this mandate. Special funding announcements related to child abuse and neglect also were issued, encouraging new investigators across multiple disciplines to apply for funding. Special topics were targeted. In 2001, for example, a program announcement targeted research on child neglect.[6] That announcement expanded support from several NIH institutes, the National Institute of Justice and Office of Juvenile Justice and Delinquency Prevention in the Office of Justice Programs at the Department of Justice, the Children's Bureau, and the Office of Special Education Programs in the Department of Education.

In 2007, a program announcement, "Research on Interventions for Child Abuse and Neglect,"[7] was developed in response to the 2005 Surgeon General's workshop on this topic. The grant was supported by the National Institute of Mental Health (NIMH), National Institute on Alcohol Abuse and Alcoholism (NIAAA), National Institute of Child Health and Human Development (NICHD), National Institute on Drug Abuse (NIDA), and National Institute of Neurological Disorders and Stroke (NINDS); the NIH Office of Behavioral and Social Services Research; the NIH Fogarty International Center; CDC's NCIPC; and the Children's Bureau. After 2010, however, NIMH withdrew from participation.[8]

NICHD detailed to its council its commitment to research on child abuse and neglect and violence in general in January 2009, stating that within the Social and Affective Development/Child Maltreatment and Violence Program of NICHD's Child Development Behavior Branch, attention to child abuse and neglect includes active involvement in trans-NIH and transagency efforts to advance the science in the field of child abuse and neglect research; this involvement includes co-chairing the NIH Child Abuse and Neglect Working Group. The Child Development Behavior Branch also

---

[6]See http://grants.nih.gov/grants/guide/pa-files/PA-01-060.html (accessed January 27, 2014).
[7]See http://grants.nih.gov/grants/guide/pa-files/PA-07-437.html (accessed January 27, 2014).
[8]See http://grants.nih.gov/grants/guide/notice-files/NOT-MH-10-006.html (accessed January 27, 2014).

worked with the Children's Bureau, supporting supplemental studies, based on the NIS-4, aimed at understanding the various definitions of child abuse and neglect used by reporting agencies and their standards for reporting suspected abuse and neglect to child protective services or to the NIS-4.[9]

Administration on Children, Youth and Families, Children's Bureau

Created in 1912, the Children's Bureau within ACYF is focused on improving the lives of children and families. With an annual budget of about $8 billion, the agency funds services in all of the states and has a research program. The Children's Bureau funds an extensive training and technical assistance network; provides a series of child abuse prevention grants; and over the years has funded some field-initiated research grants and dissertation awards, as well as the NIS and annual reports on child abuse and neglect. The Children's Bureau also funds national quality improvement centers in several areas of child welfare that conduct evaluations. Currently there are three national quality improvement centers in the research domains of differential response in child protective services, early child experiences, and representation of children in the child welfare system (Children's Bureau, 2013). The goal for these centers is to assist child welfare professionals and agencies with service delivery by generating and disseminating research and lessons learned from the field. The Children's Bureau also funds the Child Welfare Information Gateway, an online clearinghouse for relevant information and statistics that archives data from federally supported and other research projects. In addition, the Office on Child Abuse and Neglect is now a unit within the Children's Bureau. The Children's Bureau does not currently provide support for investigator-initiated research and research grants responding to requests for applications.

Agency for Healthcare Research and Quality

AHRQ is the federal agency with responsibility for improving the quality, safety, efficiency, and effectiveness of health care, and it has a grant award program in these areas. The agency's total annual budget is about $400 million. Since 1993, AHRQ has awarded seven grants in the area of child abuse or neglect, including one career development award, two R01 awards, one conference grant, and three R03 awards.[10]

---

[9]See http://www.nichd.nih.gov/publications/pubs/upload/CDBB_Council_Report_2009_rev.pdf#page=39 (accessed January 27, 2014).

[10]See http://projectreporter.nih.gov (accessed March 28, 2013).

Title IV-E Waiver Demonstration Program

Title IV-E waivers, discussed in detail in Chapter 5, were first authorized in 1994 under P.L. 103-432 and were reauthorized under the Adoption and Safe Families Act. The creation of waivers is important for several reasons. First, they give successful state applicants the opportunity to use Title IV-B and IV-E funds more flexibly—for example, to focus more on prevention, in-home supportive services, or kinship care. Second, waivers require extensive evaluation, and several of the waiver demonstrations have used rigorous randomized designs. The authorizations for the waivers expired in 2006. However, a new round was supported under the Child and Family Services Innovation and Implementation Act of 2011 (P.L. 112-34), in part as a result of their success in states and localities as revealed by evaluation results.

Private Foundations

A number of national, local, and regional foundations provide support for child abuse and neglect research initiatives. The following sections highlight the notable contributions of the Doris Duke Charitable Foundation, the Annie E. Casey Foundation, Casey Family Programs, the William T. Grant Foundation, and the Stuart Foundation, but generous support to this field of research has been provided by many others.

Doris Duke Charitable Foundation The Doris Duke Charitable Foundation has as part of its mission supporting work that advances the prevention of child abuse and neglect. The foundation supports research fellowships for doctoral students in child abuse prevention and a variety of specific prevention projects, including prevention of abusive head injury (formerly termed shaken baby syndrome).

Annie E. Casey Foundation Work supported by grants from the Annie E. Casey Foundation (AECF) aims to improve the futures of disadvantaged children in the United States through public policy, human-service reform, and community support. The AECF Child Welfare Strategy Group (CWSG) focuses on responsive systems and supportive communities to create lifelong family connections. With its use of an intensive, embedded consulting model, the CWSG collaborates with clients to strengthen agency management, operations, policy, and front-line practice in support of their efforts to improve outcomes for children and families. The AECF KIDS COUNT project is a national and state-by-state effort to track the well-being of children in the United States. The project develops and distributes reports on key areas of well-being, including the annual KIDS COUNT Data Book.

Under the category Safety and Risky Behaviors, data are collected on the numbers of child abuse and neglect cases (both reported and substantiated).

Casey Family Programs Casey Family Programs (CFP) aims to improve foster care and the child welfare system in the United States. CFP research grants support studies that meet the needs of public child welfare jurisdictions and increase their capacity for data-driven decision making, evaluation, and performance monitoring. Specific areas of interest for research funding include preventing child abuse and neglect; accelerating permanency for children in foster care; improving the well-being of the children and families who encounter the child welfare system, including long-term outcomes such as employment, education, and mental health; and understanding the experiences of older youth who exit the child welfare system. From 2000 to 2011, CFP researchers published 60 peer-reviewed articles.

William T. Grant Foundation The William T. Grant Foundation funds research that enhances the lives of youth aged 8-25 through research grants and fellowship programs. Currently, the foundation funds research examining the formal and informal settings that youth inhabit and the use of research evidence about youth in policy and practice. Roughly 33 percent of the recent and ongoing research grants awarded before 2012 have entailed examining family life, and at least five studies have addressed issues related to youth experiences of violence, trauma, and neglect. The foundation also funds two fellowship programs: the William T. Grant Scholars Program supports scholars early in their careers; the William T. Grant Distinguished Scholars Program supports mid-career researchers seeking to work in policy or practice settings and mid-career policy makers and practitioners seeking to conduct research related to the well-being of youth.

Stuart Foundation The Stuart Foundation aims to support the ability of all children to realize their potential by improving the public education and child welfare systems in the states of California and Washington. While the aim is to improve the lives of all children and youth, the foundation strategically funds efforts to reach children in vulnerable environments, whose lives may be most impacted by improved programs and policies. The Stuart Foundation funds three main activities: the development and dissemination of effective, cutting-edge strategies for meeting the needs of children and youth; contributions to effective public policies related to children and youth; and direct delivery of support services for young people. Within the context of promoting data-informed policies and programs, the Stuart Foundation invests in projects that include efforts to gather, analyze, and use data to reveal how most effectively to serve children and youth, including children who have experienced abuse and neglect.

Funding Difficulties

Despite the research support described above, funding for research on child abuse and neglect overall has been inconsistent and inadequate to support the type and extent of research necessary to sufficiently advance the field. In her keynote address for the IOM/NRC workshop "Child Abuse and Neglect Research, Policy, and Practice for the Next Decade: Reflections on the 1993 NRC Report," Cathy Spatz Widom noted the large increase in medical and psychological articles on child abuse and neglect over the intervening period (IOM and NRC, 2012). She also observed that dedicated funding for child abuse and neglect research had remained constant since 1997, when it totaled $33.7 million; in 2012, it was projected to be $32 million. In an editorial in *Pediatrics*, "The Evolution of the Child Maltreatment Literature," Christopher Greeley makes a similar observation about the enormous growth of knowledge "despite the absence of a coordinating national research body and being under resourced" (Greeley, 2012, p. 347). By this measure, child abuse and neglect researchers have been productive. Yet given the enormous social and monetary costs of child abuse and neglect, one might ask why so little funding is designated for research in the field.

Researchers in the field frequently point out that no major federal funder considers child abuse and neglect research central to its primary mission. Child abuse and neglect researchers have the impression that they are not as competitive in the NIH grant review process as researchers investigating childhood disorders with much lower prevalence. This impression is difficult to test, but methodological limitations inherent in child abuse and neglect research could in fact affect the competiveness of grant proposals in the field as compared with many childhood conditions. As discussed earlier, front-line child abuse and neglect research involving alleged or substantiated cases must be conducted in a crisis-driven atmosphere with unique legal, ethical, and organizational complexities. The high level of family dysfunction, frequent family moves or changes in the out-of-home placement of children, and quality problems with child welfare administrative data increase attrition among subjects and the amount of missing data compared with clinic-based research on middle-class families.

Child abuse and neglect research is methodologically messy (Socolar et al., 1995). Much of the investigation and child welfare process is beyond a researcher's control, and data helpful for statistical corrections generally are not readily available. Grant and journal reviewers steeped in laboratory or clinic-based research designs and methodologies that favor optimizing internal validity often fail to appreciate the severe limitations faced by the front-line child abuse and neglect researcher. The researcher's inability to control potentially critical variables and the heterogeneity of cases, together with the complexities of past histories and comorbidities, confound efforts to reduce threats to internal validity. This is especially true for multisite research that must deal with enormous variability in populations, processes, policies, and resources across agencies. External validity and its closely related construct ecological validity, however, can be enhanced under these conditions. Interventions that succeed across diverse sites are more likely to be generalizable to the field as a whole.

Yet another reason suggested for the relative paucity of designated funding for research on child abuse and neglect is that, in contrast with many serious childhood conditions, parental advocacy for such funding is sparse. A recent study looking at 53 diseases found that for every $1,000 spent on lobbying for a given disorder there was a $25,000 increase in NIH funding the following year (Best, 2012). The study also found that less research funding was allocated to disorders associated with social stigma, such as drug and alcohol abuse or smoking, than to nonstigmatized conditions on a per-death basis. Discomfort with the topic may contribute to the sparse designated funds available for child abuse and neglect research.

The considerable costs of child abuse and neglect are distributed across many sectors, including mental health, medicine, drug and alcohol programs, education, social services, unemployment, law enforcement, and the prison system. Because these costs are largely indirect, it is difficult to estimate the potential savings attributable to reducing the problem. Thus, service providers and institutions across many sectors may not fully appreciate the benefit that would accrue to them from reductions in child abuse and neglect, and therefore do not lobby separately or collectively for more effective prevention. On the other hand, a number of professional and social policy organizations and coalitions do actively lobby for child abuse and neglect prevention and changes in child welfare policy.

Training and Mentorship

To fulfill the training mission, a field must have a supply of funded investigators conducting ongoing studies in which trainees can participate and must have access to research training funds to support trainees and new investigators while they learn. Mentors must be competent, involved, and supportive, helping trainees develop new areas of investigation and novel approaches to persistent problems.

National Institutes of Health Career Development Awards

NIH's Child Abuse and Neglect Research announcement in 1999 encouraged researchers to seek K awards. Participating institutes included NIMH, NINDS, NICHD, NIDA, and NIAAA.

Centers for Disease Control and Prevention

In 1987, CDC funded five interdisciplinary Injury Control Research Centers at leading universities, providing core support and funding for specific projects. The program grew, and currently there are 11 funded centers. Another 8 universities have hosted an Injury Control or Prevention Center since the program began 25 years ago (CDC, 2012b). At least four current or past CDC-supported centers (North Carolina, Pittsburgh, University of Washington, and Washington University of St. Louis) have supported child abuse research as part of their work.

Child Welfare Researchers

Although several policy efforts have focused on enhancing the child abuse and neglect research enterprise, there still are no structured career development opportunities for child maltreatment/child welfare researchers (IASWR, 2008); the field lacks policy supporting a clear researcher development strategy or career trajectory within or across disciplines. Many university-based research centers undertaking child abuse and neglect research are populated by nontenured researchers with little job security. One important component of research capacity is a strong cadre of researchers committed to the field over the long term. To this end, certain key elements should be in place. First, career support at every level and across disciplines should target opportunities to create a sustainable child abuse and neglect research career and capitalize on early interest (in the field of social work, for example, there are doctoral students who have worked in child welfare and seek a doctoral education to build knowledge that will enhance practice and policy). Second, onsite and virtual mentorship and opportunities for networking and socialization are necessary to ensure quality professional development. Third, university/agency partnerships are needed to keep the research grounded in the complex environment of services and enable the research results to inform practice (see IASWR, 2008, regarding the development of partnerships and strategies for maintaining them[11]). Fourth, community-based participatory research is needed to ensure that the research is meaningful and useful. Finally, a multidisciplinary annual or biannual conference that brings child abuse and neglect researchers together is a good vehicle for sharing research findings (IASWR, 2008).

The Administration on Children, Youth and Families does regularly support both a Head Start research conference and a welfare research and evaluation conference,[12] and the Children's Bureau supports a biannual

---

[11]See http://www.socialworkpolicy.org/wp-content/uploads/2007/06/9-IASWR-CW-Research-Partners.pdf (accessed January 27, 2014).

[12]See http://www.acf.hhs.gov/programs/opre/conferences.html (accessed January 27, 2014).

child abuse and neglect conference and conferences for states and grantees. Although these conferences are not solely focused on dissemination of research, many of the sessions are opportunities for sharing findings from recent child maltreatment research.

Since 2009, the Children's Bureau has sponsored two National Child Welfare Evaluation Summits, providing funds for state and tribal staff to attend. These meetings have provided an opportunity to present and discuss research on child welfare/child abuse and neglect, but they have not been specific to child abuse and neglect research, nor have they focused especially on career development.

The 1993 NRC report notes that specialized research training in child abuse and neglect did not exist until the mid-1980s, when one such program became available (NRC, 1993). In the late 1980s, a number of efforts were made to develop interdisciplinary graduate programs in child abuse and neglect. Gallmeier and Bonner (1992) reviewed the 10 universities funded by NC Children and Nature Coalition (NCCAN) in 1987 for 3 years to establish interdisciplinary training programs in child abuse and neglect, finding that they trained more than 400 students, 61 percent of whom were involved in some area of child abuse and neglect. Despite recommendations that these pilot programs be continued and replicated at other institutions, no such follow-up was conducted.

Child abuse and neglect research overall lacks the educational infrastructure to create and capitalize on student interest in the field. The relatively few courses devoted exclusively to child abuse and neglect across multiple disciplines signal that it is not a mainstream subject in many areas of research (Champion et al., 2003). In the field of social work, there are large numbers of courses and concentrations geared toward practice, and although many students are interested in pursuing child welfare research, there are no funding streams to support this line of research. The extremely limited federal funding dedicated to child abuse and neglect research can be viewed as further evidence of this gap. The resulting shortage of well-funded mentors and sustainable research programs limits the availability of training for the next generation of child abuse and neglect researchers. While progress has been made since the 1993 report was issued, there remains a strong need to increase support for interdisciplinary research training in child abuse and neglect.

Finding: Child abuse and neglect research encompasses a wide range of disciplines and research problems. Each of these domains has unique research infrastructure needs, methodologies, and agendas.

Finding: Child abuse and neglect is increasingly recognized as a major public health problem. A public health approach to child abuse and neglect offers a cohesive strategy for this multifaceted problem. A high-quality national surveillance system is needed to collect and analyze data with which to detect and describe aspects of child abuse and neglect, along with attendant risk and protective factors, so as to systematically inform the planning and implementation of public health interventions.

Finding: Among the medical aspects of child abuse and neglect, adequate support is needed for rigorous research to further explore the process and outcomes of both screening and medical evaluation, to examine the validity of abusive head trauma diagnoses, to support the development of more uniform approaches to practice, and to arrive at a medical consensus regarding thresholds for reporting neglect.

Finding: Despite recent federal investments, such as Title IV-E and IV-B training funds, there has been no commensurate investment in child welfare research capacity. With few child welfare researchers being supported by major federal institutional funders, there are few mentors and reviewers in the field.

Finding: While a wide array of public and private funders have made notable contributions to child abuse and neglect research, high-level, national coordination for research in this field is lacking. Funding opportunities have been fragmented and generally insufficient to develop and sustain the capacity for a national child abuse and neglect research enterprise.

Finding: Given the increasing heterogeneity of families in the United States, there is an ongoing need to increase understanding of the role of race and ethnicity in the causes and consequences of child abuse and neglect. Culturally adapted prevention and intervention programs can be evaluated to determine cultural fit, reach, and efficacy.

Finding: Several vulnerable populations, including racial and ethnic minority children (e.g., African Americans, American Indians, Alaska Natives, Latinos), children with disabilities, children of immigrant families, and LGBT youth, are underrepresented in child abuse and neglect research. Information sharing among data systems, targeted research on vulnerable populations, and changes to population-based youth surveys (e.g., adding questions on sexual identity and behavior) could improve understanding and knowledge of the causes and consequences of child abuse and neglect among these populations.

Finding: Data from longitudinal studies are essential for identifying causal pathways between abuse- and neglect-related biological changes and later adult outcomes. Longitudinal analyses also are critical to track outcomes related to the implementation of programs and delivery of services so the planning of interventions can be improved.

Finding: Current national child abuse and neglect surveillance efforts rely heavily on data reported to child welfare agencies. The children encompassed by these reports may represent a minority of total abuse and neglect incidents and can vary based on jurisdictional reporting standards.

Finding: The infrastructure needed to support a high-quality national public health surveillance system for child abuse and neglect is currently lacking. The capacity to develop such a surveillance system will require the linking of data across multiple sources, improved standardization of definitions of child abuse and neglect, and the collection of additional information on risk and protective factors.

Finding: An opportunity to obtain more accurate information on circumstances surrounding child abuse and neglect lies in the recent growth in web technologies and applications, which has expanded the potential for linkage and analysis of survey and administrative data across multiple service sectors. Given the variety of sectors that come into contact with abused and neglected children, linkage of data across multiple sources is important for greater research, practice, and policy synthesis and for examination of risk factors, recurrence or recidivism, and prevention and intervention outcomes.

Finding: Evidence-based classification schemes have brought conceptual and practical coherence to the maturing and interdisciplinary field of prevention research and the implementation of sound prevention strategies. In the past decade, federal agencies have established a number of registries and clearinghouses with a focus on prevention of child abuse and neglect. Yet their varied institutional homes underscore the fragmentation of prevention research across federal agencies and the lack of a unified federal policy and research agenda. Universities and social science research organizations have attempted to unify the evidence base in child abuse and neglect and prevention research.

CHALLENGES IN CHILD ABUSE AND NEGLECT RESEARCH

A number of factors complicate and confound research on child abuse and neglect and the most effective ways to prevent it and treat its consequences. Many of these factors relate to the complex nature of child abuse and neglect, along with the wide array of research and service domains that have a role in the field. The differing purposes for which information on child abuse and neglect is gathered have resulted in a lack of consistency in definitions and measurement of the problem across studies. Researchers must account for a myriad of co-occurring risk and protective factors in drawing conclusions about the causes or consequences of child abuse and neglect. Research on services must take into account the effects of the various services received by abused and neglected children, which may take place across a number of venues. Occurrences of child abuse and neglect are both serious and sensitive to the parties involved, resulting in difficulties in recruitment of study participants and often necessitating the gathering of data in complex and crisis-prone situations. Finally, difficulties are encountered in coordinating research and service efforts in the field. There is no federal home to monitor and coordinate research across the many relevant domains, and the actions of various providers seldom are sufficiently coordinated. Some of the key research challenges are discussed in detail below.

Lack of Consensus on Definitions and Measurement

The 1993 NRC report (Recommendation 2-1) calls for an expert panel to develop a consensus on research definitions for each form of abuse and neglect (NRC, 1993). Two recent reviews of child abuse and neglect research strategies and priorities highlight the multiple problems created for researchers and policy makers by the failure to implement this recommendation (MacMillan et al., 2007; Whitaker et al., 2005). Both reviews note that without agreement on definitions and measures, the national epidemiologic surveillance studies necessary for the implementation of a public health approach to the prevention of child abuse and neglect are impossible.

The field's persistent inability to develop a consensus on definitions and measures likely reflects the diversity of research disciplines and domains involved. In addition, authorities note an increase in the number of types of child abuse and neglect being reported as a result of growing awareness of the pernicious effects of more "subtle" forms, such as emotional abuse and emotional neglect (Gilbert et al., 2012). Others point to data indicating that the majority of children seen in the child abuse and neglect system are victims of multiple forms of abuse and neglect (Finkelhor et al., 2009). These explanations for the persistent lack of consensus on definitions indicate that a rigid set of standard definitions would be prohibitively difficult to create and likely counterproductive for research purposes. While the child abuse and neglect research field is currently hampered by a lack of agreement on definitions and measures, consensus definitions must be flexible to be useful and relevant.

Coexisting and Confounding Risk and Protective Factors

Child abuse and neglect does not occur in a vacuum. It is associated with familial factors such as domestic violence, parental substance abuse, poverty, and parental mental illness, as well as community violence and adversity. A number of studies have found a roughly stepwise dose response of increased morbidity as a function of the number of different types of abuse and neglect and family dysfunction experienced by an individual (Appleyard et al., 2005; Flaherty et al., 2009). This cumulative increase occurs for a variety of serious physical and mental health outcomes, as well as for health risk behaviors and phenomena such as smoking, drug use, and obesity. Critiques of child abuse and neglect research frequently point to the failure to measure confounding risks factors as a major flaw in many studies (MacMillan et al., 2007; Putnam-Hornstein et al., 2013; Whitaker et al., 2005). Researchers investigating causal pathways or the effectiveness of interventions face the task of measuring and controlling for these coexisting risk factors and their cumulative and potentially synergistic impact on the outcomes of interest (Putnam et al., 2013). Expertise in the measurement of these confounding variables cuts across research disciplines, necessitating the multidisciplinary, multimodal approach to abuse and neglect research discussed earlier in this report.

Differential Receipt of Additional Services Within Study Samples

Families served by the child welfare system frequently receive other services, including drug and alcohol counseling and treatment; family support services such as home visiting; and parenting, mental health, medical, special education, and financial support. In some instances, these services are legally mandated or are required as a condition of eligibility for other benefits. In a representative sample, it is impossible for an investigator to control for the diversity of configurations of such additional services (not to mention their timing and intensity). Thus, investigators seeking to isolate the effects of their intervention have difficulty modeling these other influences.

Participant Recruitment

The 1993 NRC report expresses concern about sample selection bias in child abuse and neglect research, including overrepresentation of groups of lower socioeconomic status and reliance on clinical samples of convenience (NRC, 1993). The issue of the extent to which child abuse and neglect study samples are representative of the larger population of families affected by the problem has received little attention in the literature. However, this issue has the potential to invalidate or severely bias data derived from these studies. In a prospective, case-control study of Australian children and their families, for example, 25 percent of the 103 nonparticipating families that met criteria for child sexual abuse declined to participate in the research (Lynch et al., 1993); however, the other 75 percent were never referred to the study by their social workers, who cited family dysfunction as their primary reason for nonreferral. Based on a comparison of participants and nonparticipants, the investigators concluded that the most dysfunctional families were the least likely to participate in the research. Feehan and colleagues (1995) later challenged the conclusion that dysfunctional families are less likely to participate in research, arguing that their nonparticipation most often is the result of a social worker's decision, not the family's (Feehan et al., 1995).

The other side of this question is whether research explicitly identified as focused on trauma or abuse and neglect may selectively attract subjects who have experienced abuse and neglect (Amsel et al., 2012). A randomized trial of psychotherapies for posttraumatic stress disorder found that 17 percent of the 223 consecutive subjects applying to the study were rejected because of psychotic symptoms. These subjects were likely to be males who suffered child abuse or neglect. An earlier survey of the child abuse and neglect literature found that male subjects were included in fewer than half (47.7 percent) of the 77 articles reviewed, and only 3 studies focused on males exclusively, compared with 40, including only females (Haskett et al., 1996). Thus at least two factors—family dysfunction and male gender—have been identified as potential confounders of the representativeness of abuse and neglect research samples. It is likely that the legal jeopardy inherent in this research, with its mandated reporting of future abuse, also discourages participation by some families (Melton, 2005), although reporting of abuse experienced by children already involved in a longitudinal study has been observed to have little impact on retention (Knight et al., 2006).

Complex and Crisis-Prone Front-Line Research Settings

Allegations of child abuse and neglect require rapid responses from the child protection system. In addition to the child at the center of the allegation, there are frequently siblings or other children potentially at risk who must be evaluated and provided safety as needed. When warranted by preliminary findings, law and policy typically require that a child safety plan, possibly including out-of-home placement, be implemented within 24-48 hours of receipt of the allegation. At this early stage and under these time pressures, critical decisions often must be made on the basis of imperfect information. These decisions can affect the life trajectories of whole families—for better or for worse. Remarkably little research has been conducted on risk assessment and decision making in front-line settings.

Children and their families frequently are interviewed in busy hospital emergency rooms, intimidating police stations, schools, and other settings not conducive to research. Research needs are trumped by the tension, confusion, distress, fear, and anger experienced by parents; the pressures on child welfare and medical professionals to make the right call based on sometimes ambiguous information; and the need to document the investigative process thoroughly for possible criminal proceedings.

Nonetheless, the process and content of child protection investigations and decision making is a critical area for research. Child protection is the primary pathway into the child welfare system. Very little is known about day-to-day risk assessment and decision making in child protection agencies. Most research on factors that influence risk assessment and decision making relies on simulation studies and surveys of child protection workers responding to case vignettes (Jent et al., 2011; Proctor and Azar, 2013; Stokes and Schmidt, 2012). It is known, however, that these workers experience their jobs as stressful and show high rates of secondary post-traumatic stress disorder and job burnout (Jayaratne et al., 2004; LeBlanc et al., 2012). Research in front-line settings offers opportunities to improve the assessment of risk and reduce stress on children, families, and child protection workers.

Lack of a Federal Home for Child Abuse and Neglect Research

The 15 most published U.S. investigators in the fields of child abuse and neglect have generated a total of 790 published papers, as recorded in Web of Science.[13] Funding support is reported in just 47 of these papers. The leading supporters were five different NIH institutes; CDC; the Administration on Children, Youth and Families; and the Doris Duke Charitable Foundation. The leading funder, NIMH, supported just 1.8 percent of the 790 papers. CDC supports prevention of child abuse as part of the mission of the NCICP but has only one grant cycle per year, and in 2011 funded no new grants in child abuse. New investigators in the field have no cadre

---

[13]Accessed November 25, 2012.

of established investigators or centers to turn to for support and guidance such as exists in many laboratory sciences. Review committees have little or no expertise in child abuse among their members as there are so few experienced investigators supported by NIH who are invited to sit on study sections. The paucity of knowledgeable reviewers leads to inexpert reviews and a lack of champions for research in the field; thus, perpetuating the absence of a home for child abuse and neglect research. With little success in securing funding, the field continues to be an orphan research area. A review panel on injury and violence is needed with appropriate experience and expertise to apply the strict standards for extramural support that have become standard at NIH, and with knowledge of the field and an appreciation of the need for innovation and new information.

Difficulties of Translating Research Findings into Policy and Practice

As discussed earlier, child welfare policies often are drafted in response to a tragic case that receives widespread media coverage (Gainsborough, 2010). Although theory-driven child abuse and neglect prevention policies have been articulated (e.g., social learning theories of intergenerational violence, psychoanalytic theories of parental psychopathology, environmental theories of poverty and adversity), none of these theories has proven sufficiently successful in practice to become a dominant approach to child abuse and neglect policy (Putnam-Hornstein et al., 2013). An analysis of the impact of changes in child welfare policy on abuse and neglect trends from 1979 to 2009 in six developed nations (Australia, Canada [Manitoba], England, New Zealand, Sweden, and the United States) found little evidence that new prevention initiatives had any detectable effects (Gilbert et al., 2012).

Putnam-Hornstein and colleagues (2013) argue that the failure to develop theory-driven prevention policies for child abuse and neglect stems from the lack of empirical population-based data on family and environmental risk factors and long-term abuse and neglect outcomes. They note that current child abuse and neglect trend studies depend largely on retrospective and time-limited data derived from child protection cases and lack the broader focus and key variables, including important confounders, necessary to inform prevention policies. As a possible solution, the authors point to international efforts to enhance current child protection data by case linking the data to existing health, education, and family welfare administrative datasets. These additional data generate a larger context in which to examine family factors, demographics, socioeconomic status, and community variables as contributers to the risk for abuse and neglect and as targets for prevention policies.

Traditional Silo Nature of Child Abuse and Neglect Services

The previously presented overview of child abuse and neglect research domains reflects the many systems that interact, largely independently, with abused and neglected children and their families. In many jurisdictions, abused and neglected children and their families pass through multiple agencies as their cases are processed and they receive services. Each system has its own mission, expertise, agenda, and obligations to fulfill. The systems are staffed by different disciplines, collect different types of information, and are focused on different outcomes. Often workers in one system are only vaguely aware of what other systems and services do or how they work. Misconceptions about roles and capacities are not uncommon.

Although some coordination may exist across state or county agencies at the top leadership levels, out-of-system transfers and follow-up at the basic services level often encounter difficulties. Referrals frequently contain minimal information, requiring the receiving agency to collect duplicate information and reassess the case. In part, this duplication occurs because of concerns about protecting confidentiality or, in some instances, because a legal action may be pending. Children and families become resentful of having to tell their story multiple times and to fill out forms requesting information they have previously provided.

Conducting research that requires integrating data across multiple child- and family-serving systems is extremely difficult. In addition to the inevitable hardware and software incompatibilities, separate systems collect different types of data and code and process the data in different ways, greatly complicating case linkage. Legal restrictions, often confounded by confusion about what constitutes confidential information, inhibit data sharing. Most agencies lack the expertise in data management and statistical analysis to conduct research with their own or combined datasets. In response to this need, Chapin Hall at the University of Chicago established administrative data institutes for child welfare managers in the early 1990s. To foster the integration of research with policy and practice, Chapin Hall has since 2007 offered annual sessions in advanced analytics for child welfare administration, which focuses on the use of longitudinal administrative data in child welfare decision making, program planning, and outcome monitoring.[14] Agencies also view the value of research and its relevance to their practice differently. Thus in many jurisdictions, the integrated, cross-system research necessary to understand the causes, consequences, and prevention of child abuse and neglect cannot be conducted.

---

[14]See http://www.chapinhall.org/events/advanced-analytics-child-welfare-administration-june-2012 (accessed January 27, 2014).

Finding: The complex nature of child abuse and neglect as a topic for both services and empirical research leads to the involvement of many different systems and research domains. This multiplicity presents a number of challenges for conducting research in the field. The establishment of uniform definitions and measures for all types of child abuse and neglect has proven difficult, mainly because of the diversity of research disciplines involved and the varying sources from which data are drawn. Children and families receiving services related to child abuse and neglect often are eligible to receive services from other systems, which can pose problems for researchers as diversity in the type, timing, and intensity of such additional services can be difficult to account for in studying the effects of child abuse and neglect interventions. Further, a number of potentially important cross-disciplinary outcomes may be impacted by intervention research. However, only specific outcomes of interest often are accounted for in study designs, neglecting the influences on other, relevant outcomes.

EXISTING OPPORTUNITIES TO CREATE AN INTEGRATED CHILD ABUSE AND NEGLECT RESEARCH INFRASTRUCTURE

Fortunately, major developments have occurred since the 1993 NRC report was issued that offer opportunities to create an integrated child abuse and neglect research infrastructure that can bridge the separate systems and services discussed above. The following sections highlight several notable efforts to bring interdisciplinary collaboration to child abuse and neglect research and service delivery.

Child Advocacy Centers

The child advocacy center (CAC) model originated in the 1980s to address problems of investigational redundancy, lack of interagency coordination, and stress on children and families engendered by the confusing multiagency child protection process, in most instances for children who have experienced sexual abuse. CACs are designed to be child-friendly settings in which multidisciplinary investigational teams represent the core disciplines and services involved in child welfare. The usual CAC team consists of trained forensic interviewers and representatives of law enforcement and prosecution, social work, pediatrics, and mental health. Efforts are made to interview the child as few times as possible (usually only once) and to limit system contacts for the family to one or two key staff. The CAC team reviews cases of alleged abuse and neglect, integrating medical, social, and forensic findings with other pertinent information, as well as recommending courses of action and possible services. The decision to substantiate a finding of abuse and neglect usually is made, however, by the legally designated child protection agency, utilizing input from the CAC team.

In the past 20 years, the number of CACs has grown significantly, such that there are now more than 750 CACs in the United States.[15] A number of states are further encouraging adoption of the CAC model with legislated funding. A national membership organization, the National Children's Alliance (NCA), provides training, support, technical assistance, and leadership for local CACs and accredits programs meeting its criteria.

In general, CACs currently are not conceived of as sites for collecting data and conducting high-quality, multidisciplinary research, but they represent an opportunity to enhance the child abuse and neglect research infrastructure. In fact, in the past decade, the number of CAC-type programs affiliated with university medical centers has increased significantly. University-affiliated CACs in particular have access to the human and physical capital required for a high-quality child abuse and neglect research infrastructure. In addition, they can offer researchers from outside the child abuse and neglect field access to an infrastructure within which to conduct longitudinal, case-based, cross-system, multidisciplinary research.

The Subspecialty of Child Abuse Pediatrics

The proposal to develop a new pediatric subspecialty grew out of the Ray E. Helfer Society and a conviction of some of its members that research and research support in child abuse and neglect were limited by the paucity of investigators with both research and clinical knowledge in the field. The first application to the American Board of Pediatrics was not accepted, but after two revisions and a change in name from Forensic Pediatrics to Child Abuse Pediatrics, the new subspecialty was approved by both the American Board of Pediatrics and the American Board of Medical Specialties. The training encompasses 3 years, including a year of research training. The first board examination was offered in 2009 (Block and Palusci, 2006). Currently there are 264 board-certified child abuse pediatricians.[16] Subspecialty certification is not open to physicians in other specialties, but other certified specialists in family medicine, child psychiatry, pathology, radiology, and surgery are major investigators in the field.

---

[15]See http://www.nationalchildrensalliance.org/index.php?s=6 (accessed January 27, 2014).
[16]See http://www.abp.org (accessed November 15, 2012).

Collaboration of Child Welfare, Courts, and
Social Services and Emphasis on Evaluation

The past two decades have seen a growing emphasis on fostering co-ordination and collaboration across the legal and social service systems that serve abused and neglected children and vulnerable families. A related development has been the increasing federal emphasis on the implementation of evidence-based practices (Haskins and Baron, 2011). A by-product of these developments is an increasing emphasis on evaluation, which is often multidisciplinary.

The State Court Improvement Program (CIP), discussed in detail in Chapter 5, is one example of a mechanism for encouraging coordination and collaboration (Children's Bureau, 2007). As noted in Chapter 5, efforts toward system improvement under the State CIP include coordination activities between child welfare agencies and the courts that encompass joint agency-court training, linked agency-court data systems, one judge/one family models, time-specific docketing, and formalized relationships with the child welfare agencies.[17] Similar coordination takes place under the Tribal CIP, created in 2011.

Interagency collaboration and rigorous evaluation are central to several other programs discussed in Chapter 5. The first is a grant program, funded under the Child and Family Services Improvement Act of 2006, aimed at improving permanency outcomes for children affected by methamphetamine and/or substance abuse. As described in Chapter 5, this program awarded more than 50 regional partnership grants in FY 2007 to strengthen cross-system collaboration and service integration through a number of strategies, including family treatment drug courts, increased staffing to address short-ages in both child welfare services and substance abuse treatment systems, reconciliation of conflicting time frames across legal and treatment systems to achieve desired outcomes, and use of evidence-based practice approaches and delivery of trauma-informed services. This emphasis on collaboration has continued under the Child and Family Services Improvement and Innovation Act (P.L. 112-34), which includes a targeted grants program for regional partnership grants to improve the well-being of children affected by substance abuse. And in FY 2012, the Children's Bureau awarded 17 grants to grantees with demonstrated collaborative infrastructure in place across child welfare, substance abuse treatment and mental health agencies, and the courts. Grantees must track performance indicators that form the

---

[17]See http://www.acf.hhs.gov/programs/cb/resource/court-improvement-program (accessed January 27, 2014).

basis of an annual Report to Congress and conduct rigorous impact evaluations of child and family outcomes.[18]

The National Child Traumatic Stress Network

The National Child Traumatic Stress Network (NCTSN), also described in detail in Chapter 5, is a multidisciplinary trauma treatment services-based network that could potentially serve as a national child abuse and neglect/family trauma research infrastructure. As discussed in Chapter 5, the NCTSN has a long track record of high-quality program evaluation and a core data system with detailed trauma histories on more than 14,000 children and adolescents. This dataset and the connections established by the NCTSN among communities, systems, and academic institutions could be leveraged to enable high-quality, multidisciplinary child abuse and neglect research.

Ad Hoc Child Abuse and Neglect Research Networks

As discussed in Chapter 2, more than 3 million children are reported to child protection authorities each year, but many of these children are reported multiple times, and only one-third of reported cases are founded or confirmed. Given the wide variety of forms of abuse and neglect and the overrepresentation of some children in the data, specific forms of abuse and neglect, such as abusive head trauma, Munchausen syndrome by proxy, or inflicted burns, may be sufficiently uncommon that careful research on them may be difficult in any one setting. Important work in other areas, such as neonatal intensive care, pediatric cancer, or pediatric intensive care, for which similar issues of statistical power at a single institution exist has been supported by research networks. These networks are invaluable in advancing the science for serious but less common conditions. There are few examples of research networks in child abuse and neglect, but several are noteworthy.

Organized originally out of the University of Virginia and now at Dartmouth Medical School, the Pediatric Brain Injury Research Network, or PediBIRN, is a consortium of investigators whose aim is to develop an effective clinical prediction rule for pediatric abusive head trauma.[19] This group has published a multicenter study examining outcomes for inflicted

---

[18]The National Center on Substance Abuse and Child Welfare provides assistance to local, state, and tribal agencies to support systems and practice change for families with substance use disorders that are involved in the child welfare and family judicial systems. This resource is funded jointly by the Substance Abuse and Mental Health Services Administration's Center for Substance Abuse Treatment and the Children's Bureau.

[19]See www.pedibirn.com (accessed January 24, 2014).

and noninflicted traumatic brain injuries in infants (Hymel et al., 2007). This network remains active and continues working toward the goal of a prediction rule.

The Examining Siblings to Recognize Abuse (ExSTRA) research network is a multicenter, observational, cross-sectional network of 20 child abuse teams that have adopted a common screening protocol for the siblings and household contacts of children younger than 10 evaluated for potential physical abuse. This network has produced three studies to date.

Sharing many of the same investigators, a group of 19 collaborators with a subspecialty in child abuse formed a network of investigators to develop data prospectively regarding evaluation for abdominal trauma. The Using Liver Transaminases to Recognize Abuse (ULTRA) network enrolled 1,676 children between 2007 and 2008 who were younger than age 5 and had undergone subspecialty evaluation for suspected abuse. This network has developed important data on occult abdominal trauma related to physical abuse.

Another example of network development is the Multistate Foster Care Data Archive, maintained through Chapin Hall. This network is used by multiple states and has been encouraged by CFP because of the importance, mentioned above, of using administrative data to guide practice improvements.

Finally, the National Data Archive on Child Abuse and Neglect (NDACAN), which is hosted by Cornell University and funded by the Children's Bureau, maintains Child-Maltreatment-Research-L (CMRL).[20] CMRL is a listserv whose goal is to create space for scholarly discussion among the hundreds of subscribing child abuse and neglect researchers. This online network is used primarily for sharing information about professional events relevant to the field, new resources for research that may become available, employment opportunities for child abuse and neglect research experts, and requests for information and assistance. Direct conversation about issues and opinion sharing are explicitly discouraged.

Child Abuse and Neglect Research Centers

The 1993 NRC report recommends the development of child abuse centers to address research needs in the field (NRC, 1993). Likewise, the 2001 IOM report *Confronting Chronic Neglect*, examining training in family violence in health professions schools, calls for the development of specialized research centers in violence (IOM, 2001). In reviewing NIH's disease-focused research centers at academic institutions in 2004, the IOM

---

[20] See http://www.ndacan.cornell.edu/NDACAN/CMRLListserv.html (accessed January 27, 2014).

stated that these centers are important when "the scientific opportunities and/or public health needs that the program would address have high priority" (IOM, 2004, p. 95). The IOM argued that the centers provide a platform supportive of interdisciplinary collaborations by facilitating multi-investigator teams that can develop activities often not possible under other funding mechanisms. A similar program of extramural centers addressing injury broadly has been developed by the NCIPC. These centers have been quite successful in expanding research focused on injury and increasing the number of trainees interested in the field (Runyan et al., 2010).

The Kempe Center for the Prevention and Treatment of Child Abuse was established in 1972 with support from the Robert Wood Johnson Foundation and was an early leader in child abuse research (Krugman et al., 2013). Three years later, Dr. David Chadwick founded a clinical and research center at Rady Children's Hospital in San Diego, California.[21] Several other centers that combine clinical care for and research on child abuse have been developed around the country over the years in response to local supporters and advocates; a number of these centers have had periods of funding by the NCTSN.[22] Perhaps the most recent is a new center combining clinical care and research at Pennsylvania State University.[23] These centers have struggled to meet the potential outlined by the IOM (2004) but have suffered from a lack of support by agencies that fund research in the field of child abuse (IOM, 2004).

The Child Welfare Research Center in the School of Social Welfare at the University of California, Berkeley, conducts groundbreaking research on a variety of child welfare issues, including adoption, case management, foster care, and welfare reform, and has been a leader in the state and nationally in the use of administrative data. Its main support comes from the state and a California-based foundation, although it was originally launched when the Children's Bureau funded three interdisciplinary research centers—at Berkeley, at the Center for the Study of Social Policy, and at Chapin Hall—in the early 1990s. The work of Putnam-Hornstein cited in this report is an outgrowth of the center's important contributions.

As seen in the long-standing research collaboration between the Illinois Department of Child and Family Services and the Child and Family Research Center at the University of Illinois School of Social Work, ongoing data monitoring and analysis have facilitated system-level reform. The result has been a better understanding of risk factors for child maltreatment; monitoring of safety risk, permanency trajectories, and well-being

---

[21]See www.Chadwickcenter.org (accessed March 7, 2014).

[22]See www.nctsn.org (accessed March 7, 2014).

[23]See http://www.pennstatehershey.org/web/protection-of-children/home/about (accessed March 7, 2014).

BOX 7-3
Pediatric Acquired Brain Injury Centers

A proposal currently being considered in Congress would establish 50 state Pediatric Acquired Brain Injury Centers. These centers would support clinical care, rehabilitation services, prevention activities, and research for brain injuries in children, including those related to both child abuse and sports, as well as unintentional injuries from other sources. It is too early to know whether this proposal will succeed. It follows in the footsteps of an earlier proposal in the early 2000s, supported by the American Academy of Pediatrics, to develop a number of child abuse centers in academic medical centers. That proposal, to form Health Child Abuse Research and Evaluation Centers, never received support from any federal agency or Congress and did not move forward.

BOX 7-4
The Early Experience, Stress, and Neurodevelopment Center

The Early Experience, Stress, and Neurodevelopment Center is an example of an effective multidisciplinary infrastructure for translational research on child abuse and neglect and for training for a new generation of translational researchers. The center had its origins in a 1998 call for proposals from the National Institute of Mental Health. The center was initially directed by Megan Gunnar, who studies stress and human development, and Paul Plotsky, who studies early-life stress in rodent models. The project period for the mature center, with Director Megan Gunnar and Associate Director Philip Fisher, runs from March 2009 through February 2014.

The center has 14 faculty members representing nine universities and research centers and brings to bear a range of expertise critical to understanding the impact of early-life stress on neurobehavioral development. The center's staff includes researchers who work predominantly with animal models, both rodent and nonhuman primate, as well as researchers studying human development. Their areas of expertise range from basic neuroscience to developmental psychopathology and prevention science. The center integrates basic developmental behavioral neuroscience research using nonhuman primate and human models to increase understanding of the behavioral and neurobiological impacts of early-life stress and to identify care experiences that support recovery. Preventive intervention researchers guide the center's research so that future interventions can benefit from this more comprehensive knowledge base.

Over 14 years, this center has been influential in advancing the field toward a more integrated understanding of the developmental sequalae of neglect and outcomes; identification of disparities in system contact; mapping of client access to services and treatment; and planning initiatives in response to risk factors and needs (McEwen et al., 2011).

Box 7-3 describes a current proposal for state Pediatric Acquired Brain Injury Centers. Box 7-4 describes the Early Experience, Stress, and Neurodevelopment Center.

Finding: Various interdisciplinary collaborations focused on the delivery of child abuse and neglect services, such as those found in CACs, the state CIP, and national traumatic stress networks, have improved coordination of services and can serve as venues for interdisciplinary research. Research collaboratives, such as ad hoc child abuse and neglect research networks and various privately supported child abuse and neglect research centers, serve as a model for support of the multidisciplinary research necessary to advance the field of child abuse and neglect research.

abuse. It has faciliated communication between scientists conducting basic research and those focused on the application of that work to preventive interventions for young children and their families.

The structure of the center is depicted below. Methods used by the center include behavioral observations, electrophysiology (e.g., electroencephalogram), observation of neuroendocrine activity (hypothalamic-pituitary-adrenal axis) under basal conditions and in response to psychological and pharmacological challenges, in vivo neuroimaging (magnetic resonance imaging, diffusion tensor imaging, magnetic resonance spectroscopy), and neurobehavioral tasks of amygdala and prefrontal functioning.

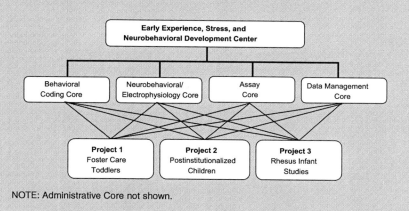

NOTE: Administrative Core not shown.

CONCLUSIONS

Child abuse and neglect research is fraught with complexities. Research in the field involves diverse independent service systems, a number of related research domains, multiple professions, ethical issues that are particularly complicated, and levels of outcome analysis ranging from the individual child to national statistics. It has been difficult to establish uniform definitions and measures for all types of child abuse and neglect, mainly because of the diversity of research disciplines involved and the varying sources from which data are drawn. Researchers also must account for a myriad of co-occurring risk and protective factors in drawing conclusions about the causes or consequences of child abuse and neglect. In addition, children and families receiving services related to child abuse and neglect often are eligible to receive services from other service systems. This can pose problems for researchers as diversity in the type, timing, and intensity of such additional services can be difficult to account for in studying the effects of child abuse and neglect interventions. Further, a number of potentially important cross-disciplinary outcomes may be impacted by intervention research.

These challenges highlight the need for a sophisticated, multidisciplinary research infrastructure. Despite notable efforts to support child abuse and neglect research by a number of public and private sources, significant components of the field's infrastructure remain inadequately developed. Future efforts need to focus on recruiting and training a dedicated and capable cadre of researchers, securing stable sources of research funding, and developing sufficient physical capital to conduct research based on sophisticated designs. Also needed are interdisciplinary collaboration and the integration of cross-disciplinary methodologies and measures to yield more robust study designs. There remains a need as well for a nationally coordinated investment in the types of research necessary to advance the field. No one federal agency provides oversight of child abuse and neglect research investments. A high-level federal mechanism to coordinate and track all federally funded research on child abuse and neglect is needed.

A high-quality population-based epidemiological surveillance system that draws on multiple data sources is critically necessary for the development of a national strategic approach to child abuse and neglect. The capacity to support more universal application of data linkage efforts among the many sources of child abuse and neglect information needs to be developed. Continued federal investment in nationally representative longitudinal studies, quality improvements in administrative data, and the timely dissemination of public-use data files are essential for understanding how the type, timing, extent, and chronicity of abuse and neglect affect children's and adolescents' psychosocial and behavioral development and for developing population- and community-level practice and policy responses to prevent and ameliorate abuse and neglect. Further, research needs to be conducted with the appropriate methodological sensitivity to adequately analyze the impact of culture and other social factors that may inform the causal pathways of child abuse and neglect, particularly for marginalized and/or underresearched populations.

Finally, the formation of child abuse and neglect research centers presents an important opportunity not only to develop and sustain a volume of high-quality interdisciplinary research related to child abuse and neglect but also to train and support a new generation of child abuse and neglect researchers to ensure the growth of the field.

REFERENCES

Amsel, L. V., N. Hunter, S. Kim, K. E. Fodor, and J. C. Markowitz. 2012. Does a study focused on trauma encourage patients with psychotic symptoms to seek treatment? *Psychiatric Services* 63(4):386-389.

Anda, R. F., J. B. Croft, V. J. Felitti, D. Nordenberg, W. H. Giles, D. F. Williamson, and G. A. Giovino. 1999. Adverse childhood experiences and smoking during adolescence and adulthood. *Journal of the American Medical Association* 282(17):1652-1658.

Anda, R. F., D. W. Brown, V. J. Felitti, J. D. Bremner, S. R. Dube, and W. H. Giles. 2007. Adverse childhood experiences and prescribed psychotropic medications in adults. *American Journal of Preventive Medicine* 32(5):389-394.

Anguksuar, L., Yup'ik, S. Jacobs, W. Thomas, and S. Lang. 1997. A postcolonial perspective on western [mis] conceptions of the cosmos and the restoration of indigenous taxonomies. *Two-Spirit People: Native American Gender Identity, Sexuality, and Spirituality* 217-222.

Appleyard, K., B. Egeland, M. H. M. van Dulmen, and L. Alan Sroufe. 2005. When more is not better: The role of cumulative risk in child behavior outcomes. *Journal of Child Psychology and Psychiatry* 46(3):235-245.

Balsam, K. F., B. Huang, K. C. Fieland, J. M. Simoni, and K. L. Walters. 2004. Culture, trauma, and wellness: A comparison of heterosexual and lesbian, gay, bisexual, and two-spirit Native Americans. *Cultural Diversity and Ethnic Minority Psychology* 10(3):287.

Barrera, M., F. G. Castro, and L. K. Steiker. 2011. A critical analysis of approaches to the development of preventive interventions for subcultural groups. *American Journal of Community Psychology* 48(3-4):439-454.

Baum, K., K. M. Blakeslee, J. Lloyd, and A. Petrosino. 2013. *Violence prevention: Moving from evidence to implementation.* http://www.iom.edu/Global/Perspectives/2013/Violence PreventionImplementation.aspx (accessed November 26, 2013).

Best, R. K. 2012. Disease politicis and medical research funding: Three ways advocay. *American Sociological Review* 77(5):780-803.

Block, R. W., and V. J. Palusci. 2006. Child abuse pediatrics: A new pediatric subspecialty. *Journal of Pediatrics* 148(6):711-712.

Bonner, B. L., S. M. Crow, and L. D. Hensley. 1997. State efforts to identify maltreated children with disabilities: A follow-up study. *Child Maltreatment* 2(1):52-60.

Brown, J., P. Cohen, J. G. Johnson, and S. Salzinger. 1998. A longitudinal analysis of risk factors for child maltreatment: Findings of a 17-year prospective study of officially recorded and self-reported child abuse and neglect. *Child Abuse & Neglect* 22(11):1065-1078.

Burton, L. 2007. Childhood adultification in economically disadvantaged families: A conceptual model. *Family Relations* 56(4):329-345.

Casanueva, C., E. Wilson, K. Smith, M. Dolan, H. Ringeisen, B. Horne, and RTI International. 2012a. *NSCAW II wave 2 report: Children and families who receive child welfare services.* Washington, DC: Office of Planning, Research and Evaluation, U.S. Department of Health and Human Services.

Casanueva, C., E. Wilson, K. Smith, M. Dolan, H. Ringeisen, B. Horne, and RTI International. 2012b. *NSCAW II wave 2 report: Children's services.* Washington, DC: Office of Planning, Research and Evaluation, U.S. Department of Health and Human Services.

CDC (Centers for Disease Control and Prevention). 2009. *CDC injury research agenda, 2009-2012.* Atlanta, GA: CDC.

CDC. 2010. *Preventing child maltreatment: Program activities guide.* http://www.cdc.gov/violenceprevention/pub/preventingcm.html (accessed November 26, 2013).

CDC. 2012a. *Cost of child abuse and neglect rival other major public health problems.* http://www.cdc.gov/violenceprevention/childmaltreatment/economiccost.html (accessed November 26, 2013).

CDC. 2012b. *Injury prevention & control: Funded programs, activities & research.* http://www.cdc.gov/injury/erpo/icrc/index.html (accessed November 27, 2012).

Champion, K. M., K. Shipman, B. L. Bonner, L. Hensley, and A. C. Howe. 2003. Child maltreatment training in doctoral programs in clinical, counseling, and school psychology: Where do we go from here? *Child Maltreatment* 8(3):211-217.

Chapin Hall. 2012. *Advance analytics for child welfare administration.* http://www.chapinhall.org/events/advanced-analytics-child-welfare-administration-june-2012 (accessed June 23, 2013).

Chapman, D. P., C. L. Whitfield, V. J. Felitti, S. R. Dube, V. J. Edwards, and R. F. Anda. 2004. Adverse childhood experiences and the risk of depressive disorders in adulthood. *Journal of Affective Disorders* 82(2):217-225.

Children's Bureau. 2007. *The national evaluation of the court improvement program: Synthesis of 2005 court improvement program reform and activities, final report.* https://docs.google.com/viewer?a=v&q=cache:2e88RgueWEQJ:www.pal-tech.com/cip/files/First Synthesis.pdf+national+CIP+evaluation+final+report&hl=en&gl=us&pid=bl&srcid =ADGEEShtnHYZqHLyzoRzJZFouKT0ZaE9BRPT_IrFnBfc5l2fLhshHU9-kxuy 5N73plkZeVTIu9WFrPaJHZ4Wq7DZX04V-m13is08bEyHm9tbdFpoZDxb7vhL_ c-yAlKxdSUZG_r_PVGA&sig=AHIEtbQKNjVeY9esdv_MeGJZ-1f1AzIVTg (accessed October 18, 2013).

Children's Bureau. 2013. *Quality improvement centers.* http://www.acf.hhs.gov/programs/cb/ assistance/quality-improvement-centers (accessed November 26, 2013).

Coulton, C. J., D. S. Crampton, M. Irwin, J. C. Spilsbury, and J. E. Korbin. 2007. How neighborhoods influence child maltreatment: A review of the literature and alternative pathways. *Child Abuse & Neglect* 31(11-12):1117-1142.

Cross, T. 2012. An overview of child maltreatment data in American Indian/Alaska native communities. Paper read at Presentation to the Committee on Child Maltreatment Research, Policy, and Practice for the Next Decade, December 10, Washington, DC.

Cross, T. L., B. J. Friesen, P. Jivanjee, L. K. Gowen, A. Bandurraga, C. Mathew, and N. Maher. 2011. Defining youth success using culturally appropriate community-based participatory research methods. *Best Practices in Mental Health* 7(1):94-114.

D'Augelli, A. R. 2005. Stress and adaptation among families of lesbian, gay, and bisexual youth: Research challenges. *Journal of GLBT Family Studies* 1(2):115-135.

D'Augelli, A. R. 2012. Panel on select populations. Paper read at Presentation to the Committee on Child Maltreatment Research, Policy, and Practice for the Next Decade, December 10, Washington, DC.

DeBruyn, L., M. Chino, P. Serna, and L. Fullerton-Gleason. 2001. Child maltreatment in American Indian and Alaska Native communities: Integrating culture, history, and public health for intervention and prevention. *Child Maltreatment* 6(2):89-102.

DeSena, A. D., R. A. Murphy, H. Douglas-Palumberi, G. Blau, B. Kelly, S. M. Horwitz, and J. Kaufman. 2005. SAFE homes: Is it worth the cost?: An evaluation of a group home permanency planning program for children who first enter out-of-home care. *Child Abuse & Neglect* 29(6):627-643.

Dong, M., S. R. Dube, V. J. Felitti, W. H. Giles, and R. F. Anda. 2003. Adverse childhood experiences and self-reported liver disease: New insights into the causal pathway. *Archives of Internal Medicine* 163(16):1949-1956.

Drake, B., and M. Jonson-Reid. 1999. Some thoughts on the increasing use of administrative data in child maltreatment research. *Child Maltreatment* 4(4):308-315.

Dube, S. R., R. F. Anda, V. J. Felitti, D. P. Chapman, D. F. Williamson, and W. H. Giles. 2001. Childhood abuse, household dysfunction, and the risk of attempted suicide throughout the life span: Findings from the adverse childhood experiences study. *Journal of the American Medical Association* 286(24):3089-3096.

Dube, S. R., V. J. Felitti, M. Dong, D. P. Chapman, W. H. Giles, and R. F. Anda. 2003a. Childhood abuse, neglect, and household dysfunction and the risk of illicit drug use: The adverse childhood experiences study. *Pediatrics* 111(3):564-572.

Dube, S. R., V. J. Felitti, M. Dong, W. H. Giles, and R. F. Anda. 2003b. The impact of adverse childhood experiences on health problems: Evidence from four birth cohorts dating back to 1900. *Preventive Medicine* 37(3):268-277.

Dubowitz, H., D. English, J. Kotch, A. Litrownik, D. Runyan, and R. Thompson. 2006. *LONGSCAN research briefs*, Vol. 2. Chapel Hill, NC: Consortium for Longitudinal Studies of Child Abuse and Neglect.

Dubowitz, H., S. Feigelman, W. G. Lane, and J. Kim. 2009. Pediatric primary care to help prevent child maltreatment: The Safe Environment for Every Kid (SEEK) model. *Pediatrics* 123(3):858-864.

Duggan, A., L. Fuddy, L. Burrell, S. M. Higman, E. McFarlane, A. Windham, and C. Sia. 2004. Randomized trial of a statewide home visiting program to prevent child abuse: Impact in reducing parental risk factors. *Child Abuse & Neglect* 28(6):623-643.

Earle, K. A., and A. Cross. 2001. *Child abuse and neglect among American Indian/Alaska Native children: An analysis of existing data*. Seattle, WA: Casey Family Programs.

Elze, D. E. 2009. Strategies for recruiting and protecting gay, lesbian, bisexual, and transgender youths in the research process. In *Handbook of research with lesbian, gay, bisexual, and transgender populations*, edited by W. Meezan and J. I. Martin. New York: Routledge. Pp. 40-68.

Evans-Campbell, T. 2008. Perceptions of child neglect among urban American Indian/Alaska Native parents. *Child Welfare* 87(3):115-142.

Fang, X., D. S. Brown, C. S. Florence, and J. A. Mercya. 2012. The economic burden of child maltreatment in the United States and implications for prevention. *Child Abuse & Neglect* 36(2):156-165.

Feehan, C. J., J. Burnham, Q. Harris, and R. Jamieson. 1995. Debate and argument who participates in child sexual abuse research? *Journal of Child Psychology and Psychiatry* 36(8):1475-1476.

Feiring, C., and M. Zielinski. 2011. Looking back and looking forward: A review and reflection on research articles published in child maltreatment from 1996 through 2010. *Child Maltreatment* 16(1):3-8.

Felitti, V. J., R. F. Anda, D. Nordenberg, D. F. Williamson, A. M. Spitz, V. Edwards, M. P. Koss, and J. S. Marks. 1998. Relationship of childhood abuse and household dysfunction to many of the leading causes of death in adults. The Adverse Childhood Experiences (ACE) study. *American Journal of Preventive Medicine* 14(4):245-258.

Ferrari, A. M. 2002. The impact of culture upon child rearing practices and definitions of maltreatment. *Child Abuse & Neglect* 26(8):793-813.

Finkelhor, D., R. K. Ormrod, and H. A. Turner. 2009. Lifetime assessment of poly-victimization in a national sample of children and youth. *Child Abuse & Neglect* 33(7):403-411.

Flaherty, E. G., R. Thompson, A. J. Litrownik, A. J. Zolotor, H. Dubowitz, D. K. Runyan, D. J. English, and M. D. Everson. 2009. Adverse childhood exposures and reported child health at age 12. *Academic Pediatrics* 9(3):150-156.

Fletcher, R., S. Fletcher, and E. Wagner. 2005. *Clinical epidemiology: The essentials*, 4th ed. Baltimore, MD: Lippincott Williams & Wilkins.

Fontes, L. A. 2002. Child discipline and physical abuse in immigrant latino families: Reducing violence and misunderstandings. *Journal of Counseling and Development* 80(1):31-40.

Fuhua, Z., and G. Qin. 2009. Child maltreatment among Asian Americans: Characteristics and explanatory framework. *Child Maltreatment* 14(2):207-224.

Gainsborough, J. F. 2010. *Scandalous politics: Child welfare policy in the states (American governance and public policy series)*. Washington, DC: Georgetown University Press.

Gallmeier, T. M., and B. L. Bonner. 1992. University-based interdisciplinary training in child abuse and neglect. *Child Abuse & Neglect* 16(4):513-521.

GAO (Government Accountability Office). 2008. *Residential facilities: Improved data and enhanced oversight would help safe-guard the well-being of youth with behavioral and emotional challenges*. Washington, DC: GAO.

GAO. 2011. *Child maltreatment: Strengthening national data on child fatalities could aid in prevention*. Washington, DC: GAO.

Germán, M., N. A. Gonzales, and L. Dumka. 2009. Familism values as a protective factor for Mexican-origin adolescents exposed to deviant peers. *Journal of Early Adolescence* 29(1):16-42.

Gilbert, R., J. Fluke, M. O'Donnell, A. Gonzalez-Izquierdo, M. Brownell, P. Gulliver, S. Janson, and P. Sidebotham. 2012. Child maltreatment: Variation in trends and policies in six developed countries. *Lancet* 379(9817):758-772.

Greeley, C. S. 2012. The evolution of the child maltreatment literature. *Pediatrics* 130(2): 347-348.

Greene, K. M., K. Hynes, and E. A. Doyle. 2011. Self-care among school-aged children of immigrants. *Children and Youth Services Review* 33(5):783-789.

Grossman, A. H., and A. R. D'Augelli. 2006. Transgender youth. *Journal of Homosexuality* 51(1):111-128.

Grossman, A. H., and A. R. D'Augelli. 2007. Transgender youth and life-threatening behaviors. *Suicide and Life-Threatening Behavior* 37(5):527-537.

Hafford, C. 2010. Sibling caretaking in immigrant families: Understanding cultural practices to inform child welfare practice and evaluation. *Evaluation and Program Planning* 33(3):294-302.

Haskett, M. E., B. Marziano, and E. R. Dover. 1996. Absence of males in maltreatment research: A survey of recent literature. *Child Abuse & Neglect* 20(12):1175-1182.

Haskins, R., and J. Baron. 2011. *Building the connection between policy and evidence: The Obama evidence-based initiatives*. London, UK: NESTA.

Heyman, R., and A. Slep. 2012. Panel on select populations. Paper read at Presentation to the Committee on Child Maltreatment Research, Policy, and Practice for the Next Decade, December 10, Washington, DC.

Hibbard, R. A., L. W. Desch, Committee on Child Abuse and Neglect, and Council on Children with Disabilities. 2007. Maltreatment of children with disabilities. *Pediatrics* 119(5):1018-1025.

Hymel, K. P., K. L. Makoroff, A. L. Laskey, M. R. Conaway, and J. A. Blackman. 2007. Mechanisms, clinical presentations, injuries, and outcomes from inflicted versus noninflicted head trauma during infancy: Results of a prospective, multicentered, comparative study. *Pediatrics* 119(5):922-929.

IASWR (Institute for the Advancement of Social Work Research). 2008. *Strengthening university/agency research partnerships to enhance child welfare outcomes: A toolkit for building research partnerships.* http://www.socialworkpolicy.org/wp-content/uploads/2007/06/9-IASWR-CW-Research-Partners.pdf (accessed November 26, 2013).

IOM (Institute of Medicine). 2001. *Confronting chronic neglect: The education and training of health professionals on family violence.* Washington, DC: National Academy Press.

IOM. 2004. *NIH extramural center programs: Criteria for initiation and evaluation.* Washington, DC: The National Academies Press.

IOM. 2011. *The health of lesbian, gay, bisexual, and transgender people: Building a foundation for better understanding.* Washington, DC: The National Academies Press.

IOM and NRC (National Research Council). 2011. *Improving access to oral health care for vulnerable and underserved populations.* Washington, DC: The National Academies Press.

IOM and NRC. 2012. *Child maltreatment research, policy, and practice for the next decade: Workshop summary.* Washington, DC: The National Academies Press.

Jayaratne, S., T. Croxton, and D. Mattison. 2004. A national survey of violence in the practice of social work. *Families in Society* 85(4):445-453.

Jent, J. F., C. K. Eaton, L. Knickerbocker, W. F. Lambert, M. T. Merrick, and S. K. Dandes. 2011. Multidisciplinary child protection decision making about physical abuse: Determining substantiation thresholds and biases. *Children and Youth Services Review* 33(9):1673-1682.

Jonson-Reid, M., and B. Drake. 2008. Multisector longitudinal administrative databases an indispensable tool for evidence-based policy for maltreated children and their families. *Child Maltreatment* 13(4):392-399.

Kaufman, J., B.-Z. Yang, H. Douglas-Palumberi, S. Houshyar, D. Lipschitz, J. H. Krystal, and J. Gelernter. 2004. Social supports and serotonin transporter gene moderate depression in maltreated children. *Proceedings of the National Academy of Sciences of the United States of America* 101(49):17316-17321.

Kaufman, J., B.-Z. Yang, H. Douglas-Palumberi, D. Grasso, D. Lipschitz, S. Houshyar, J. H. Krystal, and J. Gelernter. 2006. Brain-derived neurotrophic factor–5-HTTLPR gene interactions and environmental modifiers of depression in children. *Biological Psychiatry* 59(8):673-680.

Kellogg, N. 2005. The evaluation of sexual abuse in children. *Pediatrics* 116(2):506-512.

Kemp, A. M., F. Dunstan, S. Harrison, S. Morris, M. Mann, K. Rolfe, S. Datta, D. P. Thomas, J. R. Sibert, and S. Maguire. 2008. Patterns of skeletal fractures in child abuse: Systematic review. *British Medical Journal* 337.

Kitzman, H., D. L. Olds, C. R. Henderson, C. Hanks, R. Cole, R. Tatelbaum, K. M. McConnochie, K. Sidora, D. W. Luckey, and D. Shaver. 1997. Effect of prenatal and infancy home visitation by nurses on pregnancy outcomes, childhood injuries, and repeated childbearing. *Journal of the American Medical Association* 278(8):644-652.

Knight, E. D., J. B. Smith, H. Dubowitz, A. J. Litrownik, J. B. Kotch, D. English, M. D. Everson, and D. K. Runyan. 2006. Reporting participants in research studies to child protective services: Limited risk to attrition. *Child Maltreatment* 11(3):257-262.

Korbin, J. E. 2002. Culture and child maltreatment: Cultural competence and beyond. *Child Abuse & Neglect* 26(6):637-644.

Korbin, J. E., and J. C. Spilsbury. 1999. Cultural competence and child neglect. In *Neglected children: Research, practice, and policy*, edited by H. Dubowitz. Thousand Oaks, CA: Sage Publications. Pp. 69-88.

Korbin, J. E., C. J. Coulton, S. Chard, C. Platt-Houston, and M. Su. 1998. Impoverishment and child maltreatment in african American and European American neighborhoods. *Development and Psychopathology* 10(2):215-233.

Krugman, R. D., J. E. Korbin, and C. H. Kempe. 2013. *C. Henry Kempe: A 50 year legacy to the field of child abuse and neglect*. New York: Springer-Verlag.

Lau, A. S. 2006. Making the case for selective and directed cultural adaptations of evidence-based treatments: Examples from parent training. *Clinical Psychology: Science and Practice* 13(4):295-310.

LeBlanc, V. R., C. Regehr, A. Shlonsky, and M. Bogo. 2012. Stress responses and decision making in child protection workers faced with high conflict situations. *Child Abuse & Neglect* 36(5):404-412.

Leventhal, J. M., B. W. Forsyth, K. Qi, L. Johnson, D. Schroeder, and N. Votto. 1997. Maltreatment of children born to women who used cocaine during pregnancy: A population-based study. *Pediatrics* 100(2):e7.

Lightfoot, E. B., and T. L. LaLiberte. 2006. Approaches to child protection case management for cases involving people with disabilities. *Child Abuse & Neglect* 30(4):381-391.

Lynch, D. L., A. E. Stern, R. Kim Oates, and B. I. O'Toole. 1993. Who participates in child sexual abuse research? *Journal of Child Psychology and Psychiatry* 34(6):935-944.

MacMillan, H. L., E. Jamieson, C. N. Wathen, M. H. Boyle, C. A. Walsh, J. Omura, J. M. Walker, and G. Lodenquai. 2007. Development of a policy-relevant child maltreatment research strategy. *Milbank Quarterly* 85(2):337-374.

McEwen, E., B. George, D. Weiner, and T. Fuller. 2011. *Building and sustaining university-agency research partnerships: Lessons from the trenches in Illinois*. Paper presented at National Child Welfare Evaluation Summit, Washington, DC.

Medina, S. P., K. Sell, J. Kavanagh, C. Curtis, and J. N. Wood. 2012. *Tracking child abuse and neglect: The role of multiple data sources in improving child safety*. Philadelphia, PA: Policy Lab, Children's Hospital of Philadelphia.

Melton, G. B. 2005. Mandated reporting: A policy without reason. *Child Abuse & Neglect* 29:9-18.

The National Congress of American Indians. 2009. *Research that benefits native people: A guide for tribal leaders*. http://www.ncaiprc.org/research-curriculum-guide (accessed October 18, 2013).

National Council on Disability. 2012. *Rocking the cradle: Ensuring the rights of parents with disabilities and their children*. Washington, DC: National Council on Disability.

Nelson, H., P. Nygren, and Y. McInerney. 2004. *Screening for family and intimate partner violence systematic evidence review number 28 (contract no. 290-97-0018)*. Portland: Oregon Health and Science University Evidence-based Practice Center

NRC (National Research Council). 1993. *Understanding child abuse and neglect*. Washington, DC: National Academy Press.

Olds, D. L., C. R. Henderson, R. Chamberlin, and R. Tatelbaum. 1986. Preventing child abuse and neglect: A randomized trial of nurse home visitation. *Pediatrics* 78(1):65-78.

Olds, D. L., H. Kitzman, C. Hanks, R. Cole, E. Anson, K. Sidora-Arcoleo, D. W. Luckey, C. R. Henderson, J. Holmberg, and R. A. Tutt. 2007. Effects of nurse home visiting on maternal and child functioning: Age-9 follow-up of a randomized trial. *Pediatrics* 120(4):e832-e845.

Proctor, S. N., and S. T. Azar. 2013. The effect of parental intellectual disability status on child protection service worker decision making. *Journal of Intellectual Disability Research* 57(12):1104-1116.

Puddy, R. W., and N. Wilkins. 2011. *Understanding evidence part 1: Best available research evidence. A guide to the continuum of evidence of effectiveness.* Atlanta, GA: CDC.

Putnam, K. T., W. W. Harris, and F. W. Putnam. 2013. Synergistic childhood adversities and complex adult psychopathology. *Journal of Traumatic Stress* 26(4):435-442.

Putnam-Hornstein, E., D. Webster, B. Needell, and J. Magruder. 2011. A public health approach to child maltreatment surveillance: Evidence from a data linkage project in the United States. *Child Abuse Review* 20(4):256-273.

Putnam-Hornstein, E., B. Needell, and A. E. Rhodes. 2013. Understanding risk and protective factors for child maltreatment: The value of integrated, population-based data. *Child Abuse & Neglect* 37(2-3):116-119.

Rivera, S., and M. A. D. Arellano. 2008. Culturally modified trauma-focused treatment for hispanic children: Preliminary findings. Paper read at 22nd Annual San Diego International Conference on Child and Family Maltreatment, January, San Diego, CA.

Roditti, M. G. 2005. Understanding communities of neglectful parents: Child caregiving networks and child neglect. *Child Welfare* 84(2):277.

Rogoff, B. 2003. *The cultural nature of human development.* New York: Oxford University Press.

Runyan, D. K., P. A. Curtis, W. M. Hunter, M. M. Black, J. B. Kotch, S. Bangdiwala, H. Dubowitz, D. English, M. D. Everson, and J. Landsverk. 1998. LONGSCAN: A consortium for longitudinal studies of maltreatment and the life course of children. *Aggression and Violent Behavior* 3(3):275-285.

Runyan, C. W., S. Hargarten, D. Hemenway, C. Peek-Asa, R. M. Cunningham, J. Costich, and A. C. Gielen. 2010. An urgent call to action in support of injury control research centers. *American Journal of Preventive Medicine* 39(1):89-92.

Saewyc, E. M., C. L. Skay, S. L. Pettingell, E. A. Reis, L. Bearinger, M. Resnick, A. Murphy, and L. Combs. 2006. Hazards of stigma: The sexual and physical abuse of gay, lesbian, and bisexual adolescents in the United States and Canada. *Child Welfare* 85(2):195-213.

Sahota, P. C. 2010. *Community-based participatory research in American Indian and Alaska native communities.* http://www.ncaiprc.org/files/CBPR%20Paper%20FINAL.pdf (accessed October 18, 2013).

SAMHSA (Substance Abuse and Mental Health Services Administration). 2013. *SAMHSA's National Registry of Evidence-based Programs and Practices.* http://www.nrepp.samhsa.gov/Index.aspx (accessed November 26, 2013).

Saunders, B. E., L. Berliner, and R. F. Hanson. 2004. *Child physical and sexual abuse: Guidelines for treatment.* Charleston, SC: National Crime Victims Research and Treatment Center.

Schilling-Wolfe, D. 2010. *Using technology to improve child welfare outcomes: Pilot project completed.* Philadelphia, PA: The Field Center for Children's Policy, Practice and Research.

Schnitzer, P. G., P. Slusher, and M. Van Tuinen. 2004. Child maltreatment in Missouri: Combining data for public health surveillance. *American Journal of Preventive Medicine* 27(5):379-384.

Sedlak, A. J. 1988. *Second National Incidence Study of Children Abuse and Neglect (NIS-2).* Washington, DC: U.S. Department of Health and Human Services.

Sedlak, A. J., S. D. Broadhurst, G. Shapiro, G. Kalton, H. Goksel, J. Burke, and J. Brown. 1997. *Third National Incidence Study of Child Abuse and Neglect (NIS-3).* Rockville, MD: U.S. Department of Health and Human Services.

Sedlak, A. J., J. Mettenburg, M. Basena, I. Petta, K. McPherson, A. Greene, and S. Li. 2010. *Fourth National Incidence Study of Children Abuse and Neglect (NIS-4): Report to Congress.* Washington, DC: U.S. Department of Health and Human Services, Administration for Children and Families.

Selph, S. S., C. Bougatsos, I. Blazina, and H. D. Nelson. 2013. Behavioral interventions and counseling to prevent child abuse and neglect: A systematic review to update the U.S. Preventive Services Task Force recommendation. *Annals of Internal Medicine* 158(3): 179-190.

Silverman, W. K., C. D. Ortiz, C. Viswesvaran, B. J. Burns, D. J. Kolko, F. W. Putnam, and L. Amaya-Jackson. 2008. Evidence-based psychosocial treatments for children and adolescents exposed to traumatic events. *Journal of Clinical Child and Adolescent Psychology* 37(1):156-183.

Socolar, R. S., D. K. Runyan, and L. Amaya-Jackson. 1995. Methodological and ethical issues related to studying child maltreatment. *Journal of Family Issues* 16(5):565-586.

Stokes, J., and G. Schmidt. 2012. Child protection decision making: A factorial analysis using case vignettes. *Social Work* 57(1):83-90.

Straus, M. A., S. L. Hamby, D. Finkelhor, D. W. Moore, and D. Runyan. 1998. Identification of child maltreatment with the parent-child conflict tactics scales: Development and psychometric data for a national sample of American parents. *Child Abuse & Neglect: The International Journal* 22(4):249-270.

Testa, M. F. 2012. Fostering innovation through Title IV-E waiver demonstrations. *Policy & Practice* 70(3):28-30, 48.

Trickett, P. K., J. G. Noll, and F. W. Putnam. 2011. The impact of sexual abuse on female development: Lessons from a multigenerational, longitudinal research study. *Development and Psychopathology* 23(2):453-476.

Walters, K. L., P. F. Horwath, and J. M. Simoni. 2001. Sexual orientation bias experiences and service needs of gay, lesbian, bisexual, transgendered, and two-spirited American Indians. *Journal of Gay & Lesbian Social Services* 13(1-2):133-149.

Waters, M. C., and J. E. Sykes. 2009. Spare the rod, ruin the child. First- and second-generation West Indian childrearing practices. In *Across generations: Immigrant families in America,* edited by N. Foner. New York: New York University Press. Pp. 72-97.

Weisner, T. S. 2002. Ecocultural understanding of children's developmental pathways. *Human Development* 45(4):275-281.

Whitaker, D. J., J. R. Lutzker, and G. A. Shelley. 2005. Child maltreatment prevention priorities at the Centers for Disease Control and Prevention. *Child Maltreatment* 10(3): 245-259.

WHO (World Health Organization). 2013. *Prevention of child maltreatment: WHO scales up child maltreatment prevention activities.* http://www.who.int/violence_injury_prevention/violence/activities/child_maltreatment/en/index.html (accessed November 26, 2013).

Widom, C. S., K. G. Raphael, and K. A. DuMont. 2004. The case for prospective longitudinal studies in child maltreatment research: Commentary on Dube, Williamson, Thompson, Telitti, and Anda (2004). *Child Abuse & Neglect* 28(7):715-722.

Yang, C. Y., T. Sato, N. Yamawaki, and M. Miyata. 2013. Prevalence and risk factors of problematic Internet use: A cross-national comparison of Japanese and Chinese university students. *Transcultural Psychiatry* 50(2):263-269.

Yoshikawa, H. 2011. *Immigrants raising citizens: Undocumented parents and their young children.* New York: Russell Sage Foundation.

8

Child Abuse and Neglect Policy

Since the 1993 National Research Council (NRC) report was published, numerous changes have been made to federal and state laws and policies designed to impact the incidence, reporting, and negative health and economic consequences of child abuse and neglect. This chapter reviews the foundations for the development of child abuse and neglect law and policy and describes the current environment of laws and policies related to child abuse and neglect at both the federal and state levels. Also discussed is the evaluation and analysis of these laws and policies. Related research needs are detailed as well.

Policy change in the child protection arena frequently has resulted from a synergistic set of factors: (1) the development of and reporting on evidence that a specific practice reform has had a positive impact, (2) the existence of one or more models or demonstrations of successful implementation of such reforms, and (3) a combination of clinician and advocacy community support for legislation that further promotes the reforms. Thus, for example, it was these factors that led to federal legislative policy reform making voluntary home visiting more widely available through Section 2951 of the Patient Protection and Affordable Care Act. This Maternal, Infant, and Early Childhood Home Visiting Program is designed to strengthen and improve related programs and activities, improve coordination of services for at-risk communities, and identify and provide evidence-based home visiting programs that can improve outcomes for families residing in at-risk communities.

Although the scope of what constitutes "policy" includes both legislation and government agency regulations, protocols, and so on, this chapter addresses primarily the evolution of federal and state laws on child abuse and neglect as they affect knowledge and practice. Regulations and protocols are typical results of the process of implementing laws at the state and local levels. However, a nonstatutory "policy" reform can also be national in scope. Examples are the recommendations for policy reform issued in the early to mid-1990s by the U.S. Advisory Board on Child Abuse and Neglect.

For example, recommendation 13 of the Advisory Board's first report, *Child Abuse and Neglect: Critical First Steps in Response to a National Emergency* (U.S. Advisory Board on Child Abuse and Neglect, 1990, p. 138), calls on the Secretary of Health and Human Services (HHS) to "launch a major coordinated initiative involving all relevant components of the Department of Health and Human Services to promote the systematic conduct of research related to child abuse and neglect." The Advisory Board's second report, *Creating Caring Communities: Blueprint for an Effective Federal Policy on Child Abuse and Neglect* (U.S. Advisory Board on Child Abuse and Neglect, 1991) focuses on the broad federal government response to child abuse and neglect. The report calls for enactment of a "National Child Protection Policy," one goal of which would be to drive the child protection–related actions of all federal agencies. The report includes a nine-page "Proposed National Child Protection Policy" and a call for an appropriate federal research agency to determine the cost of implementing such a policy, as well as the cost of not doing so. To help prevent child abuse and neglect, the report's recommendations also include the first call by a blue-ribbon federal panel for national implementation of universal voluntary neonatal home visitation (what the report calls a "dramatic new federal initiative aimed at preventing child maltreatment"). Included as well are four pages of recommendations for improving federally supported research and evaluation related to child abuse and neglect.

The Advisory Board's fourth report, *Neighbors Helping Neighbors: A New National Strategy for the Protection of Children* (U.S. Advisory Board on Child Abuse and Neglect, 1993), again addresses federal research policy, calling on federal agencies to subject federally supported child protection activities to rigorous evaluation; calling on the National Institute of Mental Health to solicit research aimed at clarifying the relationships among social support, culture, and child abuse and neglect; and urging that federally supported research also assess children's, parents', neighbors', and workers' own experiences of the context in which child abuse and neglect occurs and their perceptions of systemic responses to the problem.

At its core, the debate around the development of laws and policies to help prevent child abuse and neglect involves questions of public value (Pecora et al., 2000). It also involves trade-offs entailed in law making between public benefit and private interests. For example:

- What is the balance between children's fundamental right to be safe and parents' right to raise their children as they see fit?
- Should the government's role be to offer families, on a voluntary basis, services related to the protection of their children, or to force families to accept services they could construe as unwanted government intrusion into family life?
- How can policy promote fairness in child protective interventions, recognizing, for example, that some families come from different cultures whose practices may not coincide with what is covered by child protection laws?
- What is the appropriate balance between the due process rights of parents not to have child abuse or neglect case records preserved by child protection agencies in cases that are very old or in which a report of abuse or neglect was not substantiated and the authority of states to maintain appropriate central registries of child abuse and neglect case-related data that might later be used as part of child protection efforts?

The development of child abuse and neglect laws and policies should include the application of reason, evidence, and an evaluative framework to such decisions (Pecora et al., 2000). The application of *reason* refers to public discourse by practitioners, advocates, researchers, and legislators (Pecora et al., 2000). The *evidence* for passing laws and changing public policy is derived from a variety of sources, some explicitly guided by research and scientific evidence and others reflecting social consensus about legitimate government activity. For example, even though research evidence suggests that lengthy incarceration for acts of violence is not always necessary for community safety, it is widely supported by citizens because of the societal functions of punishment for wrongdoing and justice for victims.

The *evaluative framework* for child abuse and neglect laws and policies lies with the ability to anticipate and deal with a series of predictable problems that occur as a result of the laws' and policies' implementation. Research helps answer questions when those answers are critical to effective implementation. For example:

- Is banning the behavior targeted in legislation, such as certain forms of corporal punishment that are most likely to cause serious injury to a child, likely to reduce the rate of child abuse and neglect-related fatalities?
- Are safe haven laws (permitting a mother to, without legal consequence, abandon a newborn child safely) constructed so as to reduce the number of child abandonments and even deaths of unwanted children that would have occurred in the laws' absence?

- Are there sufficient resources to educate those persons included in a law as mandated reporters of child abuse and neglect, and what is the impact of changing the requirements for who must report or what must be reported?
- Is there sufficient public support for changing the definition of what constitutes child abuse and neglect under state law?

Given these complexities, the research design needed to evaluate laws and policies is not always the same as the design one would use to evaluate *practice* interventions. Although some laws and policies can be evaluated by random assignment (e.g., studying the differential response approach of social services in responding to child abuse and neglect reports), random assignment cannot be used if it would differentially affect the legal rights of citizens, if it would subject citizens to unequal treatment under the law, or if it would place children in jeopardy. Furthermore, simply studying the incidence of child abuse and neglect in the aggregate (such as at the state or national level) is unlikely to aid in determining and attributing its potential causes.

Another difficulty in evaluating laws and policies related to child abuse and neglect is that adherence to a law, such as a mandatory reporting law, often is predicated on public knowledge, understanding, and support that frequently vary across practitioner disciplines, as well as within and among states. Finally, many of the changes in child abuse and neglect laws and policies over the last few decades have been incremental changes to existing legislation (such as the federal Child Abuse Prevention and Treatment Act [CAPTA]). In those cases, what is needed in terms of law and policy analysis or evaluation is research on the implementation and augmentation of the law or policy, rather than the core law or policy itself.

Given these difficulties in conducting analyses of laws and policies and the fact that laws and policies vary by state, the paucity of research in this area is unsurprising.

THE POLICY LANDSCAPE

Federal and state laws define what constitutes the abuse and neglect of children. They also designate those who must report suspected child abuse and neglect, or make all citizens with reason to suspect abuse and neglect mandated reporters. State laws addressing the abuse and neglect of children were passed in all 50 states following the 1962 amendments to the Social Security Act that required all states to include child protection in their child welfare systems (Myers, 2008). At the same time, the 1962 article "The Battered Child Syndrome" (Kempe et al., 1962, 1985) gave rise to public concern that many voluntary societies for the prevention of cruelty to children were disappearing, having been largely replaced by government counterparts known today as child protective services agencies.

In 1974, passage of CAPTA[1] established state responsibilities for child protection and supported the execution of these responsibilities with new federal money for state programs and national research. CAPTA has been reauthorized multiple times, most recently in 2010 (CWIG, 2011a). As discussed below, CAPTA provided a federal definition of child abuse and neglect and set into motion a series of reforms of state laws, policies, and practices.

One direct consequence of CAPTA was the establishment within HHS of a National Center on Child Abuse and Neglect. This center was subsequently made an office with, unfortunately, far fewer staff, as a part of reorganization within the department. CAPTA also created authority for the aforementioned U.S. Advisory Board on Child Abuse and Neglect,[2] a blue-ribbon expert panel, but after releasing four reports, it was disbanded and never revived.

Some support for child abuse and neglect research has continued to be provided by the Office on Child Abuse and Neglect. However, policy-related research continues to be extremely underdeveloped. Important research-appropriate policy issues affecting hundreds of thousands of children annually relate to such topics as

- mandatory reporting;
- child abuse central registries (record-keeping repositories) and related issues of constitutional rights;
- education of potential child abuse and neglect reporters, sometimes tied to health professional licensing;
- the use of safety and risk assessment instruments by child protective services agency personnel;
- training in child abuse and neglect and family violence in medical and other professional schools;
- organization of child protection service delivery at the state or county government level;
- adoption of new approaches to working with families in which child abuse and neglect is suspected, such as differential response and family group decision making;
- in increasing numbers of states, replacing the traditional process of making substantiation decisions in all cases of reported child abuse and neglect that are investigated with an assessment process that does not label parents as having abused or neglected their child;

---

[1]U.S.C. 42 § 62.
[2]U.S.C. 42 § 5102.

- use of kinship foster care as an alternative to traditional foster care;
- emphasis on the safety, permanency, and well-being of children after termination of parental rights; and
- the appropriate role for law enforcement and the courts in helping families care for their children and in helping to ensure that children's safety, permanency, and well-being needs are addressed.

Some policy changes appear never to be questioned, even in the absence of evidence to support their wisdom. These changes include instituting or broadening the scope of mandated reporting of suspected child abuse and neglect. Policy research could and should assess the likely consequences before policy changes are made—for example, when a definition of abuse or neglect is broadened to include children who are witnesses to or otherwise exposed to domestic violence in the home.

Since the 1993 NRC report was issued, a variety of controversies have arisen that strongly suggest the need for additional policy-related research. These include, for example, concerns about racial and socioeconomic bias in the making of child abuse and neglect reports (Drake and Zuravin, 1998; Drake et al., 2011; Lane et al., 2002; Magruder and Shaw, 2008) and wide variation in the interpretation of legal requirements by mandated reporters for reporting reasonable suspicion of child abuse or neglect (Levi and Brown, 2005). It is critical that legislators and program administrators support research designed to carefully examine the federal and state laws that guide responses to child abuse and neglect and build a new knowledge base to guide the implementation of policy changes.

FEDERAL LAWS AND POLICIES

This section reviews key federal laws and policies designed to address the incidence and consequences of child abuse and neglect that have been enacted over the last several decades and suggests areas in which future research is needed.

The Child Abuse Prevention and Treatment Act

In 1974, CAPTA[3] authorized, among other things, very modest funds for a state grant program focused on initial child protective intervention in cases of suspected abuse or neglect; Congress has since appropriated these funds annually. Despite the limited funding they have received, all states have made significant changes to their child abuse and neglect legislation as mandated by CAPTA's eligibility requirements. CAPTA has been reau-

[3]42 U.S.C. § 5101 et seq.

thorized every 4-8 years since 1974 (CWIG, 2011a), and reauthorizations have nearly always modified or added new eligibility conditions; as a result, the language of state laws has undergone continual changes to comply with CAPTA.

Definitions in CAPTA

CAPTA sets 18 as the age up to which states must have laws on reporting of child abuse and neglect that mandate a child protection system response. The committee knows of no research on how states and counties respond to reports of abuse or neglect involving older teens, or on what child protection agency practices best address youth aged 16 or 17 who are reported as suspected victims for the first time.

CAPTA also limits the term "abuse and neglect" to acts or failures to act by parents or caretakers. Some states do not so limit the perpetrators of abuse and neglect, but include reporting of child abuse and neglect allegedly committed by those outside of the child's home (as a recent example, sports coaches). The CAPTA limitation on who a perpetrator of abuse and neglect may be results in many states having skewed data on child abuse, especially child sexual abuse, because only intrafamilial incidents may be reported in many states. The committee knows of no research that has looked at how a state's definition of a perpetrator of abuse and neglect affects children's protection from abuse and neglect overall.

In one of its periodic congressional reauthorizations, CAPTA also gave states the option of mandating reporting of only those acts, or failures to act, of alleged abuse and neglect that are recent and that have resulted in physical or emotional harm to the child that is considered serious. Although few states have such limiting language in their definitions of what must be reported, there is no evidence on whether this limiting language results in abused and neglected children falling through the cracks or whether child protective services agencies receive large numbers of reports in which the harm to children is not considered serious.

Likewise, the committee has seen no research on how the CAPTA definition of sexual abuse, which was broadened to include acts related to the production of child pornography, statutory rape, and prostitution of children, has affected the protection of those children. Given the wider recognition of and concern about child sexual victimization, research on the impact of states having this broadened language on reportable sex crimes involving children would be most helpful.

Still another expanded definition of what is understood to be child abuse and neglect, and again one that has not to the committee's knowledge been studied, is the inclusion of a form of medical neglect, or the "withholding of medically indicated treatment of disabled infants with life-threatening conditions." These have been referred to as "Baby Doe" cases, and a great deal of attention was originally focused on a few cases of severely disabled infants in hospitals who died after allegedly being deprived of treatment (U.S. Advisory Board on Child Abuse and Neglect, 1991). The Baby Doe provision of CAPTA remains in effect, but the committee could find no research on the frequency, outcomes, or cost of handling these cases. This type of case is different from the more general "medical neglect" of a child's health needs, which sometimes leads to child protective interventions. There are occasionally religious reasons for withholding treatment (e.g., parents who refuse a blood transfusion, transplant, cancer treatment, etc., on religious grounds). CAPTA requires states to have processes in place whereby a court can order treatment in these circumstances. Another "medical neglect" issue potentially arises in cases where infants are left in neonatal intensive care units for weeks or months at a time, and their parents fail to visit. The committee is unaware of research related to any of these issues.

Title I of CAPTA

The State Grant Program under CAPTA is for "improving the child protective services system" of each state, specifically by supporting a wide range of comprehensive activities. To obtain CAPTA funding to support their child protective services programs, states must comply with congressionally mandated eligibility conditions. Not counting the Baby Doe (protection of severely disabled newborns) response requirement described above, CAPTA currently includes more than 20 requirements for state laws or statewide programs that must be met for a state to receive an annual State Grant. During the years since these provisions were incorporated into federal law, little to no investment has been made in studying how these requirements are best implemented.

State legislatures have continually added to these provisions, in different ways. For example, state legislatures have broadened the scope of who must report suspected child abuse and neglect, penalized the making of false reports of abuse and neglect, extended access to child protective services records to members of multidisciplinary child protection teams, required cross reporting of cases by child protective services to the police (and vice versa), and required that a child's guardian ad litem be an attorney. Again, little or no investment has been made in research to learn whether these changes better protect children.

Few of these changes to CAPTA have ever been examined scientifically with respect to their positive or negative impact. For example, one change to CAPTA mandated hospital referrals to child protective services when infants are born with and identified as being affected by illegal substance abuse, even though the birth of a drug-exposed newborn is generally, in and of itself, not legally considered abuse or neglect. The latest 2010 reauthorization of CAPTA added to this requirement a referral to child protective services for children born with a fetal alcohol spectrum disorder (Children's Bureau, 2011).

Research is similarly lacking on the implementation of other additions to CAPTA's eligibility requirements. They include (1) a requirement for public disclosure of findings or information in cases of child abuse and neglect-related fatalities or near fatalities, (2) prompt expungement of child protective services records for certain purposes when reports are determined to be unsubstantiated or false, (3) a mechanism for individuals who disagree with an official finding of abuse or neglect to appeal that finding, (4) a requirement for child protective services employees to advise adults accused of abuse or neglect of the allegations made against them at the time of initial contact with child protective services, (5) mandated training of child protective services caseworkers on their legal duties to protect the rights of children and families, and (6) a requirement for every child under age 3 who is substantiated as an abuse or neglect victim to be referred for early intervention services funded under Part C of the federal Individuals with Disabilities Education Act (IDEA).

Some other CAPTA eligibility requirements track emerging best practices in the field. Except for the support of the Children's Bureau in studying the implementation of differential response and some statewide studies of that practice reform, however, the committee is unaware of any investment in research to determine how these CAPTA-promoted best practices are being implemented across the country.

One eligibility requirement of CAPTA that has been studied involves important state citizen oversight of child protective services. Every state must establish and maintain "citizen review panels" to examine the policies, procedures, and practices of child protective services. Panel examination is supposed to include a review of handling of specific cases and the extent to which child protective services is effectively discharging its responsibilities. Although research has examined the impact of these panels, further study of how their recommendations have or have not resulted in positive reforms of their states' child protection systems is needed.

Discrepancies/Issues with Reported Child Abuse and Neglect Data

CAPTA mandates that states annually provide "to the maximum extent practicable" a data report that now (since the 2010 CAPTA reauthorization) includes 16 separate types of data (Children's Bureau, 2011). Some of the required data are straightforward, such as (1) the number of children reported as suspected child abuse and neglect victims; (2) the number of those reports that were substantiated, unsubstantiated, or determined to be false; (3) the number of child abuse and neglect-related deaths, both in the children's homes and in foster care; and (4) the number of child protective services personnel in different categories (e.g., intake, investigation), their average caseload, and their education and qualifications and training requirements. Compiling accurate data on other data elements is more difficult, and research is needed to determine how states can better collect these data. Examples include (1) the number of substantiated child victims receiving or not receiving services; (2) the number of children removed from their home, organized by disposition of their cases; (3) the number of families receiving "preventative services"; (4) child protective services response times, from initial investigation to provision of services; (5) the number of children reunited with their family after foster placement; and (6) cases in which a family received "family preservation services," but within 5 years was the subject of further reports of abuse or neglect or a child fatality.

Several additional data elements required by CAPTA are even more difficult to collect. They include data on (1) the number of children provided a court-appointed advocate in their abuse and neglect cases, and those advocates' average number of out-of-court contacts with their child clients; (2) the number of children under the care of the child welfare system who were transferred into the custody of the juvenile justice system (what are called "crossover youth"); (3) the number of children referred to child protective services for prenatal drug or alcohol exposure; and (4) the number of children eligible for referral to the Part C IDEA program, as well as the number actually referred. Again, a study of best practices for accurately collecting these data would be helpful to the states.

Other Components of CAPTA Needing Policy Implementation Research

Children's Justice Act CAPTA includes two additional state grant programs. The first is a program funded through the U.S. Department of Justice but implemented by the Children's Bureau. Known as the Children's Justice Act, its formal name is Grants to States for Programs Relating to Investigation and Prosecution of Child Abuse and Neglect Cases. As with the CAPTA State Grants and the State Prevention Grants (in Title II of CAPTA, discussed below), all states have been deemed eligible for, and receive, this funding. Although the legislation requires a comprehensive evaluation of the state's systems related to child maltreatment, there has been insufficient investment in examining how the goals of this part of CAPTA have or have not been adequately achieved.

CAPTA Title II Prevention Grants to states Title II of CAPTA provides grants to states in amounts greater than those provided under the Title I

State Grant Program. Called Community-Based Grants for the Prevention of Child Abuse or Neglect, the purpose of this funding is "to support community-based efforts to develop, operate, expand, enhance, and co-ordinate initiatives, programs, and activities to prevent child abuse and neglect and to support the coordination of resources and activities, to better strengthen and support families to reduce the likelihood of child abuse and neglect" and "to foster an understanding, appreciation, and knowledge of diverse populations in order to be effective in preventing and treating child abuse and neglect."

In contrast with the Title I State Grants, which lack an evaluation requirement, Title II requires that states "describe the results of evaluation, or the outcomes of monitoring, conducted under the State program to demonstrate the effectiveness of activities conducted under this title in meeting the purposes of the program." Although descriptive summaries of how some states have used these funds are available (Children's Bureau, 2013; Summers et al., 2011), the committee is unaware of any comprehensive examination/synthesis of these mandated evaluations or of any overall research on how Title II–funded programs have directly impacted the prevention of child abuse and neglect. Nor is the committee aware of any studies of how a focus on "diverse populations" may have led to improvements in preventing child abuse and neglect among different racial and ethnic groups.

CAPTA discretionary funding for demonstration projects Although it is very limited, each year CAPTA discretionary funding is used to support individual grants for state and local child abuse and neglect-related projects. CAPTA requires these discretionary grant projects "to be evaluated for their effectiveness." Funded projects must provide for such evaluations either as a stated percentage of their demonstration grant funding or as a separate grant or contract entered into by HHS for the purpose of evaluating that project or a group of projects. Because Congress has listed discrete areas for demonstration funding (and will likely add others in the future), it would be helpful to know more about whether the policy reforms suggested by prior congressionally enumerated grant areas have in fact been achieved. Therefore, it would again be helpful to the field if support were provided for a study examining these evaluations and their findings overall.

CAPTA research priorities set by Congress Congress has mandated that the Children's Bureau, "in consultation with other Federal agencies and recognized experts in the field, carry out a continuing interdisciplinary program of research, including longitudinal research, that is designed to provide information needed to better protect children from child abuse or neglect and to improve the well-being of victims of child abuse or neglect."[4] At least a portion of such research is to be field initiated. CAPTA lists the areas in which such child abuse and neglect research may be funded. This list of research areas raises two concerns. First, the extremely limited funding appropriated for research under CAPTA means that few of these areas will be topics of research grants. Second, there are many important areas on this list that have never been the subject of any CAPTA (or other federal) research grant funding, and these issues also need attention.

Need for Enhanced Research Funding

CAPTA has since 1974 been the federal law that most directly relates to, and provides very modest funding for, improved identification and intervention in cases of child abuse and neglect. However, CAPTA establishes expectations for actions by states' child protection systems that are too often largely unmet. At each periodic reauthorization of CAPTA, members of Congress have added provisions to the law requiring (through additions to State Grant eligibility requirements) that state and county child protective services systems do more, but always without providing any increased federal resources. The committee hopes the above discussion will serve as a roadmap for the administration and Congress to enhance the financial support provided under CAPTA. This enhanced funding is needed to expand the national child abuse and neglect research portfolio and provide the added knowledge required to achieve a significantly improved child protection system. (See also the detailed discussion of research funding in Chapter 7.)

The Victims of Child Abuse Act[5]

In addition to CAPTA, several other federal laws contain the words "child abuse" in their title or focus primarily on the immediate response to the identification of abused and neglected children. Originally enacted in 1990, for example, the Victims of Child Abuse Act (VCAA) has for more than two decades provided support for the work of children's advocacy centers (CACs) and enhancement of the prosecution of child abuse cases (through the National Center for the Prosecution of Child Abuse, a program of the National District Attorneys Association) (Subchapter I). The VCAA also has been a vehicle for funding of Court-Appointed Special Advocate (CASA) programs (Subchapter II) and training and technical assistance to judges who hear civil child protection (dependency) cases (through grants

---

[4]CAPTA Sec. 104, 42 U.S.C. 5105.
[5]42 U.S. Code Section 13001, et seq.

to the National Council of Juvenile and Family Court Judges) (Subchapter III). Each year since the VCAA became law, millions of dollars have been appropriated to support these activities. Although there have been evaluations of the effectiveness of CAC and CASA programs, as well as of the work of "Model Courts" supported with Subchapter III funding, there is a need for additional, independent scientific studies of the impact of these programs on the responses to child maltreatment. The VCAA has continued to be an essential funding mechanism for improvements in government reactions to reported and substantiated child maltreatment, but it is important now to allocate funds so that Congress can be better informed about the effectiveness of the reforms this law has long supported, which can best be accomplished through rigorous research.

Subchapter IV of the VCAA contains a federal requirement for reporting of child abuse (but not "neglect") that occurs on "Federal land or in a federally operated (or contracted) facility." This makes this provision, in essence, the federal lands equivalent of the state mandatory reporting law requirement of CAPTA. The VCAA language about reporting (i.e., what to report, when to report, who must report, cross-reporting obligations, immunity for reporters, penalties for failure to report, and training requirements for prospective reporters) is quite different from that in CAPTA. To the committee's knowledge, no research has been conducted on the operation or impact of this federal lands child abuse reporting law, including how the differences between its provisions and those of CAPTA impact child abuse reporting, investigation, and intervention.

The Child Victims' and Child Witnesses' Rights Law[6]

Also enacted in 1990, the Child Victims' and Child Witnesses' Rights law provides a framework for how child abuse victims who are involved in "Federal court prosecutions of offenders" are protected throughout the judicial process. The purpose of this legislation is to minimize the trauma experienced by child abuse victims as a result of their involvement in the federal criminal court system. Once again, the definitions in this law differ from the abuse definitions in CAPTA. The law authorizes federal judges to take a variety of measures to aid child victims or witnesses. These include, for example, (1) using alternatives to live in-court testimony of child victims, (2) setting limits on challenges to the competency of child witnesses, (3) providing privacy protections for child victims/witnesses, (4) describing special requirements related to child victim impact statements, (5) use of multidisciplinary child abuse teams, (6) appointment of a guardian ad litem for a child victim or witness, (7) allowing testifying children to have an

---

[6]18 U.S. Code Section 3509.

adult support person with them, and (8) establishing a procedure to ensure a speedy trial of child victim cases. Although this law was intended to reduce system-related child trauma, the committee is unaware of any studies of the implementation of its provisions.

Laws on Reporting and Responding to Child Abuse in Indian Country[7]

The Indian Child Protection and Family Violence Prevention Act of 1990 was enacted to address the perceived lack of reporting of child abuse and neglect by Indian nations. It established mandatory reporting of child abuse and neglect on Indian lands.[8] However, no regulations have ever been adopted under this act, and no funding is currently being provided for its implementation. Again, moreover, the definitions of child abuse in this act and in CAPTA differ. Unlike CAPTA, this act includes a prescribed criminal penalty for failing to report abuse and for inhibiting or preventing the making of a report (the latter is a provision not found in any of the other federal laws described). Congress also established a special procedure for dealing with these reports, required a unique database for the reports, provided for grants to improve treatment of Native American child abuse victims, and otherwise supported improvements in investigation and other interventions in these child abuse cases.

The committee is unaware of any research on the incidence of or responses to child abuse on Indian reservations. The committee urges HHS and the Department of the Interior, Bureau of Indian Affairs, to support data collection and studies that can inform Congress on how these 1990 laws have or have not reduced child abuse in Indian country or improved the reporting of and intervention in these child abuse cases.

In 1978, Congress enacted the Indian Child Welfare Act (see Chapter 5).[9] The purpose of this legislation was to "promote cultural and familial preservation for Indian children," not only in cases related to child welfare system intervention but also in other custody and adoption cases. However, only "sparse empirical research has examined the implementation of and outcomes associated with this landmark legislation" (Cross, 2006, 2008; Limb et al., 2004, p. 1279), and thus this is an area also in need of federal research attention.

> *Finding:* CAPTA provides the legal foundation for state and national child abuse and neglect prevention and treatment activities, yet many impacts of CAPTA have not been evaluated through rigorous re-

---

[7]18 U.S. Code Section 1169 and 25 U.S. Code Section 3201 et seq.
[8]P.L. 101-630, 18 U.S.C. 1169a.
[9]25 U.S.C. § 1902.

search. Topics lacking research include the effects on child protection of (1) state and county responses to first-time reports involving older teens, (2) state definitions of perpetrators, (3) the inclusion of language limiting reporting to recent and serious acts, (4) the inclusion of broadened language on reportable sex crimes, (5) various expansions of medical neglect definitions, (6) state responses to State Grant program requirements, (7) CAPTA-promoted best practices, (8) citizen review panel recommendations, (9) programs funded by Children's Justice Act grants, (10) programs funded by CAPTA Title II Prevention Grants, and (11) CAPTA discretionary grant evaluations.

Finding: To identify best practices to support state and county implementation of CAPTA requirements, research is needed on (1) responses to first-time reports involving older teens, (2) implementation of State Grant program requirements, and (3) data collection for difficult data elements that states are required to report to the Children's Bureau.

Finding: CAPTA includes research priorities identified by Congress. Nevertheless, the funding appropriated for research under the act has been too limited to address more than a few of the research priorities identified, and many key priorities have never received CAPTA or other federal research grant funding.

Finding: The VCAA funds CACs, the National Center for the Prosecution of Child Abuse, and CASA programs and sets requirements for the reporting of child abuse on federal lands. While research has examined the effectiveness of CACs and CASA programs, no research has been conducted on the operation or impact of the federal lands child abuse reporting law.

Finding: The Child Victims' and Child Witnesses' Rights law was designed to reduce the trauma experienced by child abuse and neglect victims as a result of their involvement in the federal criminal court system, but no studies have examined the effects of implementing the law's provisions.

Finding: The Indian Child Protection and Family Violence Prevention Act established mandatory reporting of child abuse and neglect on Indian lands, but no research has examined the incidence of or responses to child abuse and neglect on Indian lands.

Finding: The Indian Child Welfare Act established tribal authority over decisions to place American Indian children in out-of-home care, but little empirical research has examined how the act has been implemented and what effect it has had on the experiences of American Indian children in the child welfare system.

STATE LAWS AND POLICIES

This section reviews key state laws and policies addressing child abuse and neglect that have been enacted in recent years and suggests areas in which future research is needed.

Laws Establishing Definitions of Child Abuse and Neglect, Laws Defining Drug Use as a Form of Child Abuse and Neglect, and Laws Pertaining to Witnessing Domestic Violence

As previously discussed in this chapter, CAPTA establishes a minimum threshold for the definition of child abuse and neglect beyond which states are free to develop their own variations. These state definitions, established by state legislative and child protective departmental authority, consistently include definitions of physical abuse, sexual abuse, neglect, and emotional abuse (CWIG, 2011b). At the same time, these definitions vary, and some states specify additional types of abuse and neglect. For example, states consistently define physical abuse to include physical injury, but many (38) (CWIG, 2011b) also include situations in which the child is threatened with or is at substantial risk of harm. Failure to provide and supervisory neglect generally are included in neglect definitions, but some states also specify educational neglect (24 states) and medical neglect (7) (CWIG, 2011b).

Variation is seen as well in state definitions of child abuse and neglect-related "near fatalities." Since data on these events are not captured in the CAPTA-created national surveillance system—the National Data Archive on Child Abuse and Neglect (NDACAN)—no guidance on their definition is provided at the federal level. According to a 2011 Government Accountability Office (GAO) report that presents results of a survey of child welfare administrators in the 50 states, the District of Columbia, and Puerto Rico, 32 states have a state law or policy that defines a near fatality; however, these definitions may or may not be congruent (GAO, 2011). Partly as a result of confidentiality restrictions, coordination among jurisdictions and state agencies is limited. This limited coordination presents further challenges for reporting data on both abuse/neglect-related fatalities and near fatalities as part of national surveillance systems (GAO, 2011). Inadequate support has been provided for research that would help identify best practices in overcoming barriers to uniform identification and data collection for cases of the most severe forms of child abuse and neglect.

Exacerbating confusion over the legal definition of child abuse and neglect are differences in the guidelines or standards for defining child abuse and neglect among and within disciplines, agencies, and professional groups. For example, standards for what is considered a case of child abuse and neglect may vary among the courts, child protective services, and health care providers within a state, as well as among individuals within those groups (CWIG, 2011b). New research is critically needed to better understand how these differing standards and interpretations affect the protection of children from abuse and neglect.

Nearly all states have laws within their child protection statutes that address the issue of substance use by parents. CAPTA funding is predicated on having procedures in place for notification of child protective services when babies are born exposed to substances and on having plans in place for their safe care. States vary as to whether these procedures are formally included in their definition of child abuse and neglect or separate statutes on such referrals and care are in place. For children in the home who are exposed to drug activity of their parents, many states have expanded their civil definition of child abuse and neglect to include this situation, others address it in their criminal statutes, and still others have enacted enhanced penalties for drug crimes conducted in the presence of children. Again, this lack of uniformity in legal approaches is exacerbated by the lack of research on what approaches are best suited to addressing the problem.

Finally, although the definition of domestic violence also varies across states, many state laws consider cases in which a child witnesses violence among family members to be a form of child abuse and neglect. Currently, 23 states have laws designed to protect children from exposure to domestic violence in the home, although variation exists among these laws (CWIG, 2012a). Several states have specific definitions of witnessing such violence, including being physically present or in the vicinity or being able to see or hear the act of violence. Several state laws are explicit about the child being related to the adult victim or perpetrator; other state laws apply to any child. Legal consequences for violating these state laws include criminal penalties resulting in jail time, fines, or both; mandated counseling; removal of visitation privileges; or mandatory supervised visits of noncustodial parents. In Georgia, for example, committing an act of violence in the presence of a child is termed third-degree child cruelty and is considered a misdemeanor (CWIG, 2012a). Here also, the lack of research on the impact of these legal approaches results in policy making in a highly controversial area without evidence-based support.

Analyses

Even though state-level data collection has expanded markedly in the past three decades, no evaluations have examined the relationship between instituting laws defining child abuse and neglect and demonstrated improvements in child safety. Differences in state laws defining abuse and neglect have been summarized (e.g., CWIG, 2011b), but no evaluations have explored the relationships between differing abuse and neglect definitions and their impact on child safety. Further, no evaluations have focused on improvements in child safety or well-being associated with the inclusion of educational neglect, medical neglect, parental drug abuse, or exposure to intimate partner violence in abuse and neglect definitions.

Maintaining a safe environment for children is one of the least clear-cut elements of defining or legislating child neglect. Charges that a parent has failed to protect a child from danger (i.e., violence in the home) "exemplify the lack of clarity in this concept and related legal practices. Protection of the child from ... harm in the home might seem ... to be one of the most basic parental responsibilities ... however, there is no consensus on what constitutes a threshold of dangerousness in children's exposure" (Kantor and Little, 2003, p. 340). The federal court case of *Nicholson v. Williams*, U.S. Court of Appeals (2nd Cir. 2, 171), served as a caution to states to legislate carefully in this area. Perhaps for this reason, many states do not address domestic violence issues within their child protection laws.

Several studies have been conducted on legislative and policy shifts related to identifying children who witness domestic violence. A 2008 study of the San Francisco Police Department assessed the effectiveness of a new policy requiring officers to complete supplemental documentation for any incident or crime involving domestic violence, with the goal of identifying children who may have been exposed. Findings suggest the policy shift had a clear effect on officers' documentation of domestic violence-related incidents, resulting in improved identification of children exposed to violence in the home (Shields, 2008). Although Shields looked only at the experiences of one locality, those experiences may inform other localities on policy updates aimed at increasing rates of identification of children exposed to domestic violence.

A 2006 analysis of the Minnesota legislature's 1999 decision to amend the definition of child neglect to include exposure to domestic violence revealed that changes in legal definitions are not always the best solution for children and families experiencing violence (Edleson et al., 2006). The law was repealed during the next legislative session because of the short-sightedness of legislators who believed a "modest" language change would ensure that child welfare agencies reached children being exposed to violence in their homes; social service agencies estimated the changes would cost the state millions of dollars, for which no funds were appropriated. The language also implicated domestic violence victims as perpetrators of child abuse and neglect. Kantor and Little (2003) suggest that the problem with Minnesota's amended definition (and others like it) was ambiguity.

For example, were children considered victims if they heard the violence occurring but did not see it?

Research Needs

No rigorous studies are available with which to understand the impact of varying child abuse and neglect definitions, and in particular, the inclusion of medical neglect, substance abuse, and domestic violence, on child safety and well-being. Although data are not available with which to compare abuse and neglect rates before and after specific child abuse and neglect laws were established, the more recent passage of laws identifying substance abuse and domestic violence as child abuse and neglect related could be explored. Studies could also examine underlying mechanisms thought to explain the impact of these phenomena on untoward outcomes. Such research could intervene to reduce the elements of that risk to see whether doing so improved child and family outcomes.

For example, studies could be conducted in states that impose enhanced criminal penalties for perpetrators who commit domestic violence in the presence of a child to determine the effect, if any, of those laws and policies on deterrence and whether changes occurred in the number of victims seeking help. Cross and colleagues (2012, p. 13) recommend further research on the effects of differential response on exposure to domestic violence: "Differential response [DR] holds promise for responding to EDV [exposure to domestic violence], but the methods through which DR addresses EDV need to be articulated, and the prevalence of EDV in DR cases and the effects of DR on EDV need to be studied."

Laws on Mandatory Reporting

Mandatory reporting of child abuse and neglect has its origins in the United States, where model statutes for laws designed to introduce this process were first drafted in the early 1960s (Kalichman, 1999; Mathews and Kenny, 2008). Indeed, all states either designate specific professions whose members are mandated by law to report child abuse and neglect or have a universal mandate requiring all citizens to report child abuse and neglect. Individuals designated as mandatory reporters vary across states, and include but are not necessarily limited to social workers, teachers and other school personnel, physicians and other health care workers, mental health professionals, child care providers, medical examiners, and law enforcement personnel (CWIG, 2012b). Other professionals specified as mandated reporters in selected states include clergy, court-appointed special advocates (CASAs), animal control officers, domestic violence workers, substance abuse counselors, video and film processors, and most recently sports coaches and other adults in youth athletic programs.

States impose penalties on mandatory reporters who fail to report suspected child abuse or neglect as required by law (CWIG, 2012c). These penalties range from misdemeanors in the majority of states to felonies for more serious cases or cases with multiple violations in other states. To prevent malicious or intentionally false reporting of cases, many states also impose penalties against any person who files a report known to be false. These penalties range from a fine, to a misdemeanor, to a felony for multiple cases, to jail time, and may include the potential for civil liability for any damages resulting from the false report.

During 2012, 107 bills were introduced in 30 states and the District of Columbia on the topic of reporting child abuse and neglect. Several of these bills identified individuals who should be included as mandatory reporters, and many specified enhanced penalties for failure to report (NCSL, 2012).

Other components of the mandatory reporting process that vary across states include (1) what types of abuse or neglect are required to be reported (including emerging definitions such as exposure to domestic violence or to drug activity, discussed above), (2) standards for making a report (such as the amount of alleged harm required for a report to be mandated or whether the reporting duty includes risk of future abuse, as well as reports of past abuse), (3) specification of when a communication is privileged or inapplicable to reporting situations, and (4) anonymity or confidentiality of reporters and the reporting documents. In 2012, pursuant to a mandate in the 2010 CAPTA reauthorization, HHS began studying the issue of liability of those who assist child protective services in their investigations or otherwise become involved in the child protection process after an initial report is made.

Analyses

As a consequence of a much-publicized case involving children who had been sexually abused by a staff member of Pennsylvania State University, legislative interest has arisen across the country in broadening child abuse and neglect reporting laws to make all adults mandated reporters. The State Policy Advocacy and Reform Center (McElroy, 2012) conducted a comparative analysis of current state statutes to determine whether states with universal mandated reporting have higher reporting and/or substantiation rates. The analysis found that universal mandated reporting laws did not appear to be correlated with rates of calls coming into states' hotlines. It did find that rates of substantiation were higher in states with universal mandated reporting laws. However, whether the increased rates were a function of more professionals reporting or increased reporting from the general public was unclear. All other indicators (i.e., number of victims, rates of child abuse and neglect, rates by type) were not significantly different between reporting groups.

Several studies have indicated that professionals with mandatory reporting requirements have varying levels of knowledge and information regarding child abuse and neglect reporting (Alter et al., 2012; Alvarez et al., 2004; Davidov et al., 2012; Kenny, 2002; Khan et al., 2005; Meyerhoff et al., 2012; Sedlak et al., 2010). This issue was recently studied with regard to the reporting of children exposed to domestic violence. In one study, nurse home visitors had uneven understanding of whether they were required to report child abuse or neglect if a child was present when intimate partner violence occurred (Davidov et al., 2012). Shields (2008) observed an increase in police documentation of children exposed to domestic violence in San Francisco after the implementation of a new policy and supplemental forms required for completion.

In a survey of physicians who had completed a course on child abuse and neglect as a prerequisite to licensure in New York State, 84 percent of respondents knew the signs of child abuse and neglect (Khan et al., 2005). Physicians from different practice specialties had significantly different understanding of the procedure for reporting suspected abuse and neglect. Pediatricians, emergency physicians, and family practitioners had more knowledge of this process than surgeons and internists (Khan et al., 2005).

In Minnesota, state law requires child protective services agencies to inform mandated reporters periodically about definitions and rules and any additional definitions or criteria approved by the county board (Alter et al., 2012). The state's Office of the Legislative Auditor found that the agencies used a variety of approaches to update and inform mandatory reporters; the majority (79 percent) of mandated reporters appraised themselves as adequately informed about their responsibility to make a report, and nearly all of those mandated reporters knew whom to contact to make a report. Yet 27 percent of pediatric health professionals and 5 percent of school personnel surveyed indicated that they would make a report of suspected abuse and neglect to a designated individual in their workplace, whereas the law requires a direct report to child protective services or law enforcement (Alter et al., 2012).

Alvarez and colleagues (2004) estimate that 40 percent of professionals who are mandated reporters have failed to report child abuse or neglect at some time. They note a number of barriers to reporting abuse and neglect, including a lack of knowledge about its signs and symptoms and the ability to identify them correctly, lack of knowledge of reporting procedures, concern about negative consequences to the child or family, fear of retaliation, or a belief that child protective services will be unable to help.

In the survey of mandatory reporters in Minnesota, as many as 20 percent of mandated reporters considered not filing a report when they suspected abuse and neglect; the two most common reasons they cited were (1) they did not think their suspicions were strong enough to justify making a report, and (2) previous reports of suspected abuse and neglect had been ruled out by child protective services (Alter et al., 2012). The authors note an inherent conflict between the "reporting" mentality and the "screening" mentality that can lead to frustration on the part of reporters when their report is not screened in because of the more restrictive criteria for that process compared with reporting. While most of the mandated reporters asserted that the screening guidelines were "about right," a sizable minority said that the guidelines were too strict. The authors note that providing information on specific screening requirements needs to be balanced with the risk that individuals will "prescreen" prior to reporting or will tailor reports to meet the specific screening criteria (Alter et al., 2012).

The most recent National Incidence Study (NIS-4) provides evidence that professionals may not recognize abuse and neglect in some cases, and in other cases recognize signs of abuse and neglect but do not report it (Sedlak et al., 2010). Professionals in schools were less likely to report suspected abuse and neglect than other professionals (Sedlak et al., 2010). Sentinels who had received training on reporting laws and procedures were more likely to have reported suspected child abuse and neglect than those who had not received such training (Sedlak et al., 2010), suggesting that additional training of the general mandated reporting workforce would increase reporting.

Research Needs

McElroy (2012) suggests the need for research comparing the rates of child abuse and neglect reporting and substantiation in states across several years, focusing on variability at the state level. This research could include a careful exploration of such variables as the definition of a mandatory reporter, whether the state is a "universal" reporting state, the definitions of child abuse and neglect, poverty rates, and the presence of a differential response system. Studies of the efficacy of training programs for mandated reporters, including how different training models have more or less impact with different audiences, could provide guidance to policy makers.

Legal Standards for Substantiating Child Abuse and Neglect

Once cases of child abuse or neglect have been reported, they must be investigated and verified. All states and territories have specific requirements for the initial response by agencies receiving reports of child abuse and neglect. In most states, a screening process is used to determine whether a report will be accepted; this process includes a review of the report in the context of the state's definitions of child abuse and neglect. Every state mandates that child protective services begin an investigation within a timely manner, usually within 72 hours, and in even less time when there is reasonable cause to believe that the child is in imminent danger (CWIG, 2009b). Although the methods used to determine which reports require immediate responses vary among states, almost every state uses a type of safety assessment. States most typically have a two- or three-tiered model for substantiation, and the standard of evidence varies from state to state (CWIG, 2009a; English et al., 2002).

Analyses

The committee encountered no research on the impact on child abuse and neglect intervention of having different evidence standards for case substantiation, but a limited amount of research has examined certain aspects of substantiation across states. The Congressional Research Service reviewed all state evidence required for child abuse and neglect substantiation and ranked states according to least strict, more strict, and strictest standards. The level of evidence required was found to be correlated with reported rates of child abuse and neglect victims. For example, in fiscal year (FY) 2007, the 20 states with the least strict evidence required for substantiation reported 13.3 victims per 1,000 children, the 28 states requiring more strict evidence reported 9.4 victims per 1,000 children, and the 2 states with the strictest evidence requirements reported 1.7 cases per 1,000 children (GAO, 2011).

In Washington State, a three-tiered model for substantiation includes the categories of *founded, inconclusive,* and *unfounded* (English et al., 2002). The Washington Risk Model, a comprehensive decision-making tool established in 1987, was found by researchers not only to provide the risk information required in the central electronic data system but also to serve as an organizational framework for child protective services workers (English et al., 2002). Interviews with the workers revealed that multiple factors enter into the decision on substantiation, with determinations being based on the risk assessment as well as factors in the workers' environment. Chronicity of abuse and neglect was found to be a key factor in the substantiation decision, with 84 percent of case workers stating that chronicity was of moderate or high importance in the determination. Workers used the Washington Risk Model to evaluate the severity of the case, articulate opinions to the court, clarify borderline situations, and support decisions (English et al., 2002).

Some states have developed specialized diagnostic centers to improve determinations of child abuse and neglect. Socolar and colleagues (2001) conducted a case study of programs used for medical diagnosis of child abuse and neglect in five states.[10] Three of the states (Florida, North Carolina, and Oklahoma) had operational programs, and two (Louisiana and Kansas) were in the process of implementing such programs. These centers were established in response to concerns about the quality, availability, and/or consistency of assessments of child abuse and neglect. All of the statewide programs had made training a priority, including for physicians, nurses, social workers, and any interested party. The authors found that state funding was critical to the support of programs, particularly statewide programs, but that it was important to ensure that the funding was diversified. They also noted that beyond the funding or the quality of the individuals within the programs, the success of such centers can depend as well on the establishment of alliances, adequate reimbursement, and recognition of the political climate in which the center operates (Socolar et al., 2001).

Research Needs

The literature cited in the previous section only hints at the complexity behind substantiation decisions, from issues of chronicity and workers' concerns about child safety, to the availability of quality medical diagnoses, to sufficient training for the workforce. These issues cannot be explored in a vacuum, however, but need to be analyzed with regard to how definitions of abuse and neglect vary across states, the different models and requirements for screening reports, and the availability of services for families identified as being at risk. The issue of substantiation needs to be explored in conjunction with analyses of differential response.

Further work on substantiation also needs to be done in the context provided by the many studies showing that children involved in both substantiated and unsubstantiated abuse or neglected cases have very similar case characteristics and case outcomes (Hussey et al., 2005; Kohl et al., 2009). These findings show, quite conclusively, that this labeling decision does not effectively differentiate those children with a high likelihood of reabuse or those with a high likelihood of developmental delays from children whose reports of abuse or neglect are not substantiated.

Criminal Sentencing Laws

Criminal penalties for child physical and sexual abuse vary considerably across states, and they are presumed to be dependent on the nature

---

[10]Medical diagnosis refers to "medical assessment of suspected child abuse or neglect to arrive at a diagnosis, and systems for medical diagnosis to refer to programs that are established to foster the process of medical diagnosis" (Socolar et al., 2001, p. 443).

and severity of the abuse. Most states require convicted child sex offenders to be listed on a registry, in some states for their entire lives. Other possible penalties and/or consequences, in civil child protective court proceedings, may include termination or limitation of parental rights. An examination of the charges and penalties for one form of abuse, abusive head trauma, found weak relationships between fatality or severity and the type of felony charged. Race of the perpetrator was a stronger predictor of more serious charges (Keenan et al., 2008). Whether public knowledge of criminal and civil penalties actually helps prevent child abuse or neglect has not, to the committee's knowledge, been studied.

Disclosure of Confidential Child Abuse and Neglect Records

Federal funding through CAPTA requires states to keep records of child maltreatment confidential to protect the rights of the child and the child's parents or legal guardians. State statutes vary with respect to the persons or entities allowed access to the central registry and other child protective services agency records of abuse and neglect. Those typically allowed access include physicians; researchers; police personnel; judges and other court personnel; the person who is the subject of a report (who does not, however, have access to the identity of the reporter); a person who was an alleged child victim; and the parent, guardian, or guardian ad litem of an alleged victim who is a minor. In some states, feedback, or summaries of investigations and case outcomes, is provided to persons or agencies making the initial report, and such information may also be provided to prospective foster or adoptive parents or to other public agencies providing services to the child and family.

For most cases, public disclosure is not allowed. Some states, however, pursuant to an exception in CAPTA, allow public reporting of child protective services case information when child abuse and neglect-related fatalities or near fatalities are involved—for example, when a child in state or county custody dies, when clarification or correction of information released through other sources is needed, or when the perpetrator of abuse has been arrested or criminally charged. Several states allow access to registry or departmental records of abuse and neglect for those reviewing employment applications for the provision of child care or youth care or checking on the suitability of prospective foster or adoptive parents. The latter case falls under the federal Adam Walsh Child Protection and Safety Act of 2006,[11] which requires states to "check any child abuse and neglect registry maintained by the state for information on any prospective foster or adoptive parent." It is important to note that the committee is unaware

---

[11] P.L. 109-248, 42 U.S.C. 16990.

of any research establishing that any particular state statutory scheme for release of records in such cases is more likely to protect children than any other.

Safe Haven (Baby Moses) Laws

All U.S. states and Washington, DC, have enacted legislation to address infant abandonment and infanticide, in some respects the cruelest form of child abuse and neglect. In exchange for surrendering a baby at a safe location, safe haven laws normally allow one parent, or a representative of that parent, to maintain anonymity and to be protected from prosecution for abandonment or neglect. In most states, the laws apply to very young infants—72 hours old or younger (n = 15), 5 to 14 days old (n = 11), or 1 month old (n = 14)—but some states allow parents to drop infants off within 45 days, 60 days, or up to 1 year (CWIG, 2010). The legislation varies across states by (1) who may leave a baby at a safe haven, (2) what providers are considered safe havens, (3) how old an infant may be to be properly relinquished, (4) responsibilities of safe haven providers, (5) protections from liability afforded to providers, (6) protections for the parents in terms of anonymity, (7) protection of the father's rights, (8) awareness campaigns, and (9) parental liability.

Analyses A number of commentators have written extensively about the purpose or impact of safe haven laws, referencing mainly anecdotal evidence or unofficial state data. Some have been critical, as in a white paper by the Evan B. Donaldson Adoption Institute, which suggests that safe haven laws have not been shown to be effective in minimizing unsafe infant abandonment; that the laws are limited by their inability to address the underlying causes of infant abandonment; and that the laws can interfere with aspects of child welfare policy, particularly with adoption statutes (Evan B. Donaldson Adoption Institute, 2003). Others hold a more optimistic view. In her commentary on the subject, Ayres (2009) suggests that public awareness of safe haven laws is the key to their effectiveness. Through a qualitative review of state-level policy changes in the form of case studies, she argues that increased public awareness of the laws through well-funded media campaigns has contributed to a reduction of unlawful infant abandonment.

To the committee's knowledge, however, there have been no rigorous evaluations of the impact of save haven laws on infant abandonment or death. In fact, the tools needed to conduct an effective evaluation of these laws are not yet in place. States do not systematically collect data on infant abandonment, so it is not possible to make comparisons before and after enactment of the laws. While some notable efforts have been made to collect statistics on infant abandonment using unofficial state data (see NCSL, 2003) or news reports (Pruitt, 2008), these data have been insufficient to allow an adequate assessment of the impact of safe haven laws. Further, the anonymity provisions of the laws preclude the collection of information necessary for evaluating the laws—whether women who surrender their baby at a safe haven would otherwise have abandoned their child in an unsafe place instead of pursuing a different, legally permissible course of action such as adoption. In her commentary on the topic, Oberman (2009) suggests that without information on the mothers who abandon their children, evaluating safe haven laws is nearly impossible.

Research needs Given the unavailability of certain data discussed above, the most rigorous study designs are not feasible for addressing this issue. However, time-series analyses (see, e.g., Albert, 2001) comparing rates of abandonment, death, and infanticide before and after implementation of state safe haven laws, combined with cross-state comparison of states with different age requirements, could help shed light on the issue. Factors that should be built into this design include, at a minimum, the amount of investment made in notifying the public about the availability of safe havens through signage and social media, the range of settings that are approved as safe havens, and the availability of other resources to prevent unwanted pregnancies. Other research designs that might be used to examine the impact of safe haven laws include instrumental variable approaches (see, e.g., Doyle, 2007) and regression discontinuity designs.

Child Abuse and Neglect Central Registries

Registries that maintain statewide information on individual child abuse and neglect cases remain a needed policy-related research focus. In addition, Section 633 of the Adam Walsh Child Protection and Safety Act required HHS to establish a national child abuse registry and to conduct a feasibility study regarding implementation issues. The interim report to Congress about the registry addressed the purpose of a national child abuse registry and its availability for employment and background checks. The same issues of accuracy, standard of proof, notification, appeal, expungement, availability to law enforcement or other non-child protection systems, and due process have not been carefully examined at the state level.

Representation of Children in Child Abuse and Neglect Proceedings

All states have provisions, mandated since 1974 under CAPTA, for appointing a guardian ad litem to represent the interests of a child in a case of child abuse and neglect that results in civil child protective judicial activity. However, these provisions vary among states with respect to who is appointed, with some states appointing a lay individual, others requiring that an attorney be appointed, and others allowing volunteer CASAs to take on the role. In some states, a CASA may be appointed in addition to rather than as the guardian ad litem, while in other states, the court appoints legal counsel for the child as required by state law. There is no federally established standardized training for any of these positions, and states vary in their training requirements either through state laws, court rules, or continuing legal education obligations. While a National Quality Improvement Center on Legal Representation of Children is currently examining the impact of two different models of child representation, the committee is unaware of other rigorous comparative evaluations of different approaches taken across the country.

Child Fatalities Due to Abuse and Neglect

A number of developments have led to recent bipartisan legislation— the Protect Our Kids Act—designed to address child fatalities due to abuse and neglect. These developments include the rising number of known child abuse and neglect-related deaths even as rates of child abuse fall; a 2011 GAO report stating that such fatalities are undercounted and that states are highly inconsistent in the ways they track, count, and examine these fatalities (GAO, 2011); findings of research on children's hospital admissions (Berger et al., 2011); and the almost daily media reports of the death of children due to abuse and neglect. The Protect Our Kids Act, signed by the President on January 14, 2013, created a national commission to examine child abuse and neglect-related fatalities and to recommend actions that should be taken to evaluate current programs and prevention efforts addressing the problem, as well as a comprehensive national strategy for reducing and preventing child abuse and neglect-related fatalities nationwide. The Children's Bureau responded to concerns about rising rates of child abuse and neglect-related deaths by developing a contract for information gathering with Walter R. McDonald & Associates, as well as convening a 2012 meeting of child welfare directors and child fatality reviewers to examine their processes.

The literature in this area includes only three studies, just one of which had a quasiexperimental design. Palusci and colleagues (2010) found that in Michigan, policy changes made after an initial phase of reviews of child fatalities due to abuse and neglect appeared to have positive impacts. Decreases were seen in fatalities among children familiar to child protective services, and specific policy changes appeared to result in improved professional practice. During this same time, however, child fatalities due to unaddressed mental health needs increased, as did inaccuracies in medical examiner findings—both of which are systems-level problems that cannot be addressed solely within the child welfare system. While they hesitate to assign causality, Palusci and colleagues (2010) suggest that it is important to consider whether changes proposed by the review panel could reasonably be expected to affect child abuse and neglect-related fatalities. A number of changes in state law, policy, and procedures during this time impacted child protective services procedures, including training, supervision, and peer review. The authors theorize that the review panel's recommendations may have had an impact because of the familiarity of the panel members with the child welfare system and the formal process that exists for moving from reviews to recommendations to state action.

During its first 5 years of operation, the Arizona Child Fatality Review Program (ACFRP) identified 29 percent of deaths of children under age 18 as preventable, and 56 percent of deaths of children over age 9 (Rimsza et al., 2002). The ACFRP found that 61 percent of the child abuse-related deaths were preventable. Child protective services in Arizona were involved in 21 percent of the child abuse cases prior to the fatal injury or neglect; in two cases, out-of-state child protective services agencies were involved but did not report findings to Arizona. Additionally, the ACFRP identified two instances in which medical personnel were believed to have failed to recognize suspicious injuries. The ACFRP identified five deaths it believed were ruled incorrectly by the medical examiner as natural or accidental that should have been classified as due to child abuse or neglect (Rimsza et al., 2002).

Douglas and McCarthy (2011) report that the focus of child fatality review teams varies widely among states, although the focus of most teams includes fatalities due to child abuse and neglect. Additionally, there is little uniformity with regard to content areas in the legislation establishing such teams. The most frequent content areas included in state laws are the composition of the team (93.4 percent), confidentiality concerns (86.9 percent), review outcomes (86.9 percent), the team's purpose (95.6 percent), and the team's selection of cases (58.7 percent) (Douglas and McCarthy, 2011).

In most states (89 percent), the stated purpose of the team is to prevent future deaths, but fewer than two-thirds of states require reports from the team to the executive branch of government or the child welfare system, only half of states require public education as a result of the team's reviews and recommendations, and even fewer states require a public report from the team (although many print them) (Douglas and McCarthy, 2011). States whose establishing legislation for the teams was passed early in the development of such teams were more likely to have an investigative focus for the team. Higher crime rates marginally but significantly predicted that a state's team would focus on prevention (Douglas and McCarthy, 2011).

More rigorous research is required to assess the effectiveness of such

teams in preventing deaths due to child abuse and neglect. Given the varying scope of the teams in each state, this research would need to account for
several potentially confounding variables, including how the states define
deaths due to child abuse and neglect.

Research also is needed to better understand what are referred to as
"near fatalities" (i.e., children hospitalized for abuse and neglect who are
labeled as in serious or critical condition), as well as to look across data
systems, as in Putnam-Hornstein's (2011) examination of abuse and neglect
and birth and death records in California. The latter study provided insight
in the area of risk factors, noting that previous reports of physical abuse
were correlated with child abuse and neglect-related deaths.

Finding: State laws differ significantly in defining child abuse and neglect. Very little research has examined the impacts of state definitions
of child abuse and neglect on child safety, including the effects of instituting state definitions; changing state definitions to include educational neglect, medical neglect, parental substance abuse, or exposure
to intimate partner violence; and differences among state definitions.

Finding: Differences in state definitions of child abuse and neglect-
related "near fatalities," the exclusion of data on fatalities and near
fatalities from NDACAN, and limited coordination among jurisdictions and state agencies pose challenges to tracking and analyzing the
most severe cases of child abuse and neglect. Insufficient research has
been conducted to identify best practices for overcoming these barriers.

Finding: The guidelines and standards for defining child abuse and
neglect vary significantly within states among the various disciplines,
agencies, and professional groups involved in preventing, identifying,
and responding to the problem. No research addresses the impact of
these variations on the safety of children.

Finding: Research on state mandatory reporting laws reveals higher
rates of substantiation in states with universal mandated reporting
laws. Research on professional mandated reporters indicates that many
do not report suspected cases of child abuse and neglect because of
multiple barriers. Some evidence indicates that additional training of
the general mandated reporting workforce could increase reporting.

Finding: While no research evaluates the impact of states' different
evidence standards for case substantiation on intervention outcomes,
states with more strict evidence requirements for substantiation were

found to have lower reported rates of child abuse and neglect than states with less strict evidence requirements.

Finding: Limited research reveals that complex substantiation decisions are tied to the chronicity of abuse, workers' concerns about child safety, the availability of quality medical diagnoses, and workforce training. Furthermore, research conclusively finds that children involved in both substantiated and unsubstantiated abuse or neglect cases have very similar case characteristics and outcomes.

Finding: Criminal penalties for child physical and sexual abuse vary across states, but research has not examined whether public knowledge of criminal and civil penalties helps prevent child abuse and neglect. Furthermore, analysis of charges and penalties for abusive head trauma has found race to be a stronger predictor of more serious charges than fatality or severity.

Finding: Beyond the CAPTA requirement that states preserve the confidentiality of child abuse and neglect records to protect the rights of the child and the child's parents or legal guardians, state statutes vary with respect to the persons or entities allowed access to central registries of child abuse and neglect and other case records. No research establishes that any state's statutory scheme for releasing records leads to better protection of children.

Finding: No rigorous evaluations have examined the impact of safe haven laws on infant abandonment or death. Such evaluations are hampered by the lack of systematic collection of state-level data on infant abandonment and by anonymity provisions in the law that make it impossible to interview women placing their children in safe havens about alternative courses of action.

Finding: State CASA provisions vary significantly, but an ongoing study of two different models of child representation by the National Quality Improvement Center on Legal Representation of Children is the only known rigorous comparative evaluation of different approaches.

Finding: Recent federal action designed to address child fatalities due to abuse and neglect includes the Protect Our Kids Act, which established a national commission to examine fatalities, recommend actions for program evaluation, and develop a national strategy for prevention, and activities by the Children's Bureau.

Finding: At the state level, the focus of child fatality review teams varies widely. One successful panel review of child fatalities was conducted in Michigan by experts familiar with the child welfare system; they suggested policy changes, which were followed by decreases in child fatalities. More rigorous research is required to assess the effectiveness of such panels in preventing deaths due to child abuse and neglect. Such research would benefit from improved definitions of near fatalities and from linking of data across systems.

CONCLUSIONS

The heterogeneity of state laws on child abuse and neglect offers an opportunity for a natural experiment that could help illuminate what does and does not work. The impact of policy change could be examined by studying state variations in such areas as mandated reporters, definitions of abuse and neglect, inclusion of the witnessing of intimate partner violence, and other elements included in state laws, as well as the range of penalties. As outlined in this chapter, opportunities also exist to examine variations in reporting laws, county- versus state-administered systems, differential response, mandated nursery-based preventive education in abusive head trauma, and education of mandated reporters about abuse and neglect. New research approaches should be considered, such as propensity scoring (D'Agostino, 1998) and difference-within-difference analyses (Shafrin, 2006), which can be powerful tools for examining policy-relevant questions. Explicit requirements for policy research should be part of any newly funded and developed child abuse and neglect research centers.

REFERENCES

Albert, V. N. 2001. Using time-series analysis to evaluate the impact of policy initiatives in child welfare. *Evaluation and Program Planning* 24(2):109-117.

Alter, J., E. Bennett, V. Bombach, S. Delacueva, J. Hauer, D. Kirchner, D. Meyerhoff, J. Randall, K. J. Starr, J. Trupke-Bastidas, and J. Vos. 2012. *Evaluation report: Child protection screening.* St. Paul, MN: Office of the Legislative Auditor, State of Minnesota, Program Evaluation Division.

Alvarez, K. M., M. C. Kenny, B. Donohue, and K. M. Carpin. 2004. Why are professionals failing to initiate mandated reports of child maltreatment, and are there any empirically based training programs to assist professionals in the reporting process? *Aggression and Violent Behavior* 9(5):563-578.

Ayres, S. 2009. Kairos and safe havens: The timing and calamity of unwanted birth. *William and Mary Journal of Women and the Law* 15(227):227-289.

Berger, R. P., J. B. Fromkin, H. Stutz, K. Makoroff, P. V. Scribano, K. Feldman, L. C. Tu, and A. Fabio. 2011. Abusive head trauma during a time of increased unemployment: A multicenter analysis. *Pediatrics* 128(4):637-643.

Children's Bureau. 2011. *New legislation-Public Law 111-320, the CAPTA Reauthorization Act of 2010.* Washington, DC: U.S. Department of Health and Human Services, Administration on Children, Youth and Families.

Children's Bureau. 2013. Report to Congress on the effectiveness of CAPTA state programs and technical assistance. Washington, DC: U.S. Department of Health and Human Services, Administration on Children, Youth and Families. http://www.acf.hhs.gov/programs/cb/resource/capta-effectiveness-report-to-congress (accessed December 3, 2013).

Cross, S. L. 2006. Indian family exception doctrine: Still losing children despite the Indian Child Welfare Act. *Child Welfare* 85(4):671-690.

Cross, T. L. 2008. Disproportionality in child welfare. *Child Welfare* 87(2):11-20.

Cross, T. P., B. P. Mathews, L. Tonmyr, D. Scott, and C. Ouimet. 2012. Child welfare policy and practice on children's exposure to domestic violence. *Child Abuse & Neglect* 36(3):210-216.

CWIG (Child Welfare Information Gateway). 2009a. *Child witnesses to domestic violence: Summary of state laws.* Washington, DC: U.S. Department of Health and Human Services, Children's Bureau.

CWIG. 2009b. *Making and screening reports of child abuse and neglect: Summary of state laws.* Washington, DC: U.S. Department of Health and Human Services, Children's Bureau.

CWIG. 2010. *Infant safe haven laws: Summary of state laws.* Washington, DC: U.S. Department of Health and Human Services, Children's Bureau.

CWIG. 2011a. *About CAPTA: A legislative history.* Washington, DC: U.S. Department of Health and Human Services, Children's Bureau.

CWIG. 2011b. *Definitions of child abuse and neglect.* Washington, DC: U.S. Department of Health and Human Services, Children's Bureau.

CWIG. 2012a. *Child witnesses to domestic violence.* Washington, DC: U.S. Department of Health and Human Services, Children's Bureau.

CWIG. 2012b. *Mandatory reporters of child abuse and neglect.* Washington, DC: U.S. Department of Health and Human Services, Children's Bureau.

CWIG. 2012c. *Penalties for failure to report and false reporting of child abuse and neglect.* Washington, DC: U.S. Department of Health and Human Services, Children's Bureau.

D'Agostino, R. B. 1998. Propensity score methods for bias reduction in the comparison of a treatment to a non-randomized control group. *Statistics in Medicine* 17(19):2265-2281.

Davidov, D. M., S. M. Jack, S. S. Frost, and J. H. Coben. 2012. Mandatory reporting in the context of home visitation programs: Intimate partner violence and children's exposure to intimate partner violence. *Violence Against Women* 18(5):595-610.

Douglas, E. M., and S. C. McCarthy. 2011. Child fatality review teams: A content analysis of social policy. *Child Welfare* 90(3):91-110.

Doyle, J. J. 2007. Child protection and child outcomes: Measuring the effects of foster care. *American Economic Review* 97(5):1583-1610.

Drake, B., and S. Zuravin. 1998. Bias in child maltreatment reporting: Revisiting the myth of classlessness. *American Journal of Orthopsychiatry* 68(2):295-304.

Drake, B., J. M. Molley, P. Lanier, J. Fluke, R. P. Barth, and M. Johnson-Reid. 2011. Racial bias in child protection? A comparison of competing explanations using national data. *Pediatrics* 127:471-478.

Edleson, J. L., J. Gassman-Pines, and M. B. Hill. 2006. Defining child exposure to domestic violence as neglect: Minnesota's difficult experience. *Social Work* 51(2):167-174.

English, D. J., D. B. Marshall, L. Coghlan, S. Brummel, and M. Orme. 2002. Causes and consequences of the substantiation decision in Washington state child protective services. *Children and Youth Services Review* 24(11):817-851.

Evan B. Donaldson Adoption Institute. 2003. *Unintended consequences: "Safe haven" laws are causing problems, not solving them.* New York: Evan B. Donaldson Adoption Institute.

GAO (Government Accountability Office). 2011. *Child maltreatment: Strengthening national data on child fatalities could aid in prevention.* Washington, DC: GAO.

Hussey, J. M., J. M. Marshall, D. J. English, E. D. Knight, A. S. Lau, H. Dubowitz, and J. B. Kotch. 2005. Defining maltreatment according to substantiation: Distinction without a difference? *Child Abuse & Neglect* 29(5):479-452.

Kalichman, S. C. 1999. *Mandated reporting of suspected child abuse: Ethics, law, and policy,* 2nd ed. Washington, DC: American Psychology Association.

Kantor, G. K., and L. Little. 2003. Defining the boundaries of child neglect: When does domestic violence equate with parental failure to protect? *Journal of Interpersonal Violence* 18(4):338-355.

Keenan, H. T., M. Nocera, and D. K. Runyan. 2008. Race matters in the prosecution of perpetrators of inflicted traumatic brain injury. *Pediatrics* 121(6):1174-1180.

Kempe, C. H., F. Silverman, B. Steele, W. Droegmueller, and H. Silver. 1962. The battered child syndrome. *Journal of the American Medical Association* 181(1):17-24.

Kempe, C. H., F. N. Silverman, B. F. Steele, W. Droegmueller, and H. K. Silver. 1985. The battered-child syndrome. *Child Abuse & Neglect* 9:143-154.

Kenny, M. C. 2002. Compliance with mandated child abuse reporting. *Journal of Offender Rehabilitation* 34(1):9-23.

Khan, A., D. H. Rubin, and G. Winnik. 2005. Evaluation of the mandatory child abuse course for physicians: Do we need to repeat it? *Public Health* 119(7):626-631.

Kohl, P. L., M. Jonson-Reid, and B. Drake. 2009. Time to leave substantiation behind: Findings from a national probability study. *Child Maltreatment* 14(1):17-26.

Lane, W. G., D. M. Rubin, R. Monteith, and C. W. Christian. 2002. Racial differences in the evaluation of pediatric fractures for physical abuse. *Journal of the American Medical Association* 288(13):1603-1609.

Levi, B. H., and G. Brown. 2005. Reasonable suspicion: A study of Pennsylvania pediatricians regarding child abuse. *Pediatrics* 116(1):e5-e12.

Limb, G. E., T. Chance, and E. F. Brown. 2004. An empirical examination of the Indian Child Welfare Act and its impact on cultural and familial preservation for American Indian children. *Child Abuse & Neglect* 28(12):1279-1289.

Magruder, J., and T. V. Shaw. 2008. Children ever in care: An examination of cumulative disproportionality. *Child Welfare* 87(2):169-188.

Mathews, B., and M. C. Kenny. 2008. Mandatory reporting legislation in the United States, Canada, and Australia: A cross-jurisdictional review of key features, differences and issues. *Child Maltreatment* 13(1):50-63.

McElroy, R. 2012. *Analysis of state laws regarding mandated reporting of child maltreatment with appendix.* http://childwelfaresparc.com/2012/09/20/new-policy-brief-an-analysis-of-state-laws-regarding-mandated-reporting-of-child-maltreatment (accessed August 26, 2013).

Meyerhoff, C., K. J. Starr, and M. Schroeder. 2012. *Child protection screening: Evaluation report.* St. Paul: Office of the Legislative Auditor, State of Minnesota, Program Evaluation Division.

Myers, J. E. B. 2008. A short history of child protection in America. *Family Law Quarterly* 42(3):449-463.

NCSL (National Council of State Legislatures). 2003. *Update: Safe havens for abandoned infants.* http://www.ncsl.org/issues-research/human-services/update-safe-havens-for-abandoned-infants.aspx#laws (accessed February 13, 2013).

NCSL. 2012. *Mandatory reporting of child abuse and neglect: 2012 introduced state legislation.* http://www.ncsl.org/issues-research/human-services/2012-child-abuse-mandatory-reporting-bills.aspx (accessed February 11, 2013).

NRC (National Research Council). 1993. *Understanding child abuse and neglect.* Washington, DC: National Academy Press.

Oberman, M. 2009. Judging Vanessa: Norm setting and deviance in the law of motherhood. *William and Mary Journal of Women and the Law* 15(2):337-359.

Palusci, V. J., S. Yager, and T. M. Covington. 2010. Effects of a citizens review panel in preventing child maltreatment fatalities. *Child Abuse & Neglect* 34(5):324-331.

Pecora, P. J., J. K. Whittaker, A. N. Maluccio, R. P. Barth, and R. D. Plotnick. 2000. *The child welfare challenge: Policy, practice, and research,* 2nd ed. Piscataway Township, NJ: Transaction Publishers.

Pruitt, S. L. 2008. The number of illegally abandoned and legally surrendered newborns in the state of Texas, estimated from news stories, 1996-2006. *Child Maltreatment* 13(1):89-93.

Putnam-Hornstein, E. 2011. Report of maltreatment as a risk factor for injury death: A prospective birth cohort study. *Child Maltreatment* 16(3):163-174.

Rimsza, M. E., R. A. Schackner, K. A. Bowen, and W. Marshall. 2002. Can child deaths be prevented? The Arizona child fatality review program experience. *Pediatrics* 110(1):e11.

Sedlak, A. J., J. Mettenburg, M. Basena, I. Petta, K. McPherson, A. Greene, and S. Li. 2010. *Fourth National Incidence Study of Children Abuse and Neglect (NIS-4): Report to Congress.* Washington, DC: U.S. Department of Health and Human Services, Administration for Children and Families.

Shafrin, J. 2006. *Difference in difference estimation.* http://healthcare-economist.com/2006/02/11/difference-in-difference-estimation (accessed February 20, 2013).

Shields, J. P. 2008. An evaluation of police compliance with domestic violence documentation policy reform: Improving the identification of exposed children. *Best Practice in Mental Health* 4(1):65-73.

Socolar, R. R., D. D. Fredrickson, R. Block, J. K. Moore, S. Tropez-Sims, and J. M. Whitworth. 2001. State programs for medical diagnosis of child abuse and neglect: Case studies of five established or fledgling programs. *Child Abuse & Neglect* 25(4):441-455.

Summers, S. J., C. Abdullah, and J. Sharp. 2011. Community-Based Child Abuse Prevention: Accomplishments and New Directions 2011. Chapel Hill, NC: FRIENDS National Resource Center for Community-Based Child Abuse Prevention. http://friendsnrc.org (accessed December 3, 2013).

U.S. Advisory Board on Child Abuse and Neglect. 1990. *Child abuse and neglect: Critical first steps in response to a national emergency.* Washington, DC: U.S. Departmant of Health and Human Services and Office of Human Developmental Services.

U.S. Advisory Board on Child Abuse and Neglect. 1991. *Creating caring communities: Blueprint for an effective federal policy on child abuse and neglect: Second report.* Washington, DC: U.S. Department of Health and Human Services, Administration for Children and Families.

U.S. Advisory Board on Child Abuse and Neglect. 1993. *Neighbors helping neighbors: A new national strategy for the protection of children.* Washington, DC: U.S. Department of Health and Human Services.

9

Recommendations

The 1993 National Research Council (NRC) report notes that "Child maltreatment is a devastating social problem in American society" (NRC, 1993, p. 1). The committee responsible for the present report, armed with research findings gleaned during the past 20 years that document the deleterious impact of child abuse and neglect on the health, well-being, and social constructs of populations across the United States, regards child abuse and neglect not just as a social problem but as a serious public health issue. Child abuse and neglect affects not only children but also the adults they become. Its effects are broad and deep, affecting every aspect of human functioning, and costing American taxpayers considerable federal and state investments in programs and services to address the resulting cascade of problems.

The committee deliberated on recommendations whose implementation can respond to this public health problem while remaining realistic about the nature of actions that can be taken in these challenging political and economic times. The intent of the recommendations presented in this chapter is to capitalize on existing opportunities whenever possible, and at the same time to urge new actions the committee deems essential.

Existing research and service system infrastructures are not sufficient for responding to this public health challenge. The committee's bold goal is that in the near future, significant and recognizable changes will have been accomplished, changes that will make a difference for children and families and represent measurable, substantive improvement in the many systems that support them.

GUIDING PRINCIPLES

In developing recommendations to advance child abuse and neglect research, the committee identified several cross-cutting, guiding principles. These are not independent recommendations, but are part of the rationale for the actions recommended by the committee and are important considerations for their implementation. The following principles are critical to advancing understanding and knowledge of child abuse and neglect:

- disentangle the roles of cultural processes, social stratification influences, ecological variations, and immigrant/acculturation status;
- apply multidisciplinary, multimethod, and multisector approaches; and
- leverage and build upon the existing knowledge base of child abuse and neglect research and related fields, as well as research definitions, designs, and opportunities.

Disentangle the Roles of Cultural Processes, Social Stratification Influences, Ecological Variations, and Immigrant/Acculturation Status

Efforts to address child abuse and neglect must be informed by an understanding of the complex roles of culture, social stratification, and associated contextual factors in the causes, consequences, prevention, and treatment of the problem, particularly in light of the increasing heterogeneity of families in the United States. A focus on cultural processes, social stratification influences, ecological variations, and immigrant/acculturation status is pertinent to understanding the causes and consequences of child abuse and neglect and involvement with child protective services or other social service systems. These factors also matter in developing and testing the effectiveness of prevention and intervention strategies and replicating and adapting evidence-based practices for distinct populations or groups so as to ensure cultural fit, reach, efficacy, and adoption (Barrera et al., 2011), as well as social validity and practical application.

While an increasing body of research has been dedicated to examining differential experiences based on race, ethnicity, and social context, the level of methodological sensitivity required to parse the roles and interrelationships of these factors accurately has not been adequately incorporated across child abuse and neglect research. Further, these factors tend to be omitted from the major considerations driving current research and programmatic development.

In designing studies that consider and evaluate the impact of social and economic factors on child abuse and neglect, it is important for researchers to adopt a critical stratification lens and to avoid the error of equating domains of stratification with the attributes and practices of culture. Understanding cultural factors related to risk and protective factors or the effectiveness of interventions for child abuse and neglect calls for the complementary use of qualitative and quantitative research methodologies. The use of methods and approaches that are culturally sensitive and responsive to diverse and vulnerable populations is also critical to understanding the interplay of micro- and macro-level processes and establishing the evidence base.

Apply Multidisciplinary, Multimethod, and Multisector Approaches

As noted in Chapter 7, child abuse and neglect research domains reflect the many systems that interact, largely independently, with abused and neglected children and their families. In many jurisdictions, abused and neglected children and their families pass through multiple agencies as their cases are processed and they receive services. Each system has its own mission, expertise, agenda, and obligations to fulfill. The various systems are staffed by different disciplines, collect different types of information, and are focused on different outcomes. Definitions of what is considered an act of child abuse and neglect also differ according to systemic priorities and variations in the state legislation that mandates child abuse and neglect reporting. For research purposes, differences in the way child abuse and neglect is identified, documented, and handled create difficulties for obtaining an accurate picture of its incidence and surrounding circumstances. Further, agencies place different values on research and its relevance to their practice. Thus in many jurisdictions, the integrated, cross-system research necessary to understand causes, consequences, prevention, intervention, and treatment for child abuse and neglect cannot be conducted.

There is a pressing need to overcome these barriers and to undertake multidisciplinary research that spans systems. Such efforts would link research to the many locations where abused and neglected children receive services and in so doing, bring together the expertise and perspectives of the many interrelated fields that can assist in understanding the multiple, complex facets of child abuse and neglect. Steps to overcome these barriers include developing a discrete set of definitions and methodology for question design for use in specific types of research; investing in the capacity to link data across systems; conducting multidisciplinary, multimodal research to capture the different and interrelated impacts of the many services received by abused and neglected children, including a more comprehensive array of intervention outcomes; and applying multimethod research designs, including those that incorporate qualitative approaches and use methodologies that better reveal the dynamics of the impacts of community and organizational structure on outcomes.

Leverage and Build on the Existing Knowledge Base of Child Abuse and Neglect Research and Related Fields, as Well as Research Definitions, Designs, and Opportunities

The conclusions and recommendations presented in this report call for dramatic improvements to the knowledge base and the capacity to conduct research in the field of child abuse and neglect. As stakeholders prepare to invest in such research capacity, it is important to note the opportunities offered by notable past and current empirical and services research efforts among the many disciplines associated with child abuse and neglect, as well as related fields. In an era of fiscal constraints, leveraging such existing resources and opportunities is critical to avoid duplication of effort and to support necessary research in an efficient manner.

Thus in preparing an agenda for future child abuse and neglect research, it is important to draw upon what is currently known so as to identify critical gaps in the collective understanding of the problem. The review of evidence presented in this report, along with the attendant findings, should provide guidance in this regard.

Opportunities also exist to leverage existing research infrastructures and mechanisms so as to efficiently build the proper supports for large-scale, sustainable child abuse and neglect research efforts. Longitudinal studies present a tremendous opportunity to collect the data necessary to advance understanding of the causes and consequences of child abuse and neglect, as well as the effectiveness of services for its prevention and treatment, but are often costly to initiate and require the sustained commitment of study sponsors. The addition of child abuse and neglect variables to existing population-based, longitudinal studies of children, such as the National Children's Study, offers a way to leverage existing large-scale data collection efforts and research agendas. In addition, systematic secondary analyses of child abuse and neglect data from existing longitudinal studies, such as the Longitudinal Studies of Child Abuse and Neglect (LONGSCAN) and the National Survey of Child and Adolescent Well-Being (NSCAW), would make valuable and efficient contributions to research, policy, and practice discussions.

A significant opportunity to supplement current research efforts also lies in the creation of sustainable infrastructure for the conduct of research at the various service locations where abused and neglected children and their families are seen on a daily basis. Linking researchers to service providers would allow for readily available, community-based research samples, and those research efforts could in turn contribute to the improvement of services provided by these entities.

RECOMMENDATIONS

The following recommendations represent an actionable framework that can guide and support future child abuse and neglect research reflecting the needs and knowledge gaps detailed throughout this report. Recommendations 1, 2, and 3 urge the development of a national strategic plan to initiate the process of federal coordination and resource allocation that is necessary to support the field of child abuse and neglect research, with a focus on the research priorities set forth in this report. Recommendations 4 through 7 represent critical steps toward the creation of a sustainable infrastructure for child abuse and neglect research. While these infrastructure recommendations should be considered in the implementation of a national strategic plan, they are actions of considerable importance that merit separate and specific consideration from the agencies and institutions targeted as key actors. Finally, Recommendations 8 and 9 provide for the evaluation of federal and state policies related to child abuse and neglect.

It is important to note that the committee's charge called for identifying child abuse and neglect research priorities. Therefore, the focus of these recommendations is on needed components of future research in the field, to the exclusion of specific actions for providers in the delivery of prevention and treatment services. The actions of service providers are obviously of critical importance to the well-being of children impacted by child abuse and neglect, but encompass an area of inquiry that falls outside the purview of this report. It is the committee's hope that this report's discussion of research needs related to the effective provision of services and the structure of the systems in which they are delivered will lead to improvements in the prevention of child abuse and neglect and the care of those it affects.

A National Strategic Plan for Child Abuse and Neglect Research

This report has described the current landscape of child abuse and neglect research and presented the body of knowledge that can serve as a foundation for the future growth of the field. Advances in knowledge, technology, and research implementation tools have helped bring about substantial improvements in the collective understanding of the consequences of child abuse and neglect, as well as the efficacy of prevention and treatment approaches to mitigating this devastating societal problem. Innovation in linking data across multiple sources has provided access to means of developing more accurate assessments of the community-level prevalence of child abuse and neglect. Dramatic advances in both neural and genomic sciences have offered new insights into the neural and biological processes associated with abuse and neglect. The development of prevention and treatment models has presented service providers with a range of viable program options, and the testing of such models has shown that child abuse and neglect can be both preventable and manageable through informed approaches.

The findings presented in this report also identify challenges to be overcome and opportunities to be explored in the field, providing guidance on research areas most in need of further development. Despite the many advances in child abuse and neglect research over the past two decades, significant gaps in knowledge remain. Improved surveillance of child abuse and neglect is needed to identify unexplored risk factors and to better depict and examine the significance of national and state incidence trends. Research on the causes of child abuse and neglect needs to move beyond correlational designs and analyses to test causal models. The consequences of child abuse and neglect need to be better understood in terms of the behavioral and neurobiological mechanisms that mediate the association between exposure to abuse and neglect and its behavioral and neurobiological sequelae. Research on intervention and treatment services needs to move beyond the development of model programs to devise effective strategies for the implementation and replication of programs in varying community settings. Work needs to be initiated on a body of research to examine the effects of changes to the ever-shifting laws and policies related to child abuse and neglect at the federal, state, and local levels. And throughout all domains of child abuse and neglect research, the roles of race, ethnicity, and culture need to be adequately explored, with increased attention to children in underserved and underresearched populations.

Chapter 7 of this report highlights the benefits of applying a public health framework to guide empirical research on child abuse and neglect, as well as associated research on interventions, services, and policy. Doing so will require a holistic approach to a problem that spans many spheres of academic and programmatic disciplines and encompasses many systems. New, cross-disciplinary partnerships and support structures are needed to permit advances in the implementation of a coordinated, rigorous, scientific approach and make significant progress in the field. To this end, a shift is needed toward a well-coordinated, properly directed, adequately supported, multidisciplinary scientific enterprise.

The field of child abuse and neglect research currently is lacking a core, national-level priority-setting body that can reach all of the many associated disciplines and that has the capacity to allocate the resources necessary to develop a sustainable, accountable research infrastructure. Research support needs to be substantially increased and stable to allow for more complete investigations of specific topics and to provide for long-term studies. Mechanisms need to be implemented to facilitate the cohesive interaction of individuals and institutions across varied disciplines and sectors. The committee therefore makes the following three recommendations to support the development of a national process for coordinating and prioritizing investment in child abuse and neglect research.

A Coordinated National Agenda for Child Abuse and Neglect Research

A critical component of a national strategic plan will be a comprehensive research agenda for child abuse and neglect. This research agenda will examine factors related to both children and adults across physical, mental, and behavioral health domains; include issues that encompass child welfare, economic support, criminal justice, education, and health and behavioral health care systems; and assess the differential needs of a variety of subpopulations. Research needs to be directed at the areas of greatest need, and priority setting will require the input of stakeholders across disciplines and systems. On a national scale, this agenda will necessarily involve coordination and collaboration across a variety of federal agencies, as well as partnerships with state agencies, tribes, private entities, and universities that are at the forefront of innovation.

> **Recommendation 1: Federal agencies, in partnership with private foundations and academic institutions, should implement a research agenda designed to advance knowledge and understanding of the causes and consequences of child abuse and neglect, as well as the identification and implementation of effective services for its treatment and prevention. The research priorities listed in Figure 9-1 should be considered in this agenda.**

In formulating a national research agenda, it will be critical to identify the most pressing needs and the most significant gaps in knowledge. The findings and conclusions presented throughout this report should be used to guide a national strategy for setting priorities in child abuse and neglect research. To further distill these messages, the committee has identified key research priorities that should be included in a national research agenda and should be considered by all entities concerned with supporting the advancement of the empirical knowledge base on child abuse and neglect, as well as efforts to prevent and ameliorate its deleterious effects. These research priorities, summarized in Figure 9-1, fall into three major categories: research on the causes and consequences of child abuse and neglect, services research in complex systems, and child abuse and neglect policy research.

In its statement of task, the committee was asked to identify research areas that are no longer a priority for funding. However, the committee could not find support for either scaling back or discontinuing research funding in any specific topic area related to child abuse and neglect. Whereas research in the field of child abuse and neglect has made tremendous progress over

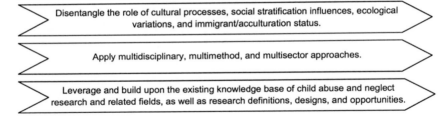

Causes and Consequences

- Improve understanding of the separate and synergistic consequences of different forms of child abuse and neglect.
- Initiate high-quality longitudinal studies of child abuse and neglect.
- Target innovative research on the causes of child abuse and neglect.
- Improve understanding of the behavioral and neurobiological mechanisms that mediate the association between child abuse and neglect and its sequelae.

Services in Complex Systems and Policy

- Explore highly effective delivery systems.
- Develop and test new programs for underserved children and families.
- Identify the best means of replicating effective interventions and services with fidelity.
- Identify the most effective ways to implement and sustain evidence-based programs in real-world settings.
- Investigate the longitudinal impacts of prevention.
- Encourage research designed to provide a better understanding of trends in the incidence of child abuse and neglect.
- Evaluate the impact of laws and policies that address prevention and intervention systems and services for child abuse and neglect at the federal, state, and local levels.

Disentangle the role of cultural processes, social stratification influences, ecological variations, and immigrant/acculturation status.

Apply multidisciplinary, multimethod, and multisector approaches.

Leverage and build upon the existing knowledge base of child abuse and neglect research and related fields, as well as research definitions, designs, and opportunities.

FIGURE 9-1 Research priorities in child abuse and neglect.

the past two decades, more rigorous and coordinated research and evaluations, particularly those utilizing cross-disciplinary research designs and high-quality longitudinal data, are needed to establish a complete understanding of the causes and consequences of child abuse and neglect and the programs, services, and policy mechanisms designed to prevent and treat its effects. As federal agencies, private foundations, and academic institutions work toward the implementation of a national research agenda, it will be important to monitor future progress in research in specific topic areas with an eye toward identifying cases in which additional research will no longer produce tangible benefits for the child abuse and neglect knowledge base.

A National Plan for Implementing and Sustaining Child Abuse and Neglect Research

The committee that developed the 1993 NRC report identified as a key priority federal leadership to guide, plan, and coordinate child abuse and neglect research. Based on its review of the current federal infrastructure supports for child abuse and neglect research, the present committee found that high-level, federal coordination of research in this field is still lacking. Notable progress has been made in understanding the problem and efforts to remediate its effects and prevent its occurrence; however, much more could be accomplished if emerging research occurred within a coordinated framework. Support for child abuse and neglect research remains fragmented across a number of federal agencies, private foundations, and academic centers, with little coordination. Further, the small aggregate research budget for this major public health problem, coupled with the episodic and scattered nature of funding opportunities, discourages scientists from pursuing child abuse and neglect research as a sustainable career path. Also lacking is accountability for progress in the field of child abuse and neglect research as a whole. To create a robust portfolio of child abuse and neglect research opportunities directed at areas of urgent need and to sustain the consistent pursuit of knowledge in this field, a mechanism for high-level, federal coordination, priority setting, and resource allocation should be implemented.

Currently, the Federal Interagency Work Group on Child Abuse and Neglect does provide a convening forum at the federal level, with representation from more than 40 different federal agencies, including nearly all agencies with a major stake in child abuse and neglect research. The group's stated mission is as follows:

- to provide a forum through which staff from relevant federal agencies can communicate and exchange ideas concerning child abuse and neglect-related programs and activities,
- to collect information about federal child abuse and neglect activities, and
- to provide a basis for collective action through which funding and resources can be maximized.

The Federal Interagency Work Group on Child Abuse and Neglect is thus in a unique position that allows it to readily assess the needs, capabilities, and available resources of a large number of federal stakeholders. It also presents an opportunity to explore and strengthen interagency cooperation on issues that are relevant to the missions of multiple organizations.

Recommendation 2: The Federal Interagency Work Group on Child Abuse and Neglect, under the auspices of the assistant secretary of the Administration for Children and Families, should develop a strategic plan that details a business plan, an implementation strategy, and departmental accountability for the advancement of a national research agenda on child abuse and neglect.

The aim of the strategic plan should be to implement the research agenda formulated in accordance with Recommendation 1 by developing the capability to conduct the research necessary to explore rigorously the areas of greatest need, as well as areas that present an opportunity to achieve significant advances in knowledge in the field. The plan should detail specific actions tailored to support research in key areas of need identified in this report. It should also include components of an implementation strategy and a business plan. An implementation strategy will be needed to specify mechanisms required to conduct the necessary research, including but not limited to research grants, cooperative agreements, or contracts; data collection; and staffing requirements. A business plan will be needed to target specific agency resources that will be used to support the implementation strategy.

Within the Federal Interagency Work Group on Child Abuse and Neglect is a research subcommittee that provides the group with support and guidance for research initiatives. The group also has been involved in collaboration with the National Institutes of Health's (NIH's) Child Abuse and Neglect Working Group, which is tasked with reporting on current NIH efforts, accomplishments, and future plans for research in child abuse and neglect. Both the research subcommittee and the NIH working group should have critical roles in the Federal Interagency Work Group on Child Abuse and Neglect's shaping of a strategic plan for the implementation of a national research agenda on child abuse and neglect. In the course of its work, the Federal Interagency Work Group on Child Abuse and Neglect should also draw upon the diverse perspectives of its constituents and should engage researchers conducting work throughout the many disciplines associated with child abuse and neglect to ensure the requisite support for the types of research needed to advance knowledge in the field. Opportunities for interagency and interdisciplinary collaboration should be identified so that challenges can be approached with a diversity of perspectives, resources can be shared, and duplication of effort can be avoided.

In this context, it is important to note that the work of these groups depends on the leadership and resources of various research funding agencies. The development of a national strategic plan will depend on the ongoing support of the Administration for Children and Families (ACF), NIH, and many other member agencies of the Federal Interagency Work Group on Child Abuse and Neglect.

Accountability for Implementation of the Strategic Plan

To ensure accountability, the strategic plan for child abuse and neglect research should designate specific responsibilities of federal agencies and corresponding program offices, directed according to agency mission and relative availability of resources.

> **Recommendation 3: The assistant secretary of the Administration for Children and Families should convene senior-level leadership of all federal agencies with a stake in child abuse and neglect research to discuss and assign accountability for the implementation of a strategic plan to advance a national research agenda on child abuse and neglect.**

This convention of high-level federal leadership should take place in several stages and have the specific intent of assigning accountability for implementation of the strategies devised by the Federal Interagency Work Group on Child Abuse and Neglect, as well as generally improving federal coordination for the continuous support of child abuse and neglect research endeavors.

As noted, child abuse and neglect research spans a number of academic and professional spheres, and it accordingly has received support from a wide array of federal agencies. Therefore, participants invited to this discourse should be representative of the multiple agencies whose missions touch upon the many facets of child abuse and neglect research. Representation should include but not be limited to the following agencies and offices:

- Office of the Assistant Secretary for Planning and Evaluation;
- Institute of Education Sciences of the Department of Education;
- Indian Health Service;
- Office of Planning, Research and Evaluation;
- Office of Minority Health;
- NIH (including Office of Behavioral and Social Sciences Research, National Institute on Alcohol Abuse and Alcoholism, National Institute of Child Health and Human Development, National Institute of Dental and Craniofacial Research, National Institute on Drug Abuse, National Institute of Mental Health, and National Institute of Neurological Disorders and Stroke);
- Substance Abuse and Mental Health Services Administration;
- Maternal and Child Health Bureau;
- Centers for Disease Control and Prevention;

- National Institute of Justice;
- Office of Juvenile Justice and Delinquency Prevention; and
- Agency for Healthcare Research and Quality.

The committee recognizes the importance of on-the-ground experience in assembling the appropriate balance of expertise and authority to foster the success of the convening effort. Therefore, the committee urges the assistant secretary of ACF to use his discretion to identify and include the appropriate participants.

As a first step, the assistant secretary of ACF should convene the relevant federal leadership before the strategic plan assigned to the Federal Interagency Work Group on Child Abuse and Neglect under Recommendation 2 is completed. The focus of this meeting should be to identify specific departments, agencies, program offices, and federal leadership staff that should receive the incipient strategic plan. The assistant secretary should then direct the Federal Interagency Work Group on Child Abuse and Neglect to disseminate the strategic plan to the identified designees upon its completion. After the strategic plan has been completed and distributed, the assistant secretary should once again convene the leadership of relevant federal agencies to review its contents and to designate responsibilities and allocate resources according to the plan's directives. All elements of the strategic plan should be assigned to specific departments, agencies, or program offices.

To provide for future monitoring of performance under the strategic plan, the Federal Interagency Work Group on Child Abuse and Neglect should be directed and empowered to provide an annual report to the assistant secretary that contains an assessment of its member agencies' accomplishments in achieving the plan's goals and identifies new issues that may necessitate revisions to the plan. If necessary, the assistant secretary should reconvene relevant federal leadership to ensure that agencies are meeting their objectives under the plan and to assign revisions to the plan.

The committee's recommendations to develop a national strategic plan call for a convening of diverse federal agency leadership resulting in coordinated and robust support for child abuse and neglect research across the many associated disciplines. Given that there currently is no federal home for research on child abuse and neglect, however, barriers will likely remain to adequate implementation of a comprehensive and coordinated research agenda. Accordingly, Box 9-1 presents additional suggestions for implementation strategies to ensure interagency commitment to support for child abuse and neglect research.

BOX 9-1
Suggested Implementation Strategies

- Grant authority to the Federal Interagency Work Group on Child Abuse and Neglect for oversight and enforcement of a national strategic plan for child abuse and neglect research.
- Create a Children's Policy Council through executive order of the White House Office on Child Abuse and Neglect that includes staffing from the Domestic Policy Council.*
- Include children and youth among the Domestic Policy Council's issue area focus on family.
- Prescribe an interagency, coordinated approach to child abuse and neglect research, practice, and policy through either congressional legislation or presidential mandate. A recent model for action of this nature is the U.S. Government Action Plan on Children in Adversity. The impetus for that action plan was the fragmented nature of the activities of the wide array of U.S. government agencies with a stake in protecting vulnerable children globally. Requirements for a comprehensive, coordinated, and effective response on the part of the U.S. government to the world's most vulnerable children as part of an interagency strategy were codified in P.L. 109-95. That statute also authorized presidential action to monitor and evaluate actions taken under the interagency strategy. The resulting action plan contains six delineated objectives and outlines specific activities assigned to a set of agency actors for advancement toward corresponding outcomes.

---

*This policy council could be modeled after the White House Rural Council, which was created by Executive Order and includes representation of all federal agencies with a mission of addressing challenges in rural America, building on the administration's rural economic strategy, and improving the implementation of that strategy. It is staffed by the Domestic Policy Council and the National Economic Council and is chaired by the secretary of agriculture. The Policy Council has a specific focus on increasing coordination and collaboration to best serve rural communities.

A Research Infrastructure to Build and Sustain a Field of Child Abuse and Neglect Research

The nature of the research needs identified in this report provides the underlying rationale for the resources and infrastructure that will be needed to support progress. To build a field of research focused on child abuse and neglect, it will be essential to adequately develop the infrastructure components required to sustain a national, multidisciplinary research enterprise. As discussed in Chapter 7, productive, high-quality scientific research on child abuse and neglect requires a particularly sophisticated infrastructure because of complexities involving diverse independent service systems, multiple professions, ethical issues that are especially complicated, and levels of outcome analysis ranging from the individual child to national statistics. Critical components of such an infrastructure generally include a dedicated and capable cadre of researchers, stable sources of research funding, and sufficient physical capital to conduct research based on sophisticated designs.

Optimism for the attainment of such a goal can be found in the fact that the field does not have to be built from the ground up. The efforts of ACF, NIH, and other federal research funding agencies, as well as the work of private foundations and academic institutions, have all helped lead to dramatic advances in research on this topic. A key catalyst for the development of a strong, national research infrastructure for the field of child abuse and neglect will be leveraging existing resources, knowledge, and opportunities presented by the work conducted within the field thus far. Through national coordination, dedicated funding support, and the commitment of key stakeholders, a foundation can be built from which child abuse and neglect research endeavors will flourish.

It is the committee's hope that the lessons learned presented in this report will provide a framework for the various entities that support child abuse and neglect research to combine their efforts and contribute to the formation of the necessary infrastructure in a stable and sustainable fashion. Through the following recommendations, the committee provides several discrete, actionable steps whose implementation would greatly contribute to the capacity to conduct child abuse and neglect research. However, the research infrastructure necessary to sustain a robust, national child abuse and neglect research enterprise will require a broad array of commitments across all of the various disciplines associated with this field.

National Surveillance for Child Abuse and Neglect

A high-quality, population-based, epidemiological surveillance system that draws on multiple data sources is critically necessary to the development of a national strategic approach to child abuse and neglect. Such a system would improve knowledge of the scope of child abuse and neglect to allow for a better understanding of the magnitude of the problem, identification of populations at greatest risk, and changes in prevalence over time. A more accurate reporting of the incidence of child abuse and neglect could also help in tracking the effectiveness of prevention programs and thus identifying the types of activities that should be replicated. In addition, a comprehensive surveillance system would provide for the collection of data on myriad potential environmental, community, and societal risk factors to guide the direction of effective prevention activities.

Recommendation 4: The Centers for Disease Control and Prevention, in partnership with the Federal Interagency Work Group on Child Abuse and Neglect, should develop and sustain a national surveillance system for child abuse and neglect that links data across multiple systems and sources.

Critical steps toward developing an effective national surveillance system include movement toward more standardized use of child abuse and neglect definitions, further exploration of the context in which child abuse and neglect occurs, and linking of multiple data sources.

Standardization of child abuse and neglect definitions The identification of children exposed to child abuse and neglect for research purposes often draws on sources that characterize experiences of abuse and neglect in dissimilar ways. For example, child abuse and neglect is reported to child protective services agencies differently depending on the state in which the agency is located, and surveys designed to elicit recall of abuse and neglect experiences often approach the task with divergent question methodologies. The result can be great variability and inconsistency in reporting on the incidence of child abuse and neglect. One of the first steps toward creating a national surveillance system should be to develop an approach to standardizing definitions of child abuse and neglect across sources from which national data are to be drawn.

Based on the committee's review of definitional work in the field over the past two decades, the use of single, uniform definitions for the different types of child abuse and neglect throughout the field is neither feasible nor optimal. Given that child abuse and neglect represents a diverse set of behaviors with implications relevant to many research domains, definitions must be flexible enough to accommodate a variety of specific research questions. Within the parameters of these constraints, however, the standardization of child abuse and neglect definitions can be improved by the development of a discrete set of definitional elements and a methodology for question design that can be selected for use in specific types of research. This set of definitional elements should be based on items proven to elicit an accurate assessment of the incidence of abuse and neglect and should be designed to best allow for comparison across studies.

Linking of data across multiple sources To provide accurate and effective surveillance of child abuse and neglect, data must be drawn from a variety of sources. Because abused and neglected children come in contact with multiple systems (e.g., mental and physical health care, education, law enforcement, child death reviews), aggregating data across multiple independent sources can improve identification of cases that were not referred to child welfare agencies. Linking case-based data from multiple sources allows for better identification of the scope of child abuse and neglect, including fatalities (Gibbs et al., 2013; Schnitzer et al., 2008); the development of profiles of children at risk, such as high-risk infants through a birth match process (Shaw et al., 2013); and planning and implementation of community-level prevention strategies (Putnam-Hornstein and Needell, 2011; Putnam-Hornstein et al., 2011). Multisectoral datasets allow for real-time examination of pressing research, practice, and policy questions at multiple levels of analysis (i.e., individual, familial, agency, and geographic), such as the intersection of drug market activity, changing neighborhood conditions, and substantiated child abuse and neglect (Freisthler et al., 2012).

There are many logistical difficulties involved in creating such linkages of data across systems, and agency capacity for the data management and statistical analysis required for the purpose is often lacking. In addition to the inevitable hardware and software incompatibilities, separate systems collect different types of data and code and process the data in different ways, greatly complicating case linkage. Legal restrictions, often compounded by confusion about just what is confidential information, inhibit data sharing. Most agencies lack the expertise in data management and statistical analysis to conduct research with their own or combined datasets. Investment in the capacity to link data across the many systems that encounter abused and neglected children is therefore a priority for advancing knowledge in the field.

Research Cadre for Child Abuse and Neglect

One of the strengths of the scientific enterprise is the expectation that its members will provide training, mentorship, and support for new investigators. To fulfill this mission, a field must have a supply of funded investigators conducting ongoing studies in which trainees can participate. The field must have access to research training funds to support trainees and new investigators while they learn. Mentors must be competent, involved, and supportive, helping trainees develop new areas of investigation and novel approaches to persistent problems. Strengthening the next generation of child abuse and neglect researchers will require a communication system and learning collaborative that can link these young scholars throughout their careers with those exploring similar and complementary research questions. To bolster the workforce with knowledgeable and dedicated researchers, the field also needs support to elevate its institutional relevance as a legitimate and highly important field of academic pursuit.

Recommendation 5: Federal agencies, in partnership with private foundations and academic institutions, should invest in developing and sustaining a cadre of researchers who can examine issues of child abuse and neglect across multiple disciplines.

To support and develop opportunities to train researchers in this field, a commitment across the various multisectoral entities that support child abuse and neglect research will be necessary. Such training opportunities must be available to develop researchers at all stages of their careers, including programs targeted toward graduate and undergraduate students as well as early and midcareer research professionals. A specific focus on interdisciplinary training programs is necessary, to reflect the breadth of fields related to child abuse and neglect research. There are a number of examples and models of successful child abuse and neglect research training initiatives that should be replicated and implemented broadly across disciplines and their affiliated public and private institutions.

Various multidisciplinary professional societies have been formed to advance research in child abuse and neglect. In 1977, the International Society for the Prevention of Child Abuse and Neglect was incorporated in Denver to enhance professional education in and recognition of child abuse and neglect around the world (ISPCAN, 2013). Most recently, in 2005, the Academy on Violence and Abuse was founded to support health professionals making violence and abuse core components of health care education (AVA, 2010).

Among federal agencies, NIH Career Development Awards provide a mechanism for training and developing researchers at different career stages. These awards are designed to provide support and protected time for an intense career development experience. They could be used to target child abuse and neglect researchers, and similar mechanisms could be developed at other relevant federal agencies to support workforce development in this field.

Among private foundations, the Doris Duke Charitable Foundation's Fellowships for the Promotion of Child Well-Being, implemented through Chapin Hall at the University of Chicago, serve as a model for the type of comprehensive, multidisciplinary training opportunities that need to be developed in the field of child abuse and neglect research. The stated goal of these fellowships is to "identify and develop a new generation of leaders interested in and capable of creating practice and policy initiatives that will enhance child development and improve the nation's ability to prevent all forms of child maltreatment" (Chapin Hall at the University of Chicago, 2013). The fellowships support grantees' research efforts at their respective academic institutions and provide academic as well as policy or program mentors to guide the fellows in their work and professional development. Fellows are recruited from a variety of disciplines associated with child abuse and neglect research, and a peer learning network is being developed to encourage communication and collaboration among the multidisciplinary fellows along with their associated mentors.

Multidisciplinary Research Centers on Child Abuse and Neglect

The call for child abuse and neglect research centers is not new. The 1993 NRC report called for the establishment of such centers, a message that was echoed with regard to family violence in the 2001 Institute of Medicine (IOM) report *Confronting Chronic Neglect*. To date, however, there has been no movement toward federal support for such centers in the manner envisioned by those earlier committees, and the need for the centers has not diminished. In a field in which research opportunities are often fragmented and inconsistent, these centers would provide a stable home for child abuse and neglect research endeavors, allow the research to be guided by a multidisciplinary perspective, and help train a new generation of child abuse and neglect researchers to ensure a dedicated workforce for the future.

A key benefit of the creation of research centers is the ability to bring together partners with a diversity of perspectives and strategic resources. Successful research centers in other fields, including the Alzheimer's Disease Centers, the Harvard Youth Violence Prevention Center, and the Geriatric Education Centers, have shown how such centers can leverage diversity and resources to advance their areas of inquiry in unique ways (IOM, 2001). These research centers have provided funding for innovative lines of research; strengthened multidisciplinary work by enabling researchers to coordinate their efforts; and established stable, continuous funding streams for major research projects that would not be feasible for individual researchers to undertake. Furthermore, research centers have demonstrated their effectiveness in disseminating new knowledge to key professional and lay communities.

> **Recommendation 6: Federal agencies, in partnership with private foundations and academic institutions, should provide funding for new multidisciplinary education and research centers on child abuse and neglect in geographically diverse locations across the United States.**

In the field of child abuse and neglect, the establishment of dedicated research centers would allow entities with the infrastructure capacity to conduct high-quality research, such as academic institutions and private foundations, to access community settings where abused and neglected children are seen regularly, such as child protective services, the courts, child advocacy centers, and community health centers. This interdisciplinary collaboration could lead to the creation of a more robust research portfolio. Specific efforts that could be undertaken by such centers include

- conducting child abuse and neglect research in the specific areas of need identified in this report;
- developing new lines of investigator-initiated research;
- providing an interdisciplinary forum for the exchange of ideas and the formation of partnerships;
- supporting professional development in the field of child abuse and neglect research through training programs and mentorship opportunities; and
- conducting research on the impact of policies that address child abuse and neglect prevention and intervention systems, as well as services at the federal, state, and local levels.

National Institutes of Health Child Maltreatment, Trauma, and Violence Study Section

Housed within NIH's Center for Scientific Review, study sections provide for the review and initiation of investigator-initiated research related to the section's specified areas of interest. A stable mechanism for evaluating and supporting new areas of investigator-initiated research is critically important for the development and progression of the field of child abuse and neglect research. This mechanism would allow researchers with a concrete understanding of child abuse and neglect research needs to help shape the direction of the field.

> **Recommendation 7: The National Institutes of Health should develop a new child maltreatment, trauma, and violence study section under the Risk, Prevention, and Health Behavior Integrated Review Group.**

Research developed through a study section on child abuse and neglect, trauma, and violence would fit within areas of interest specific to the Risk, Prevention, and Health Behavior Integrated Review Group. Most notably, child abuse and neglect research would advance knowledge related to the review group's interest in behavioral and interpersonal interventions; risk and protective processes and models; and social, cognitive, and affective conditions and processes that influence disease and disorder across the life span. The review panel of the proposed study section should comprise a wide range of cross-disciplinary expertise to reflect the spectrum of disciplinary perspectives needed to adequately assess the variety of research needs associated with the field of child abuse and neglect. The panel should represent key fields in research on child abuse and neglect such as psychology, psychiatry, child and adolescent development, neuroscience, genetics, social work, criminology, criminal justice, pediatrics, family medicine, nursing, and surgery, among others.

Evaluation of Child Abuse and Neglect Laws and Policies

As discussed in Chapter 8, numerous federal policy changes have been designed to impact the incidence, reporting, and negative health and economic consequences of child abuse and neglect. However, little work has been done to evaluate the impact of these changes. Such research is needed to determine the effectiveness of policies and in turn to influence future legislative action at both the federal and state levels. Research also is needed to understand the impact of regulatory policies on not only the populations they target but also the systems in which they are implemented. Explicit requirements for the support of policy research should be part of any new legislation related to child abuse and neglect so as to also spur the development of this body of research and guide the future actions of policy makers.

> **Recommendation 8: To ensure accountability and effectiveness and to encourage evidence-based policy making, Congress should include support in all new legislation related to child abuse and neglect, such as reauthorizations of the Child Abuse Prevention and Treatment Act, for evaluation of the impact of new child abuse and neglect laws and policies and require a review of the findings in reauthorization discussions.**

While a number of federal statutes, such as the Child Abuse Prevention and Treatment Act, dictate minimum federal standards for child abuse and neglect policy, many of the laws and policies affecting how child abuse and neglect is handled in the United States are developed and carried out at the state level. As with federal policies in this area, little research has been conducted on the impact of law and policy changes at the state level. Such research is needed to support future laws and policies that are grounded in sound evidence and to explore the impact of those changes at the individual, community, and system levels.

> **Recommendation 9: To ensure accountability and effectiveness, to support evidence-based policy making, and to allow for exploration of the differential impact of various state laws and policies, state legislatures should include support in all new legislation related to child abuse and neglect for evaluation of the impact of new child abuse and neglect laws and policies and require a review of the findings in reauthorization discussions.**

Also clearly needed is support for policy-relevant research that takes advantage of the variations among states in laws, policies, and programs to enhance knowledge of what works. Opportunities exist to examine, for example, variations in reporting laws, inclusion of children's exposure to intimate partner violence as reportable, county- versus state-administered child protection systems, differential response, mandated nursery-based prevention education in abusive head trauma, and mandated reporter education on abuse and neglect.

FINAL THOUGHTS

The recommendations presented in this chapter represent immediate and groundbreaking actions whose implementation would significantly advance the capacity to conduct research on child abuse and neglect in areas of tremendous value. However, the necessary support for this research will not be attainable without the ongoing commitment of the many stakeholders with ties to this work. Furthermore, concerted action of these stakeholders based on the findings, conclusions, and recommendations presented in this report needs to be initiated now. The immediate need for such widespread action can be distilled into three major points.

The benefits are tangible. Various estimates of the societal costs of child abuse and neglect reveal a significant burden across populations within the United States. At the same time, the science of prevention and treatment, along with the testing of associated programs and services, has shown that the incidence of child abuse and neglect can be reduced, and its deleterious effects that cascade throughout the life course can be mitigated. Investments in child abuse and neglect research provide a clear path to improving the nation's population health, as well as other metrics of well-being. Additionally, one of the frequently overlooked benefits of conducting research on child abuse and neglect issues is that progress can be translated to the many interrelated fields of study. Domains such as child development, child welfare, education, social work, pediatrics, and criminology all stand to benefit from advances in child abuse and neglect research.

Opportunities are present. By leveraging existing resources and building upon the knowledge base derived from previous research, the task of building a sustainable child abuse and neglect research infrastructure becomes less daunting than it may appear.

The timing is urgent. In addition to the exigency of the societal burden imposed by child abuse and neglect, immediate action is warranted by the fact that building the proper supports to sustain a national child abuse and neglect research enterprise will take a considerable amount of time. A shift in organizational culture, the creation of a sustainable infrastructure, the development of a new generation of dedicated researchers, the collection of longitudinal data, and effective dissemination and implementation research are examples of necessary endeavors that will require time before the associated benefits can be realized.

It is the committee's hope that the messages of this report will result in swift and effective action at the federal, state, and community levels across the many and varied sectors with a role in child abuse and neglect research.

REFERENCES

AVA (Academy on Violence and Abuse). 2010. *Welcome to the Academy on Violence and Abuse.* http://www.avahealth.org (accessed November 27, 2012).

Barrera, M., F. G. Castro, and L. K. Steiker. 2011. A critical analysis of approaches to the development of preventive interventions for subcultural groups. *American Journal of Community Psychology* 48(3-4):439-454.

Chapin Hall at the University of Chicago. 2013. *Doris Duke fellowships for the promotion of child well-being.* http://www.chapinhall.org/fellowships/doris-duke-fellowships (accessed June 25, 2013).

Freisthler, B., N. J. Kepple, and M. R. Holmes. 2012. The geography of drug market activities and child maltreatment. *Child Maltreatment* 17(2):144-152.

Gibbs, D. A., L. Rojas-Smith, S. Wetterhall, T. Farris, P. G. Schnitzer, R. T. Leeb, and A. E. Crosby. 2013. Improving identification of child maltreatment fatalities through public health surveillance. *Journal of Public Child Welfare* 7(1):1-19.

IOM (Institute of Medicine). 2001. *Confronting chronic neglect: The education and training of health professionals on family violence.* Washington, DC: National Academy Press.

ISPCAN (International Society for Prevention of Child Abuse and Neglect). 2013. *ISPCAN history.* http://www.ispcan.org/?page=History (accessed November 27, 2012).

NRC (National Research Council). 1993. *Understanding child abuse and neglect.* Washington, DC: National Academy Press.

Putnam-Hornstein, E., and B. Needell. 2011. Predictors of child protective service contact between birth and age five: An examination of California's 2002 birth cohort. *Children and Youth Services Review* 33(8):1337-1344.

Putnam-Hornstein, E., D. Webster, B. Needell, and J. Magruder. 2011. A public health approach to child maltreatment surveillance: Evidence from a data linkage project in the United States. *Child Abuse Review* 20(4):256-273.

Schnitzer, P. G., T. M. Covington, S. J. Wirtz, W. Verhoek-Oftedahl, and V. J. Palusci. 2008. Public health surveillance of fatal child maltreatment: Analysis of 3 state programs. *American Journal of Public Health* 98(2):296-303.

Shaw, T. V., R. P. Barth, J. Mattingly, D. Ayer, and S. Berry. 2013. Child welfare birth match: Timely use of child welfare administrative data to protect newborns. *Journal of Public Child Welfare* 7(2):217-234.

Appendix A

Workshop Open Session Agendas

**First Meeting of the Committee on Child Maltreatment
Research, Policy, and Practice for the Next Decade: Phase II**

Keck Center
500 Fifth Street, NW
Washington, DC 20001

OPEN SESSION

1:30-3:00	Charge to the Committee from the Sponsors
3:00-3:30	Open Comments from the Public

**Third Meeting of the Committee on Child Maltreatment
Research, Policy, and Practice for the Next Decade: Phase II**

National Academy of Sciences Building
2101 Constitution Avenue, NW
Washington, DC 20001

OPEN SESSION

1:00 pm	Welcome *Anne Petersen, Research Professor, University of Michigan (Committee Chair)*
1:10-2:10	**Panel on Select Populations** *Introduced by Charles Nelson, Professor of Pediatrics and Neuroscience, Harvard Medical School (Committee Member)* Anthony D'Augelli, Professor of Human Development, Department of Human Development and Family Studies, The Pennsylvania State University Terry Cross, Executive Director, National Indian Child Welfare Association Richard Heyman, Co-Director, Family Translational Research Group, New York University Amy Slep, Co-Director, Family Translational Research Group, New York University
2:10-2:50	Discussion, moderated by Charles Nelson
2:50-3:00	Break
3:00-4:20	**Panel on Research Funding and Infrastructure** *Introduced by Mary Dozier, Unidel Amy E. du Pont Chair of Child Development, University of Delaware (Committee Member)* Valerie Maholmes, Director, Social and Affective Development/Child Maltreatment and Violence Program, National Institute of Child Health and Human Development, National Institutes of Health

Beverly Fortson, Behavioral Scientist, Research and Evaluation Branch, Division of Violence Prevention, Centers for Disease Control and Prevention

Mary Bassett, Director for Child Abuse Prevention and for the African Health Initiative, Doris Duke Charitable Foundation

Carrie Mulford, Social Science Analyst, National Institute of Justice

4:20-5:00   Discussion, moderated by Mary Dozier

5:00-5:30   Comments from the Public

5:30   Adjourn Open Session

Appendix B

Research Recommendations and Priorities from the 1993 National Research Council Report *Understanding Child Abuse and Neglect*

IDENTIFICATION AND DEFINITIONS

2-1: Recognizing that the absence of consistent research definitions seriously impedes the development of an integrated research base in child abuse and neglect, a series of expert multidisciplinary panels should be convened to review existing work and to develop a consensus on research definitions of each form of abuse and neglect.

2-2: Sound clinical-diagnostic and research instruments for the measurement of child maltreatment are needed to operationalize the definitions discussed under Recommendation 1.

2-3: Research should be conducted on the detection processes that lead to the definition of cases identified in child protective services records and other social agencies that handle child maltreatment.

2-4: Empirical research that builds on existing medical knowledge of the physical indicators of child sexual and physical abuse would assist physicians in the identification of child maltreatment. Such identification would also be facilitated by the development of training programs that integrate research findings from child maltreatment studies into the education of health professionals.

SCOPE OF THE PROBLEM

3-1: State data systems should be improved so that high-quality research on service systems can be conducted.

3-2: Standardized measures and methodological research should be developed for use in epidemiologic studies of child abuse and neglect.

3-3: Data collection efforts should capitalize on future national survey efforts to include questions on child abuse and neglect.

3-4: Research should encourage secondary analyses of existing data available from multiple national surveys for questions about abuse and neglect.

3-5: After considerable work on instrumentation, including investigations into the most effective questioning strategies, the panel recommends the funding of a series of full-scale epidemiologic studies on the incidence and prevalence of child abuse and neglect.

ETIOLOGY OF CHILD MALTREATMENT

4-1: Research using multivariate models and etiological theories that integrate ecological, transactional, and developmental factors will improve our understanding of the causes of child maltreatment. Rather than focusing on specific factors (such as depression, unemployment, or history of abuse), the interactions of variables at multiple ecological levels should be examined.

4-2: Similarities and differences among the etiologies of different forms of child maltreatment should be clarified in order to improve the quality of future prevention and intervention efforts.

4-3: Studies of similarities and differences in the etiologies of various forms of maltreatment across various social class, cultural, and ethnic populations should be supported.

PREVENTION

5-1: Research on home visiting programs focused on the prenatal, postnatal, and toddler periods has great potential for enhancing family functioning and parental skills and reducing the prevalence of child maltreatment.

5-2: Research on child sexual abuse prevention needs to incorporate knowledge about appropriate risk factors as well as the relationship between cognitive and behavioral skills, particularly in situations involving known or trusted adults. Sexual abuse prevention research also needs to integrate knowledge of factors that support or impede disclosure of abuse in the natural setting, including factors that influence adult recognition of sexual abuse or situations at risk for child abuse.

5-3: Research evaluations are needed to identify the extent to which community-based prevention and intervention programs (such as school-based violence or domestic violence prevention programs, Head Start, etc.) focused on families at risk of multiple problems may affect the likelihood of child maltreatment. Research is also needed on these programs to identify methodological elements (such as designs that successfully engage the participation of at-risk communities) that could be incorporated into child maltreatment prevention programs.

5-4: Evaluations of school-based programs designed to prevent violence and to improve parental skills are needed to identify the subpopulations most likely to benefit from such interventions and to examine the impact of school-based programs on the abusive behaviors of young parents.

5-5: Research should be conducted on values and attitudes within the general public that contribute to, or could help discourage, child maltreatment. The role of the media in reinforcing or questioning cultural norms in areas important to child maltreatment, such as corporal punishment, deserves particular attention.

CONSEQUENCES OF CHILD ABUSE AND NEGLECT

6-1: Research that simultaneously assesses consequences across multiple outcomes for multiple types of maltreatment should be supported.

6-2: The consequences of child abuse and neglect should be examined in a longitudinal developmental framework that examines the timing, duration, severity, and nature of effects over the life course in a variety of cultural environments.

6-3: Intergenerational studies require support to identify relevant cycles and key factors that affect intergenerational transmission of child maltreatment.

6-4: Research needs to consider the co-occurrence of multiple forms of child victimization in the social context of child maltreatment behaviors.

6-5: Research on the role of protective factors, including gender differences in vulnerability and manifestations of subsequent problem behaviors, needs further examination.

6-6: Research is needed to improve the methodological soundness of child maltreatment studies, to test hypotheses, and to develop relevant theories of the consequences of childhood victimization.

INTERVENTIONS AND TREATMENT

7-1: Research on the operation of the child protection system, including an evaluation of the sequential stages by which children receive treatment following reports of maltreatment, is a priority need. The factors that influence different aspects of case handling decisions, factors that improve the delivery of case services, and alternatives to existing arrangements for providing services to children and families in distress need to be described and evaluated.

7-2: Controlled group outcome studies are needed to develop criteria to assess the effects of treatment interventions for maltreated children. Adequate measures need to be developed to assess outcomes of treatment for victims of abuse and neglect, and methods by which developmental, social, and cultural variations in abuse symptomatology can be integrated into treatment goals and assessment instruments need to clarified. The criteria that promote recovery and treatment modalities appropriate for children depending on their sex, age, social class, cultural background, and type of abuse need to be identified.

7-3: Well-designed outcome evaluations are needed to assess whether intensive family preservation services reduce child maltreatment and foster the well-being of children in the long-term.

7-4: Studies of foster care that examine the conditions and circumstances under which foster care appears to be beneficial or detrimental to the child are urgently needed.

7-5: Large-scale evaluation studies of treatments for perpetrators of sexual and physical abuse and neglect (familial as well as extrafamilial), with lengthy follow-up periods and control groups of untreated or less intensively treated offenders, need to be designed to compare different treatment modalities. Because of their relatively low costs, evaluations of self-help and support programs may be particularly beneficial. Early intervention through the treatment of adolescent offenders also deserves special consideration at this time.

7-6: Effective interventions for neglectful families need to be identified. Large-scale evaluation studies of child neglect should be developed to determine types of interventions that can mitigate chronic neglectful behaviors among offending parents and improve outcomes for children victimized by neglect.

HUMAN RESOURCES, INSTRUMENTATION, AND RESEARCH INFRASTRUCTURE

8-1: Better measures are needed to assess the strengths and weaknesses of the available pool of researchers who can contribute to studies of child maltreatment. A directory of active research investigators, identifying key fields of research interests, should be developed in collaboration with professional societies and child advocacy organizations, whose members have research experience on child abuse and neglect.

8-2: Governmental agencies and foundations that sponsor research in child maltreatment need to recognize the importance of strengthening research resources in the disciplines that contribute to understanding of child abuse and neglect. In particular, efforts to cross-fertilize research across and within disciplines are necessary at this time.

8-3: The creation of a corps of research-practitioners familiar with studies of child maltreatment, especially in the fields of law, medicine, psychology, social work, sociology, criminal justice, and public health, should be an explicit goal of federal, state, and private agencies that operate programs in areas of child welfare, child protection, maternal and child health, and family violence.

8-4: The cultural and ethnic diversity of the corps of research investigators concerned with child maltreatment studies is not broad enough to explore the importance of culture and ethnicity in theories, instrumentation, and other aspects of research on child abuse and neglect. Special efforts are needed at this time to provide educational and research support for researchers from ethnic and cultural minorities to strengthen the diversity of human resources dedicated to this topic.

8-5: The interdisciplinary nature of child maltreatment research requires the development of specialized disciplinary expertise as well as opportunities for collaborative research studies. Postdoctoral training programs designed to deepen a young scientist's interests in research on child abuse and neglect should be given preference at this time over graduate student dissertation support, although both training efforts are desirable in the long term.

8-6: Federal agencies should develop mechanisms to provide continuing support, in collaboration with state agencies, for interdisciplinary training programs that can provide graduate and post-graduate education in the examination of child maltreatment issues.

8-7: Research agencies should give priority attention to the development and dissemination of research instruments that have been shown to be effective in improving the quality of data collected in child maltreatment studies. Particular attention should be given in the near term to instruments that improve the identification of child maltreatment in order to lessen research dependence on reported cases of child abuse and neglect. Attention should be given to the development of instruments that are sensitive to ethnic and cultural differences and that can improve the quality of etiology and consequences studies in selected subgroups.

8-8: Several multidisciplinary centers should be established to encourage the study of child maltreatment and to integrate research in the training of service providers. The purpose of these centers should be to assemble a corps of faculty and practitioners focused on selected aspects of child abuse and neglect, and to provide a critical mass in developing long-term research studies, evaluating major demonstration projects to build on and expand the existing base of empirical knowledge, and building a research-based curriculum for the law, medical, and social service schools.

8-9: The level of financial support currently available for research on child maltreatment is poorly documented. The Congress should request that the General Accounting Office conduct a thorough review of all ongoing federally supported research on child abuse and neglect to identify and categorize research programs that are directly or indirectly relevant to this area, particularly if their primary goal is in support of a related objective, such as the reduction of family violence, injuries, infant mortality, and so forth.

8-10: Very small amounts of research funds are available for in-depth, prospective, long-term studies of child maltreatment. The research budgets for the National Center on Child Abuse and Neglect (NCCAN), the National Institute of Mental Health, the National Institute of Child Health and Human Development, the Centers for Disease Control and Prevention, and the Department of Justice as the primary funders of child maltreatment studies, should be reviewed to identify sources of support that might be pooled for longitudinal studies of interest to several agencies.

8-11: State agencies have an important role in developing and disseminating knowledge about factors that affect the identification, treatment, and prevention of child maltreatment. NCCAN should encourage the development of a state consortium that can serve as a documentation and research support center, allowing the states to collaborate in child maltreatment studies and facilitating the dissemination of significant research findings to state officials and service providers.

8-12: As best as can be determined, the federal government currently spends about $15 million per year on research directly related to child maltreatment. Recognizing that fiscal pressures and budgetary deficits diminish prospects for significant increases in research budgets generally, special efforts are required to develop new funds for research on child abuse and neglect. In addition, governmental leadership is required to identify and synthesize research from related fields that offers insights into the causes, consequences, treatment, and prevention of child maltreatment.

8-13: Effective incentives and dissemination systems should be developed to convey empirical findings to individuals who are authorized to make social welfare decisions on behalf of children. We need to strengthen the processes by which science is used to inform and advise legislative and judicial decision makers. And we need effective partnerships among scientists, practitioners, clinicians, and governmental officials to encourage the use of sound research results in formulating policies, programs, and services that affect the lives of thousands of children and their families.

ETHICAL AND LEGAL ISSUES IN CHILD MALTREATMENT RESEARCH

9-1: The disclosure of unreported incidents of abuse by research subjects requires greater analysis to clarify the circumstances that foster such disclosures, the methods by which researchers respond to subject disclosures, and the outcomes for research subjects who disclose incidents of maltreatment.

9-2: Methodological research is needed to develop design procedures and resources that can resolve ethical problems associated with recruitment, informed consent, privacy and confidentiality, and assignment of experimental and control groups.

9-3: Research is needed to determine the impact of debriefings both on subjects' post-project perceptions as well as on research results. This research will have ethical implications for the inclusion or omission of such interviews in research designs.

9-4: Research on the institutional research board process should be done to improve the quality of the process by which studies of child abuse and neglect are initiated and approved.

PRIORITIES FOR CHILD MALTREATMENT RESEARCH

Research Priority 1: A consensus on research definitions needs to be established for each form of child abuse and neglect. (See Recommendations 2-1 and 2-3)

Research Priority 2: Reliable and valid clinical-diagnostic and research instruments for the measurement of child maltreatment are needed to operationalize the definitions discussed under Research Priority 1. (See Recommendations 2-2 and 2-4)

Research Priority 3: Epidemiologic studies on the incidence and prevalence of child abuse and neglect should be encouraged, as well as the inclusion of research questions about child maltreatment in other national surveys. (See Recommendations 3-1 through 3-5)

Research Priority 4: Research that examines the processes by which individual, family, community, and social factors interact will improve understanding of the causes of child maltreatment and should be supported. (See Recommendation 4-1)

Research Priority 5: Research that clarifies the common and divergent pathways in the etiologies of different forms of child maltreatment for diverse populations is essential to improve the quality of future prevention and intervention efforts. (See Recommendations 4-2 and 4-3)

Research Priority 6: Research that assesses the outcomes of specific and combined types of maltreatment should be supported. (See Recommendations 6-1 through 6-4)

Research Priority 7: Research is needed to clarify the effects of multiple forms of child victimization that often occur in the social context of child maltreatment. The consequences of child maltreatment may be significantly influenced by a combination of risk factors that have not been well described or understood. (See Recommendation 6-5)

Research Priority 8: Studies of similarities and differences in the etiologies and consequences of various forms of maltreatment across various cultural and ethnic groups are necessary. (Recommendations 6-6 and 6-7)

Research Priority 9: High-quality evaluation studies of existing program and service interventions are needed to develop criteria and instrumentation that can help identify promising developments in the delivery of treatment and prevention services. (See Recommendations 5-1, 5-2, 5-3, 7-2, 7-3, 7-5, and 7-6)

Research Priority 10: Research on the operation of the existing child protection and child welfare systems is urgently needed. Factors that influence different aspects of case handling decisions and the delivery and use of individual and family services require attention. The strengths and limitations of alternatives to existing institutional arrangements need to be described and evaluated. (See Recommendation 7-1)

Research Priority 11: Service system research on existing state data systems should be conducted to improve the quality of child maltreatment research information as well as to foster improved service interventions. (See Recommendation 3-1)

Research Priority 12: The role of the media in reinforcing or questioning social norms relevant to child maltreatment needs further study. (See Recommendation 5-4)

Research Priority 13: Federal agencies concerned with child maltreatment research need to formulate a national research plan and provide leadership for child maltreatment research. (See Recommendations 8-2 and 8-6)

Research Priority 14: Governmental leadership is needed to sustain and improve the capabilities of the available pool of researchers who can contribute to studies of child maltreatment. National leadership is also required to foster the integration of research from related fields that offer significant insights into the causes, consequences, treatment, and prevention of child maltreatment. (See Recommendations 8-1, 8-3, 8-4, 8-5, and 8-7)

Research Priority 15: Recognizing that fiscal pressures and budgetary deficits diminish prospects for significant increases in research budgets generally, special efforts are required to find new funds for research on child abuse and neglect and to encourage research collaboration and data collection in related fields. (See Recommendations 8-9, 8-10, and 8-12)

Research Priority 16: Research is needed to identify organizational innovations that can improve the process by which child maltreatment research findings are disseminated to practitioners and policy makers. The role of state agencies in supporting, disseminating, and utilizing empirical research deserves particular attention. (See Recommendation 8-11)

Research Priority 17: Researchers should design methods, procedures, and resources that can resolve ethical problems associated with recruitment of research subjects; informed consent; privacy, confidentiality, and autonomy; assignment of experimental and control research participants; and debriefings. (See Recommendations 9-1 through 9-4)

Appendix C

Biosketches of Committee Members

Anne C. Petersen, Ph.D., M.S. (*Chair*), is founder and president of Global Philanthropy Alliance, a foundation making grants in Africa. She also is research professor, Center for Human Growth and Development, and faculty associate, Center for Global Health, University of Michigan, among other affiliations at the university. Dr. Petersen serves on several voluntary boards or committees for government, foundations, and scientific or community-based organizations. She is co-chair of the Advisory Board for CALIT2, an organization created a decade ago to move information technology advances from the University of California system to industry in California. Dr. Petersen previously held positions as professor of psychology at Stanford University, deputy director of the Center for Advanced Study in the Behavioral Sciences, senior vice president for programs and corporate officer at the W.K. Kellogg Foundation, and department head and founding dean of the College of Health and Human Development at Penn State University. She was the first vice president for research at the University of Minnesota, as well as graduate dean and professor (Institute for Child Development and Department of Pediatrics). Previously, Dr. Petersen was University of Chicago faculty and associate director of the MacArthur Foundation Health Program. She has authored numerous articles and books. Her honors include election to the Institute of Medicine (IOM) and fellow in several scientific societies, including the American Association for the Advancement of Science (AAAS) and the American Psychological Association (APA) (three divisions), as well as founding fellow of the Association for Psychological Science (APS). She co-founded the Society of Research on Adolescence, was president of several scientific societies, and is past president of the International Society for the Study of Behavioral Development. Dr. Petersen received her B.A. in mathematics, her M.S. in statistics, and her Ph.D. in measurement, evaluation, and statistical analysis from the University of Chicago.

Lucy Berliner, M.S.W., is director of the Harborview Center for Sexual Assault and Traumatic Stress and clinical associate professor at the University of Washington School of Social Work, Department of Psychiatry and Behavioral Sciences. Her activities include clinical practice with child and adult victims of trauma and crime, research on the impact of trauma and the effectiveness of clinical and societal interventions, and participation in local and national social policy initiatives designed to promote the interests of trauma and crime victims. Ms. Berliner is on the editorial boards of leading journals concerned with interpersonal violence; has authored numerous peer-reviewed articles and book chapters; and has served/serves on local and national boards of organizations, programs, and professional societies. She also served on the IOM-National Research Council (NRC) Workshop Committee on Child Maltreatment Research, Policy, and Practice for the Next Generation (Phase One) and the IOM Panel on Research on Violence Against Women. Ms. Berliner received her M.S.W. from the University of Washington.

Linda Marie Burton, Ph.D., M.A., is James B. Duke professor of sociology and Center for Child and Family Policy (CCFP) faculty fellow at Duke University. Her research is conceptually grounded in life-course, developmental, and ecological perspectives and focuses on three themes concerning the lives of America's poorest urban, small town, and rural families: (1) intergenerational family structures, processes, and role transitions; (2) the meaning of context and place in the daily lives of families; and (3) childhood adultification and the accelerated life course. The comparative dimension of her research comprises in-depth within-group analysis of low-income African American, white, and Hispanic/Latino families, as well as systematic examination of similarities and differences across groups. She is principally an ethnographer, but integrates survey and geographic and spatial analysis in her work. Dr. Burton was one of six principal investigators involved in a multisite, multimethod collaborative study of the impact of welfare reform on families and children (Welfare, Children, and Families: A Three-City Study). She also directed the ethnographic component of the Three-City Study and was principal investigator for an ethnographic study of rural poverty and child development (The Family Life Project). Dr. Burton received her Ph.D. in sociology from the University of Southern California.

Phaedra S. Corso, Ph.D., M.P.A., is professor of health policy in the College of Public Health at the University of Georgia (UGA). Her research interests include economic evaluation of public health interventions; quality-of-life assessment for vulnerable populations; evaluation of preferences for health risks; and the prevention of violence, injury, and substance use. Prior to joining the faculty at UGA, Dr. Corso worked for 15 years at the Centers for Disease Control and Prevention, most notably as an economic analyst in the area of violence prevention. She received her Ph.D. in health policy from Harvard University.

Deborah Daro, Ph.D., M.C.P., is a senior research fellow at Chapin Hall at the University of Chicago. She has more than 30 years of experience in evaluating child abuse treatment and prevention programs and has directed some of the largest multisite program evaluations completed in the field. Currently, she is leading the development of the Doris Duke Fellowships for the Prevention of Child Abuse and Neglect, whose aim is to identify and nurture promising leaders and innovative approaches to child abuse prevention. Most recently, Dr. Daro has focused on developing reform strategies that embed individualized, targeted prevention efforts within more universal efforts to alter normative standards and community context. She is also examining strategies for creating more effective partnerships among public child welfare agencies, community-based prevention efforts, and informal support systems. Prior to joining Chapin Hall, Dr. Daro served as director of the National Center on Child Abuse Prevention Research, a program of the National Committee to Prevent Child Abuse. She has published and lectured widely, and her commentaries and findings are frequently cited in the rationale for numerous child abuse prevention and treatment reforms. She has served as president of the American Professional Society on the Abuse of Children and as treasurer and executive council member for the International Society for the Prevention of Child Abuse and Neglect. Dr. Daro received her Ph.D. in social welfare and a master's degree in city and regional planning from the University of California, Berkeley.

Howard Davidson, J.D., is director of the American Bar Association's (ABA's) Center on Children and the Law. The center has been responsible for many nationwide activities of the ABA related to children and the legal system. Mr. Davidson directs a large staff of attorneys and social scientists engaged in consulting, technical assistance, training, and writing projects on many legal topics, which have included children in the courts; legal representation issues; children's legal rights; child protection-related legislative reforms; parental rights and responsibility laws; domestic violence and its impact on children; child sexual abuse; family preservation, foster care, and legal permanency; parental kidnapping of children; child pornography and prostitution; adoption; legal planning for parents with HIV/AIDS; and a range of child/adolescent health law issues. Throughout his tenure, Mr. Davidson has provided consultation to courts, attorneys, organizations, and other professionals across the country on child welfare and child protection legal issues. He is on the board of the International Centre for Missing and Exploited Children and was appointed as a member of the U.S. Delegation, 1st World Congress Against the Commercial Sexual Exploitation of Children. Mr. Davidson received his J.D. from Boston College Law School.

Angela Díaz, M.D., M.P.H., is a professor in the Department of Pediatrics and Department of Preventive Medicine at Mount Sinai School of Medicine, where she is responsible for the Division of Adolescent Medicine. She is also director of the Mount Sinai Adolescent Health Center. Dr. Diaz served as a White House fellow in 1994-1995, examining health care policies in the U.S. territories in the Pacific and the Caribbean. She has been involved in issues of international health, as well as advocacy issues and policy in the United States. Her research has covered adolescent sexual and reproductive health, childhood sexual victimization, and human papilloma virus (HPV). Dr. Diaz is a member of the IOM and has served on multiple committees. She received her M.D. from Columbia University College of Physicians and Surgeons and her M.P.H. from Harvard University.

Mary Dozier, Ph.D., is Unidel Amy E. du Pont Chair of Child Development at the University of Delaware. She is principal investigator for the school's Infant Caregiver Project. Her interest in understanding connections among childhood experience, brain development, and behavior has led to the development of intervention techniques that are a practical application of findings from decades of research. Since 1994, Dr. Dozier has studied the development of young children who are neglected and in foster care and has developed training programs for the caregivers of these children, with efficacy trials funded by the National Institute of Mental Health. Her work has been supported by the National Institute of Mental Health continuously since 1989. She is the recipient of the Bowlby-Ainsworth Award for Translational Research on Adoption and the National Institute of Mental Health Innovation Nomination. Dr. Dozier served on the IOM-NRC Workshop Committee on Child Maltreatment Research, Policy, and Practice for the Next Generation (Phase One). She received her Ph.D. in clinical psychology from Duke University.

Fernando A. Guerra, M.D., M.P.H., is clinical professor of pediatrics at the University of Texas Health Science Center in San Antonio. He also serves as an adjunct professor in public health at the Air Force School of

Aerospace Medicine at Brooks Air Force Base in San Antonio and in management, policy, and community health at the University of Texas School of Public Health in Houston. He recently retired as director of health for the San Antonio Metropolitan Health District after 23 years of service. He oversaw the operation of 32 health locations throughout San Antonio and several areas of Bexar County. Dr. Guerra has held top leadership positions in local, regional, and national organizations that include serving as a member of the Federal Advisory Committee for the National Children's Study. He has received numerous awards for his service and contributions to public health, including the Job Lewis Smith Award of the American Academy of Pediatrics and most recently the Alumni Award of Merit from the Harvard School of Public Health. Dr. Guerra is currently serving as a consultant to the Public Health Department of the City of San Antonio in public health and health policy. He is a member of the IOM, the Public Health Accreditation Board, and the Urban Institute Board of Trustees. Dr. Guerra earned his M.D. from the University of Texas Medical Branch at Galveston and his M.P.H. from the Harvard University School of Public Health, where he was also a Kellogg fellow.

Carol Hafford, Ph.D., is a principal research scientist at NORC at the University of Chicago in the Economics, Labor, and Population Studies department. She leads federally sponsored studies on human services for vulnerable children and families that address housing needs, food security, self-sufficiency, and child maltreatment and elder abuse prevention interventions. Prior to joining NORC in 2010, Dr. Hafford was a senior research associate at James Bell Associates in the child welfare practice area. There, she conducted studies on evidence-based child neglect prevention, implementation of tribal family preservation programs, foster care and adoption services, court–child welfare–community collaborations for infants and toddlers in foster care, independent living for emancipated youth, family dependency court reforms, tribal TANF and Indian child welfare coordination, organizational and systems change across state and tribal family services, implementation of federal child welfare legislation, and monitoring of state child welfare systems through the Child and Family Services Reviews. A fellow of the Society for Applied Anthropology, Dr. Hafford has conducted longitudinal ethnographic research on runaway and homeless youth in transitional living programs and the socialization of the children of immigrants into local and transnational social support networks. She is the author of *Sibling Caretaking in Immigrant Families: Understanding Cultural Practices to Inform Child Welfare Practice and Evaluation*. Dr. Hafford earned her Ph.D. in applied anthropology from Columbia University.

Charles A. Nelson, Ph.D., is professor of pediatrics at Harvard Medical School and Richard David Scott chair in pediatric developmental medicine research at Children's Hospital, Boston. Dr. Nelson's research interests are broadly concerned with developmental cognitive neuroscience, an interdisciplinary field that requires expertise in developmental neuroscience and developmental psychology. He studies both typically developing children and children at risk for neurodevelopmental disorders, and he employs behavioral, electrophysiological (event-related potential), and metabolic (magnetic resonance imaging) tools in his research. Dr. Nelson chaired the John D. and Catherine T. MacArthur Foundation Research Network on Early Experience and Brain Development and served on the National Academy of Sciences panel that wrote *From Neurons to Neighborhoods.* His specific interests are focused on the effects of early experience on brain and behavioral development, particularly as such experience influences the development of memory and of the ability to recognize faces. Dr. Nelson received his Ph.D. in developmental and child psychology from the University of Kansas.

Ellen E. Pinderhughes, Ph.D., is associate professor in the Eliot-Pearson Department of Child Development at Tufts University. Her research examines the contextual and cultural influences on family socialization processes among families with children at risk for problematic outcomes. She also conducts research on adoption and foster care. She currently has a grant from the National Science Foundation, working as a co-investigator on Excavating Culture in Parenting Practices and Socialization among Diverse Families: A Working Conference. She is a member and serves on the governing board of the Society for Research in Child Development and is a member of the research advisory committee at the Evan B. Donaldson Adoption Institute. She is also serving as a member of the research and evaluation working group at the Safe Schools/Healthy Students Action Center, located in Alexandria, Virginia. Dr. Pinderhughes received her Ph.D. in psychology from Yale University.

Frank W. Putnam, Jr., M.D., is professor of psychiatry at the University of North Carolina at Chapel Hill. He is an adjunct professor of pediatrics and child psychiatry and former director of the Mayerson Center for Safe and Healthy Children at Children's Hospital Medical Center in Cincinnati. Previously he was scientific director of Every Child Succeeds, a home visitation program in Ohio, and later served as deputy director. Prior to his move to Cincinnati in 1999, Dr. Putnam worked with the intramural research program at the National Institute of Mental Health, where he held the positions of chief of the Unit on Developmental Traumatology (1995-1999), senior clinical investigator in the Laboratory of Developmental Psychology

(1986-1995), and staff psychiatrist in the Neuropsychiatry Branch (1982-1985). He has received numerous honors, including the Morton Prince Scientific Achievement Award in 1985, the Cornelia Wilbur Clinical Service Award in 1990, the U.S. Public Health Service Medal of Commendation in 1992, the Pierre Janet Scientific Writing Award in 1993, and the Ohio Martin Luther King Health Equity Award in 2006. His recent publications include research on the impact of trauma on child development, the experience of mothers in discussing sensitive issues in home visitation programs, and the development of quality infrastructure to support home visiting programs in a tristate area. Dr. Putnam served on the NRC-IOM Committee on Depression, Parenting Practices, and the Health Development of Young Children. He received his M.D. from Indiana University, conducted his residency in adult psychiatry at Yale University, and completed a fellowship in child psychiatry at the Children's National Medical Center in Washington, DC.

Desmond K. Runyan, M.D., Dr.P.H., is executive director of the Kempe Center for the Prevention and Treatment of Child Abuse and Neglect in Denver, Colorado. He is also national program director for the Robert Wood Johnson Foundation Clinical Scholars Program. Prior to coming to Kempe in 2011, he was professor of social medicine and pediatrics at the University of North Carolina School of Medicine. His work focuses on the application of clinical epidemiology to the problem of violence against children and the impact of societal intervention on the mental health functioning of child victims. He has examined the impact on children of the foster care system, court testimony, and the medical examination. His work has touched on all aspects of abuse, including sexual abuse, physical abuse, Munchausen's syndrome by proxy, and failure to thrive. He is currently in the twenty-first year of a multistate longitudinal study of the impact of abuse. He also is involved in a 5-year effort to assess the effectiveness of a specific parenting education program, The Period of Purple Crying, aimed at reducing or eliminating the problem of shaken baby syndrome for an entire state. He is a consulting pediatrician at the Colorado Children's Hospital and head of the section on child abuse in the Department of Pediatrics of the University of Colorado. Dr. Runyan received his Dr.P.H. from the University of North Carolina at Chapel Hill School of Public Health, and he received his M.D. and completed his residency in pediatrics at the University of Minnesota Medical School.

Cathy Spatz Widom, Ph.D., is distinguished professor in the Department of Psychology at John Jay College and a member of the Graduate Center faculty, City University of New York. A former faculty member at Harvard, Indiana, the State University of New York at Albany, and New Jersey Medical School, she is co-editor of the *Journal of Quantitative Criminology* and has served on the editorial boards of psychology and criminology journals. She is a fellow of the American Psychological Association (Division 41, Law and Psychology), the American Psychopathological Association, and the American Society of Criminology. She is a frequent consultant on national review panels and has been invited to testify before congressional and state committees. Dr. Widom has published extensively on the long-term consequences of child abuse and neglect, including numerous papers on the cycle of violence. She served on the Committee on Law and Justice of the NRC's Commission on Behavioral and Social Sciences and was co-chair of the NRC Panel on Juvenile Crime, Juvenile Justice. Dr. Widom has received numerous awards for her research, including the 1989 American Association for the Advancement of Science Behavioral Science Research Prize for her paper on the "cycle of violence." Since 1986, she has been engaged in a large study to determine the long-term consequences of early childhood abuse (physical and sexual) and neglect, and she is currently completing research on the intergenerational transmission of violence. Dr. Widom received her Ph.D. in psychology from Brandeis University.

Joan Levy Zlotnik, Ph.D., A.C.S.W., is director of the Social Work Policy Institute at the National Association of Social Workers. Previously, she served as executive director of the Institute for the Advancement of Social Work Research. She was also director of special projects and special assistant to the executive director at the Council on Social Work Education. She is the editor of a book series, *Building Social Work Research Capacity*, published in 2012 by Oxford University Press, and is co-author of the volume *Building Research Culture and Infrastructure*. Among her other publications, she is the author of *Preparing the Workforce for Family-Centered Practice: Social Work Education and Public Human Services Partnerships*; co-editor of several books, including *Charting the Impacts of University-Child Welfare Collaboration* and *Preparing Helping Professionals to Meet Community Needs: Generalizing from the Rural Experience*; and co-editor of the fall 2009 special issue of *Child Welfare*. Dr. Zlotnik is a fellow of the Gerontological Society of America and a National Association of Social Workers (NASW) Social Work Pioneer®. She also received the Association of Gerontology Education in Social Work Leadership Award and the Association of Baccalaureate Social Work Program Director's Presidential Medal of Honor. She was recognized by the National Institutes of Health's (NIH's) Social Work Research Working Group for her efforts on behalf of social work research at NIH. Dr. Zlotnik received her Ph.D. in social work from the University of Maryland.